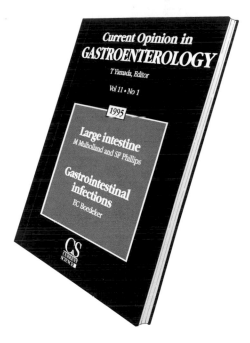

# Current Opinion in
# GASTROENTEROLOGY

## Subscribe now and stay up-to-date

### KEEP UP-TO-DATE WITH CURRENT OPINION

• Every year it is the most reliable source of information in the field.

• Every year the whole field is covered in 6 bi-monthly issues, broken down into 11 subjects.

• Every year within each subject, all the latest developments, expert comment and opinion, and recommended reading are featured.

• Every year Current Opinion in Gastroenterology is the only reference you need to keep fully informed.

### PRICES FOR ANNUAL SUBSCRIPTION

£84.95 - $134.95 Personal

£169.95 - $269.95 Institutional

£45 - $55 Pre-reg doctors/Residents

Postage: £10 UK   £15.75 Eur   $11 N Am   $37 S Am   £25 RoW

### EDITOR

**T Yamada**

### 1995 SECTIONS AND EDITORS

**January**
LARGE INTESTINE *M Mulholland & SF Phillips*
GASTROINTESTINAL INFECTIONS *EC Boedeker*

**March**
SMALL INTESTINE *DH Alpers, WF Stenson & RC Spiller*
NUTRITION *RL Fisher*

**May**
LIVER *N Gitlin & J Fevery*

**July**
INFLAMMATORY BOWEL DISEASE *DK Podolsky*
ESOPHAGUS *GNJ Tytgat*

**September**
BILIARY TRACT *RH Moseley*
PANCREAS *C Owyang*

**November**
STOMACH AND DUODENUM *ML Schubert*
IMMUNOLOGY *WA Walker*

**TO SUBSCRIBE IN N & S AMERICA CONTACT:**
CURRENT SCIENCE LTD, SUITE 700, 400 MARKET STREET,
PHILADELPHIA, PA 19106, USA.
TEL: 215-574-2210, OR TOLL FREE: 800-552-5866
FAX: 215-574-3533

**TO SUBSCRIBE IN REST OF WORLD CONTACT:**
CURRENT SCIENCE LTD, MIDDLESEX HOUSE,
34-42 CLEVELAND STREET, LONDON W1P 6LB, UK.
TEL: +44 (0)171 323 0323, OR FREEPHONE: 0800 212530
FAX: +44 (0)171 636 6911.

# European Journal of GASTROENTEROLOGY & HEPATOLOGY

## OFFICIAL JOURNAL OF THE EUROPEAN ASSOCIATION FOR GASTROENTEROLOGY AND ENDOSCOPY

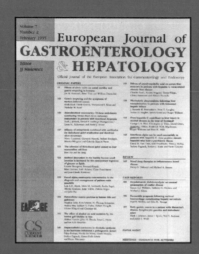

Established as a major platform for the dissemination of original research, the European Journal of Gastroenterology & Hepatology maintains consistently high standards via a combination of:

•

Outstanding original papers by experts in the fields of basic research and clinical investigation:

How does *Helicobacter pylori* infection disease increase gastric cancer risk? P Correa

Intestinal metaplasia and *Helicobacter pylori* in patients with non-ulcer dyspepsia: more arguments for the natural history RJLF Loffeld & AG Balk

•

Reviews in depth of selected major topics, edited by world authorities:

Oesophageal cancer A Watson
Management of gallstones T Northfield
Gastric carcinogenesis D Forman

IN NORTH & SOUTH AMERICA RETURN TO:
CURRENT SCIENCE LTD, SUITE 700, 400 MARKET STREET, PHILADELPHIA PA 19106
TEL: 215 574 2210   TOLL FREE: 800 552 5866 (N AM ONLY)
FAX: 215 574 3533

IN THE REST OF THE WORLD RETURN TO :
CURRENT SCIENCE LTD, 34-42 CLEVELAND STREET, LONDON W1P 6LB, UK.
TEL: +44 (0) 171 323 0323. FREEPHONE: 0800 212530 (UK ONLY).
FAX: +44 (0) 171 636 6911.

---

☑ YES! I want to subscribe to the European Journal of Gastroenterology & Hepatology (Vol 7, 1995, 12 issues)

☐ PERSONAL £94.50 / $144.95

☐ INSTITUTIONAL £194.50 / $295.00

☐ PRE-REG DOCTORS/RESIDENTS*
£65.00 / $99.95

ADD POSTAGE £18.00 (UK), £26.50 (EUROPE), $20.00 (N AM), $57.75 (S AM), £36.00 (ROW)

*MUST PROVIDE PROOF OF STATUS AND MAY ONLY SUBSCRIBE AT THE DISCOUNTED RATE WITHIN 2 YEARS OF QUALIFYING.

PRICE.....................

PLUS POSTAGE.....................

TOTAL AMOUNT PAYABLE.....................

CANADIAN SUBSCRIBERS ADD 7% GST

☐ AM EX ☐ VISA ☐ MASTERCARD

CARD NO.....................

EXP DATE.....................

SIGNATURE.....................

DATE.....................

☐ CHEQUE / EUROCHEQUE PAYABLE TO CURRENT SCIENCE LTD

☐ PLEASE INVOICE ME

☐ BANK TRANSFER

(THERE IS A 20% SURCHARGE FOR CUSTOMERS USING THIS FACILITY) CURRENT SCIENCE LTD, ACCT NO: 0056750 / SORT: 309368 LLOYDS BANK PLC, GT PORTLAND ST, LONDON W1A 4LN, UK. PLEASE INCLUDE DETAILS OF NAME AND ADDRESS WITH PAYMENT ADVICE

YOUR VAT REGISTRATION NUMBER.....................
OUR VAT REGISTRATION NUMBER GB466247723
EC SALES TAX WILL BE CHARGED WHERE NECESSARY

**NO RISK GUARANTEE**: YOUR MONEY WILL BE REFUNDED IN FULL IF YOU WRITE CANCELLING YOUR ORDER WITHIN 30 DAYS OF RECEIPT AND RETURN ALL GOODS RECEIVED UNDAMAGED.

TITLE.....................

SURNAME.....................

FIRST NAME.....................

ADDRESS.....................

.....................

.....................

.....................

COUNTRY.....................

POSTCODE/ZIPCODE.....................

TEL.....................

FAX.....................

# Annual of
# Gastrointestinal Endoscopy

*illustrated in colour*

# Annual of
# Gastrointestinal Endoscopy
## *illustrated in colour*

## Editors

### PB Cotton
Digestive Disease Center
Medical University of South Carolina
Charleston, USA

### GNJ Tytgat
Academic Medical Centre,
Amsterdam, The Netherlands

### CB Williams
St Mark's and St Bartholomew's Hospitals,
London, UK

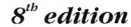

## *8ᵗʰ edition*

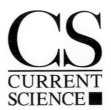

CURRENT
SCIENCE ■

British Library Cataloguing-in-Publication Data.
A catalogue record for this publication is available from the British Library.

ISBN 1-85922-187-4 ISSN 0952-6293

Although every effort has been made to ensure that drug doses and other
information are presented accurately in this publication, the ultimate
responsibility rests with the prescribing physician. Neither the publishers nor
the authors can be held responsible for errors or for any consequences
arising from the use of the information contained herein. Any product
mentioned in this publication should be used in accordance with the
prescribing information prepared by the manufacturers. No claims or
endorsements are made for any drug or compound at present under clinical
investigation.

Cover illustration: Santorinicele: balloon inflation of the minor papilla.
Courtesy of P.B. Cotton

# Contents

**Literature scanner**

Sandro Lanzon-Miller

**Current Science**

Neil Morris and Deborah Russell (Project Editors); Ben Perkins (Production Editor);
Daniel Simmons (Illustrator); Neelam Shah (Database); Patricia Harrington (Production);
Neil Morris (Typesetting)

# Preface

As in previous years, the Editors owe the appearance of this edition of the *Annual of Gastrointestinal Endoscopy* to the personal time sacrificed by all of the expert contributors. The *Annual* appears, once again, to be a stimulating compendium combining personal viewpoints with summaries of the recent world literature on endoscopy-related topics. However, 'beauty lies in the eye of the beholder' and feedback (critical or otherwise) from you, the reader, would be very welcome.

Does the *Annual* adequately reflect the world scene? In producing the *Annual*, we try to maintain a reasonably international approach. However, the exigencies of rapid publication and the impossibility of covering all languages means that we ask contributors to cover English-language articles and major case reports, but eschew abstracts and some lesser articles. More glaringly, the voluminous Japanese-language literature is not covered at present — to say nothing of German- and Latin-language articles — on the assumption that, in most cases, anything of great originality or importance is also likely to appear in English. Perhaps we should spread the net wider?

Does the *Annual* meet your needs? Whether reassuringly on the shelf, glossed over as a whole for areas of current interest, or delved into when necessary for particular topics, we hope that it lives up to expectations. Please let us know.

In particular, we will be pressing our highly innovative publishers, Current Science, to consider producing each year a companion CD-ROM covering past *Annuals* and the current update. This would have the benefit of allowing users to 'lift' selected figures or to transfer references and annotations electronically to their own database or word processor; it should also facilitate the process of making selective searches of the ever expanding past literature. Is this of interest to you?

In the meantime, we commend to you, on behalf of all the production team, our 1995 *Annual of Gastrointestinal Endoscopy* and remind you that the 1995 *Slide Atlas of Gastrointestinal Endoscopy* is also available.

*Peter B. Cotton*
*Charleston*
*USA*

*Guido N.J. Tytgat*
*Amsterdam*
*The Netherlands*

*Christopher B. Williams*
*London*
*UK*

© Current Science Ltd ISBN 1-85922-187-4 ISSN 0952-6293

# Endoscopic technology assessment in the 1990s: the role of decision analysis

## Dawn Provenzale

Department of Medicine, Duke University, Durham, North Caroline, USA

Our ability to perform endoscopic procedures and to develop new endoscopic technologies has advanced dramatically over the last decade. We have demonstrated that we can perform these procedures but in this era of health-care reform we will be called upon to demonstrate that we should do them. In other words, we, as gastroenterologists, will be required to establish that our procedures are effective: that they increase the length and/or quality of life of our patients and that they are cost-effective, in other words that they are worth the investment made to perform them. What tools are available to assist us? Certainly, randomized, controlled trials comparing new modalities to existing practices would provide the strongest scientific evidence of the effectiveness of a new technique, but randomized trials frequently require large numbers of patients with long periods of follow-up and, thus, are impractical. In the absence of controlled trials, the options are few. Clinicians could turn to professional societies to develop guidelines for practice. These recommendations, however, may not reflect individual patient preferences and local practice considerations, such as the incidence of the disorder under study and local pathology and surgical expertise in the area. We could allow policy analysts to determine our future, but policy analysts might promote the least expensive practice, without regard to its effectiveness. Finally, the clinician and the policy maker could base the decisions about a new practice or technology on analytical methods that integrate published data, and identify the critical parameters in the decision-making process. This commentary will illustrate the use of decision analysis, an explicit approach to decision making under conditions of uncertainty, and how it was applied to examine the effectiveness and cost-effectiveness of a common endoscopic practice–endoscopic surveillance of patients with Barrett's oesophagus.

Barrett's oesophagus (columnar metaplasia of the distal oesophagus due to chronic gastro-oesophageal reflux) affects nearly 700 000 people in the United States, and carries a risk of oesophageal adenocarcinoma that is 30–125 times that of an age matched population [1–10]. Patients who develop high-grade dysplasia are at greatest risk. Current recommendations are for endoscopic surveillance to detect dysplasia and to diagnose carcinoma while in an early and possibly treatable stage [2,11,12]. In addition, some authorities recommend oesophagectomy for high-grade dysplasia, while others reserve oesophagectomy only for those with cancer [6]. There are no controlled trials demonstrating that surveillance increases life expectancy in patients with Barrett's oesophagus. Furthermore, endoscopic surveillance of this large group with Barrett's oesophagus may be costly and associated with considerable morbidity [13].

Decision analysis can be used to examine the effectiveness of this recommended cancer surveillance programme with a computer model. If the effectiveness of surveillance can be established, in other words that it reduces cancer mortality, the cost-effectiveness of this practice can be evaluated. We created a computer cohort simulation of hypothetical 55-year-old men with Barrett's (the mean age of patients diagnosed with Barrett's oesophagus [14]) and no evidence of dysplasia by biopsy to examine these issues, and applied decision analysis to answer them. The decision analysis requires several steps. The first step involves framing the clinical problem into a question. The following questions were posed:

- Does endoscopic surveillance increase life expectancy in patients with Barrett's oesophagus?
- Should oesophagectomy be performed for patients diagnosed with high-grade dysplasia?
- Should oesophagectomy be reserved for patients diagnosed with cancer?

The second step involves identifying the possible strategies and determining their associated risks and benefits. We considered 12 strategies for this cohort (Fig. 1):

A: No endoscopic surveillance but endoscopy is performed for the development of new or worsened dysphagia, and oesophagectomy is performed only if cancer is diagnosed.

B: No endoscopic surveillance but endoscopy is performed for the development of new or worsened dysphagia, and oesophagectomy is performed if high-grade dysplasia is diagnosed.

$C_1$–$C_5$: Endoscopic surveillance every 1–5 years, with biopsies, and oesophagectomy only if cancer is diagnosed.

**No surveillance**

A: No surveillance: oesophagectomy for cancer

B: No surveillance: oesophagectomy for high-grade dysplasia

**Surveillance**

$C_5$: Surveillance every 5 years: oesophagectomy for cancer

$C_4$: Surveillance every 4 years: oesophagectomy for cancer

$C_3$: Surveillance every 3 years: oesophagectomy for cancer

$C_2$: Surveillance every 2 years: oesophagectomy for cancer

$C_1$: Surveillance every 1 year : oesophagectomy for cancer

$D_5$: Surveillance every 5 years: oesophagectomy for high-grade dysplasia

$D_4$: Surveillance every 4 years: oesophagectomy for high-grade dysplasia

$D_3$: Surveillance every 3 years: oesophagectomy for high-grade dysplasia

$D_2$: Surveillance every 2 years: oesophagectomy for high-grade dysplasia

$D_1$: Surveillance every 1 year : oesophagectomy for high-grade dysplasia

**Fig. 1.** Twelve possible strategies for the management of patients with Barrett's oesophagus.

$D_1$–$D_5$: Endoscopic surveillance every 1–5 years, with biopsies, and oesophagectomy if high-grade dysplasia is diagnosed (aggressive surveillance). Implicit in our model is that patients who develop high-grade dysplasia either undergo oesophagectomy, or undergo endoscopic surveillance every 3 months. A patient diagnosed with low-grade dysplasia would undergo endoscopic surveillance every 6 months [13].

The next step in the analysis involves quantifying the probability of each of the critical events that may impact on the decision for surveillance and oesophagectomy (the risk of cancer, the risks and benefits of endoscopy and oesophagectomy, and the prognosis of those who develop cancer). Probabilities for each of these critical events are obtained from published literature and are shown in Figure 2. When published data are not available, the estimates for these critical parameters are obtained from experts in the field (gastroenterologists and surgeons with extensive experience in caring for patients with Barrett's oesophagus who have undergone surveillance and oesophagectomy). Endoscopic reports from the last decade suggest that the incidence of cancer is 1 per 75 patient-years [4–10] (Fig. 2). This critical parameter in decisions about surveillance, along with the test characteristics of endoscopy for diagnosing dysplasia and cancer, is included. The complications of endoscopy, including the risk of death from a non-surgical complication and the risk of a perforation requiring surgery, are integrated into the model as well [15]. The model also includes estimates for the mortality for repair of an oesophageal perforation and the prognosis of patients who are treated for oesophageal cancer [13,16–23] (Fig. 2).

The parameters that have been included thus far relate to the biology of the disorder, the characteristics of the surveillance test for detecting adenocarcinoma, and the risks and benefits associated with surveillance. The next step examines the patient's perspective. How do patients view surveillance, and what is the impact of surveillance on quality of life? In this step, a value or utility is assigned to each outcome in the model. The outcomes considered in this model are life expectancy, and quality-adjusted life expectancy. The model calculates the average remaining life expectancy for each strategy, based on the likelihood of events such as the development of cancer, or an endoscopic complication, and on data from life-tables from the general population which provide age-, sex- and race-specific mortality rates. The results allow us to compare the effectiveness of each strategy and to determine if surveillance reduces cancer mortality and improves survival in patients with Barrett's oesophagus. The quality-adjusted life expectancy considers the impact of a surveillance programme on the quality of life of patients with Barrett's oesophagus. In order to consider quality of life, the model accounts for the inconvenience and discomfort associated with surveillance, and the morbidity of hospitalization and surgery associated with endoscopic complications. In addition to these short-term events, the long-term disability associated with oesophagectomy is incorporated into the model as well (Fig. 2) [13].

These quality adjustments assume that patients may be willing to forgo some portion of the remainder of their life to avoid the morbidity of endoscopy, an endoscopic complication or oesophagectomy. Thus, a portion of the patient's remaining life expectancy is subtracted to adjust for the short-term morbidity of the procedures. In order to adjust for long-term morbidity after an oesophagectomy, it is estimated that patients would regard living 10 years with an oesophagectomy to be equivalent to living 8 years in perfect health. A long-term quality-adjustment for an oesophagectomy of 0.8 is assigned, so that living a year of life post-oesophagectomy equals 0.8 'quality-adjusted' years [13]. In the next step of the analysis, the decision tree is evaluated. The results are listed in Figure 3. For reference, 55-year-old men from the general population have an average life expectancy of 24.5 years. For patients with Barrett's oesophagus who do not undergo surveillance, our model predicts an average life expectancy of 20.6 years. Surveillance with oesophagectomy for high-grade dysplasia provides the greatest gain in life expectancy — up to 2.4 years compared to no surveillance, and up to 1.4 years compared to surveillance with oesophagectomy for cancer. Considering only length of life (life expectancy), the optimal surveillance interval is every year. When quality of life is considered, surveillance every 2–3 years with oesophagectomy for high-grade dysplasia would provide the greatest quality-adjusted life expectancy, a gain of up to 1.2 years compared with

| A. Natural history | | Sources |
|---|---|---|
| 1. On average, the cumulative incidence of adenocarcinoma in patients with Barrett's oesophagus is 1.3% per year (1/75 patient years) | | [4–10] |
| 2. On average, the time period from endoscopically detectable oesophageal cancer to symptomatic cancer is 4–5 years | | [29] |

**B. Test characteristics**

The following represent the accuracy of endoscopic biopsy and pathologist's interpretation for detecting Barrett's mucosa, low-grade dysplasia, high-grade dysplasia and cancer. The true biologic condition of the mucosa is listed first, on the left, and the biopsy results are listed on the right.

| | | |
|---|---|---|
| **False-negative rates** | | |
| Barrett's mucosa interpreted as normal mucosa | 12.5% | * |
| Low-grade dysplasia interpreted as Barrett's mucosa | 17.5% | * |
| High-grade dysplasia interpreted as low-grade dysplasia | 11.5% | * |
| Cancer interpreted as high-grade dysplasia | 17.5% | * |
| **False-positive rates** | | |
| Normal mucosa interpreted as Barrett's mucosa | 7.5% | * |
| Barrett's mucosa interpreted as low-grade dysplasia | 14.5% | * |
| Low-grade dysplasia interpreted as high-grade dysplasia | 8.3% | * |
| High-grade dysplasia interpreted as cancer | 11.0% | * |

**C. Endoscopic and surgical procedures**

| | | |
|---|---|---|
| **Endoscopy** | | |
| Complications (perforation, respiratory arrest, myocardial infarction) | 13/10 000 procedures | [15] |
| Mortality (perforation not requiring surgery, respiratory arrest, myocardial infarction) | 0.21/10 000 procedures | [15] |
| Perforation requiring surgery | 1.6/10 000 procedures | [15] |
| **Surgical mortality** | | |
| *Repair of oesophageal perforation:* | | |
| Cancer | 19% | [23] |
| No cancer | 9.5% | [23] |
| Elective oesophagectomy | 9.5% | [16–22] |
| *Inoperable patients:* | | |
| Cancer inoperable because of other illnesses | 33% | [30] |

**D. Mortality from oesophageal cancer**

| | | |
|---|---|---|
| *Probability of complete resection of oesophageal cancer:* | | |
| Cancer detected by surveillance | 75% | [16–22,29] |
| Cancer detected when symptomatic | 49% | [16–22,29] |
| *Oesophageal cancer: relative 5-year survival:[§]* | | |
| Surveillance | 64% | [16–22,29] |
| No surveillance (complete resection) | 17% | [16–22,29] |
| Partial resection | 0.6% | [16–22,29] |
| No treatment | 0% | [16–22,29] |

**E. Short- and long-term morbidity**

| | | |
|---|---|---|
| *Short-term morbidity:* | | |
| Endoscopy | –1 day | [31] |
| Endoscopy with complication | –1 week | [31] |
| Elective surgery | –2 weeks | [31] |
| Emergency surgery | –4 weeks | [31] |
| *Long-term morbidity:* | | |
| Quality adjustment for oesophagectomy | 0.8 | ** |

**F. Costs**

| | | |
|---|---|---|
| Endoscopy | $500 | † |
| Endoscopy with complication | $2000 | † |
| Oesophagectomy | $8500 | † |
| Perforation requiring surgery: | | |
| Cancer | $17 700 | † |
| No cancer | $14 200 | † |
| Annual follow-up post-oesophagectomy | $900 | † |
| *Costs for terminal care of the patient with oesophageal cancer:* | | |
| Gastrostomy tube | $800–1300 | † |
| Hospice care per year | $35 000 | ‡ |

*Antonioli DA, Upton MP, personal communication; [§]Adjusted for deaths from other causes; **Expert opinion; †Actual variable costs and fees (New England Medical Center Clinical Cost Manager, 1990); ‡Estimates from hospice charges, Massachusetts, 1990 (Keeping S, personal communication).

**Fig. 2.** Quantifying the probability of each of the critical events: Parameters Surveillance model.

no surveillance and of up to 0.6 years compared with surveillance with oesophagectomy for cancer. Compared with the non-surveillance strategies, patients who undergo surveillance will, on average, have 4–10 times more endoscopies and endoscopic complications and twice the number of surgeries [13] (Fig. 3). These results suggest that endoscopic surveillance of patients with Barrett's oesophagus is effective in reducing mortality from oesophageal cancer and providing an increase in both length and quality of life. Because of variation in both the literature values and the opinions of experts in the field, the next step in a decision analysis is to examine the effect of changing the value of each parameter; this is called sensitivity analysis. Sensitivity analysis is performed on all parameters in the model to assess the stability of the results to variations in probability and outcome estimates. In sensitivity analyses, each parameter is varied over a broad range of values. If the preferred strategy is altered, then the analysis is said to be sensitive to the value of that parameter. Sensitivity analysis identifies the critical parameters for the decisions in the model. The identification of these critical parameters highlights areas that require future study. The sensitivity analysis targeted the incidence of cancer and the quality of life after oesophagectomy as areas requiring further inquiry. Thus, by systematically weighing the risks and benefits of diagnostic and

therapeutic options, the decision analysis provides information that can be used to determine the effectiveness of an endoscopic practice or technology and to guide future related research. If the endoscopic practice is determined to be effective, the next step in its assessment is to determine if it is cost-effective compared to other common medical practices. The decision model can incorporate costs to examine this issue.

Actual variable costs for endoscopic surveillance are included in the model. Costs reflect the economic resources consumed to provide medical services, including depreciation of equipment, building costs and professional and non-professional labour costs. This is in contrast to charges which reflect not only resources consumed, but profit or loss to the institution and may, therefore, be inflated to compensate for institutional losses [24]. The costs for endoscopy, endoscopy with a complication, the costs for elective and urgent oesophagectomy, and the costs for follow-up of post-oesophagectomy patients and of those with oesophageal cancer (Fig. 2) are included. The model records the costs as they occur during the lifetime of the patient, for example, as procedures and surgery are performed, and calculates the average lifetime cost per patient for each strategy. The analysis considers the direct costs of procedures and their subsequent complications, the

| Strategies | Procedures for 10 000 patients | | | | | |
| --- | --- | --- | --- | --- | --- | --- |
| | Cumulative incidence of cancer | Remaining life expectancy* | Quality-adjusted life expectancy | Endoscopies | Endoscopic complications | Surgeries |
| **No surveillance** | | | | | | |
| A: Oesophagectomy for cancer | 27.48 | 20.63 | 20.47 | 48 100 | 63 | 2300 |
| B: Oesophagectomy for high-grade dysplasia | 24.23 | 20.93 | 20.64 | 34 600 | 45 | 2600 |
| **Endoscopic surveillance: oesophagectomy for cancer** | | | | | | |
| $C_5$: Surveillance every 5 years | 18.11 | 21.62 | 21.04 | 200 900 | 260 | 3000 |
| $C_4$: Surveillance every 4 years | 17.34 | 21.72 | 21.08 | 223 200 | 290 | 3100 |
| $C_3$: Surveillance every 3 years | 16.59 | 21.82 | 21.12 | 253 500 | 330 | 3200 |
| $C_2$: Surveillance every 2 years | 15.92 | 21.92 | 21.15 | 296 200 | 390 | 3300 |
| $C_1$: Surveillance every 1 year | 15.37 | 22.01 | 21.15 | 360 000 | 470 | 3500 |
| **Endoscopic surveillance: oesophagectomy for high-grade dysplasia** | | | | | | |
| $D_5$: Surveillance every 5 years | 7.33 | 22.65 | 21.60 | 149 600 | 200 | 4000 |
| $D_4$: Surveillance every 4 years | 6.00 | 22.78 | 21.64 | 167 800 | 220 | 4200 |
| $D_3$: Surveillance every 3 years | 4.73 | 22.90 | 21.67 | 192 800 | 250 | 4400 |
| $D_2$: Surveillance every 2 years | 3.67 | 23.01 | 21.67 | 228 700 | 300 | 4600 |
| $D_1$: Surveillance every 1 year | 2.96 | 23.06 | 21.59 | 283 400 | 370 | 4800 |

Strategies with oesophagectomy for high-grade dysplasia result in fewer endoscopic complications and surgeries than those with oesophagectomy for cancer. Over time, more patients in the former strategies undergo oesophagectomy and, therefore, these patients do not undergo further endoscopies or suffer further endoscopic complications, resulting in fewer procedures and complications overall in these strategies. *Average remaining life expectancy for a healthy 55-year-old man is 24.5 years.

**Fig. 3.** Results of the evaluation of the decision tree.

costs of hospitalization and outpatient follow-up, and hospice costs for the care of the terminally ill patient with oesophageal cancer. The cost-effectiveness analysis is performed from the perspective of a health maintenance organization.

Cost-effectiveness analysis calculates the cost for each additional life year gained for a particular strategy, permitting comparison with other medical practices [25–27]. For example, in a high-risk patient (an asymptomatic 40-year-old man with a first-degree relative with colorectal cancer), screening for colorectal cancer (using yearly faecal occult blood testing, with flexible sigmoidoscopy and air-contrast barium enema every 3 years) costs $286 and increases life expectancy by 69 days compared to no screening. The incremental cost-effectiveness ratio, or the additional cost for each additional life year gained is the increase in cost of screening (with yearly faecal occult blood testing, and flexible sigmoidoscopy and air-contrast barium enema every 3 years) compared with no screening ($286 – $0) ÷ (69 days – 0 days) = $1513/life year gained (Fig. 4) [28]. Our model calculates incremental cost-effectiveness ratios for each strategy. For example, the incremental cost-effectiveness ratio for surveillance every 5 years with oesophagectomy for high-grade dysplasia (strategy D5) is the increase in cost for surveillance every 5 years with oesophagectomy for high-grade dysplasia compared with no surveillance with oesophagectomy for cancer (strategy A), divided by the increase in life expectancy of strategy D5 compared with strategy A.

Calculated incremental cost-effectiveness ratios permit comparison to the costs of other health-care programmes (Fig. 4). Thus, these incremental cost-effectiveness ratios and the results of this analysis can be used to identify the most cost-effective practices for the allocation of limited resources.

| | Costs per life year gained ($) | Source |
|---|---|---|
| Yearly faecal occult blood test, flexible sigmoidoscopy and barium enema every 3 years | 1513 | [28]* |
| Screening blood donors for HIV infection | 10 900 | [32]* |
| CABG for coronary disease | 20 000 | [24]** |
| Haemodialysis | 24 500 | [33] |
| Therapy for hypertension | 33 750 | [24]** |
| *Discount rate = 3%; **Discount rate = 5%. | | |

**Fig. 4.** Incremental cost-effectiveness ratios. CABG = coronary artery bypass grafting; HIV = human immunodeficiency virus.

In addition, cost-effectiveness analysis considers that future dollars are worth less than present dollars. Therefore, future costs are discounted to make them comparable to present dollars, and because life years are valued relative to dollars, they too are discounted in the cost-effectiveness analysis [28]. The standard (annual) discount rate of 5% was used. Figure 5 presents the results for strategies that consider only oesophagectomy for high-grade dysplasia. Strategies in which oesophagectomy is deferred for the development of cancer are not shown because they are clearly inferior, costing more and yielding a lower life expectancy than surveillance with oesophagectomy for high-grade dysplasia. The horizontal axis displays discounted quality-adjusted life expectancy in years, and the vertical axis displays the average lifetime cost per patient (discounted at the rate of 5%). Each of the bullets represents the results for a particular strategy. On the bottom left, no surveillance costs $5750 and provides 11.81 discounted years of life. Moving to the right, surveillance every 5 years costs $13 430 and provides 12.09 years of life. Thus, surveillance every 5 years increases life expectancy by 0.28 years at an additional cost of $7680. The incremental cost-effectiveness ratio for this strategy is calculated by dividing the additional cost by the increase in life expectancy ($7680 ÷ 0.28 years = $27 400 per additional life year gained) and is shown by the line connecting the two strategies (Fig. 5).

Figure 5 also shows that the incremental cost-effectiveness ratio for surveillance every 4 years rises quickly to $276 700 per quality-adjusted life year gained. As the surveillance interval decreases, costs increase, but life expectancy increases minimally. Thus, the incremental cost-effectiveness ratios rise rapidly as the surveillance interval decreases. Strategies with surveillance every 1, 2 or 3 years are inferior because they cost more and yield a lower discounted life expectancy than surveillance at less frequent intervals [13]. How can the policy maker use these results to determine if endoscopic surveillance of patients with Barrett's oesophagus is cost-effective compared to common medical practices? The policy maker can compare the incremental cost-effectiveness ratios for surveillance to the incremental cost-effectiveness ratios of common medical practices such as screening for colorectal cancer in high-risk populations and treatment of hypertension (Fig. 4). For the policy maker with a health-care budget of $10 000 000, surveillance every 5 years would increase the life expectancy of patients with Barrett's oesophagus by 365 years ($10 000 000 ÷ $27 400/life year gained). For comparison, $10 000 000 spent on screening for colorectal cancer would increase the life expectancy of the high-risk population by 6609 years ($10 000 000 ÷ $1513/life year gained), and $10 000 000 spent on therapy for hypertension would increase life expectancy of this group by 296 years ($10 000 000 ÷ $33 750/life year gained). These incre-

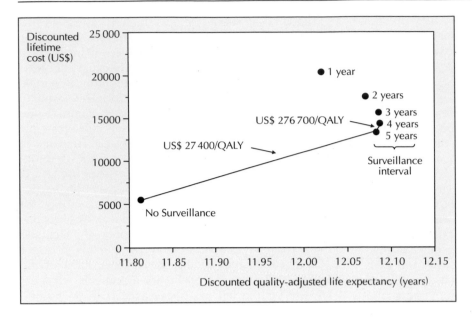

**Fig. 5.** Cost-effectiveness analysis. The results for strategies that consider only oesophagectomy for high-grade dysplasia. QALY = quality-adjusted life years.

mental cost-effectiveness ratios and the results of our analysis can be used to identify the most cost-effective practices for the allocation of limited resources.

Thus, the techniques of decision analysis and cost-effectiveness analysis are powerful tools for endoscopic practice and technology assessment. The methods described in this commentary provide data for the critical evaluation of our endoscopic practices, and for the development of policy recommendations. In an era of managed care, we can use these tools to provide policy makers with the crucial information needed to establish the effectiveness and cost-effectiveness of our practices. Our own critical appraisal of our practices can empower us to remain active participants in decisions that will determine our future.

# References

1. Talley NJ, Zinsmeister AR, Schleck C, Melton LJ: **The natural history of gastroesophageal reflux [abstract].** *Gastroenterology* 1992, **102**:A28.

2. Spechler J: **Barrett's esophagus: What's new and what to do.** *Am J Gastroenterol* 1989, **84**:220–223.

3. U.S. Bureau of the Census: *Statistical Abstract of the United States: 1991 (111th edition).* Washington DC, 1991.

4. Robertson CS, Mayberry JF, Nicholson DA, James PD, Atkinson M: **Value of endoscopic surveillance in the detection of neoplastic change in Barrett's oesophagus.** *Br J Surg* 1988, **75**:760–763.

5. Hameeteman W, Tytgat GNJ, Houthoff HJ, van den Tweel JG: **Barrett's esophagus: Development of dysplasia and adenocarcinoma.** *Gastroenterology* 1989, **96**:1249–1256.

6. Spechler SJ, Robbins AH, Rubins HB, Vincent ME, Heeren T, Doos WG, *et al.*: **Adenocarcinoma and Barrett's esophagus: an overrated risk?** *Gastroenterology* 1984, **87**:927–933.

7. Skinner DB: **The incidence of cancer in Barrett's esophagus varies according to series.** In *Benign Lesions of the Esophagus and Cancer: Answer to 210 Questions.* Edited by Giuli R, McCallum RW. New York: Springer-Verlag; 1989:764–765.

8. Ovaska J, Miettinen M, Kivilaakso E: **Adenocarcinoma arising in Barrett's esophagus.** *Dig Dis Sci* 1989, **34**:1336–1339.

9. Sampliner RE, Kogan FJ, Morgan RT, Tripp M: **Progression–regression of Barrett's esophagus.** *Gastroenterology* 1985, **88**:1567.

10. Williamson WA, Ellis FH, Gibb SP, Shahian DM, Aretz HT, Heatley GJ, *et al.*: **Barrett's esophagus: Prevalence and incidence of adenocarcinoma.** *Arch Intern Med* 1991, **151**:2212–2216.

11. ASGE: *The role of endoscopy in the surveillance of premalignant conditions of the upper gastrointestinal tract. Guidelines for clinical application.* Manchester: American Society for Gastrointestinal Endoscopy; 1986.

12. Spechler SJ: **Endoscopic surveillance for patients with Barrett's esophagus: Does the cancer risk justify the practice?** *Ann Intern Med* 1987, **106**:902–904.

13. Provenzale D, Kemp JA, Arora S, Wong JB: **A guide for surveillance of patients with Barrett's esophagus.** *Am J Gastroenterol* 1994, **89**:670–680.

14. Spechler SJ, Goyal RK: **Barrett's esophagus.** *N Engl J Med* 1986, **315**:362–371.

15. Silvis SE, Nebel O, Rogers G, Sugawa C, Mandelstam P: **Endoscopic complications. Results of the 1974 American society for gastrointestinal endoscopy survey.** *JAMA* 1976, **235**:928–930.

16. Cederqvist C, Nielsen J, Berthelsen A, Hansen HS: **Cancer of the esophagus, II. Therapy and outcome.** *Acta Chir Scand* 1978, **144**:233–240.

17. Skinner DB: **En bloc resection for neoplasms of the esophagus and cardia.** *J Thorac Cardiovasc Surg* 1983, **85**:59–71.

18. Ellis FH, Gibb SP, Watkins E: **Esophagogastrectomy — a safe, widely applicable and expeditious form of palliation for patients with carcinoma of the esophagus and cardia.** *Ann Surg* 1983, **198**:531–540.

19. Galandiuk S, Hermann RE, Cosgrove DM, Gassman JJ: **Cancer of the esophagus. The Cleveland Clinic experience.** *Ann Surg* 1986, **198**:101–108.

20. DeMeester TR, Zaninotto G, Johansson KE: **Selective therapeutic approach to cancer of the lower esophagus and cardia.** *J Thorac Cardiovasc Surg* 1988, **95**:42–54.

21. Wu YK, Huang KC: **Chinese experience in the surgical treatment of carcinoma of the esophagus.** *Ann Surg* 1979, **190**:361–365.

22. Earlam R. Cunha-Melo JR: **Oesophageal squamous cell carcinoma: I. A critical review of surgery.** *Br J Surg* 1980, **67**:381–390.

23.  Sabiston DC: *Textbook of surgery.* Thirteenth Edition. New York, Philadelphia: WB Saunders Co.; 1986:749–753.

24.  Weinstein MC, Fineberg HV, Elstein AS, Frazier HS, Neuhauser D, Neutra RR, *et al.*: *Clinical Decision Analysis.* Philadelphia: WB Saunders Co; 1980.

25.  Weinstein MC, Stason WB: **Foundations of cost-effectiveness for health and medical practices.** *N Engl J Med* 1977, **296**:716–721.

26.  Detsky AS, Naglie IG: **A clinician's guide to cost-effectiveness analysis.** *Ann Intern Med* 1990, **113**:147–154.

27.  Eisenberg JM: **Clinical economics: A guide to the economic analysis of clinical practices.** *JAMA* 1989, **262**:2879–2886.

28.  Eddy DM, Nugent FW, Eddy JF, Coller J, Gilbertsen V, Gottlieb LS, *et al.*: **Screening for colorectal cancer in a high-risk population: Results of a mathematical model.** *Gastroenterology* 1987, **92**:682–692.

29.  Guanrei Y, Songliang Q, He H, Guizen F: **Natural history of early esophageal squamous carcinoma and early adenocarcinoma of the gastric cardia in the People's Republic of China.** *Endoscopy* 1988, **20**:85–98.

30.  van Andel JG, Dees J, Dijkhuis CM, Fokkens W, van Houten H, de Jong PC, *et al.*: **Carcinoma of the esophagus: results of treatment.** *Ann Surg* 1979, **190**:684–689.

31.  United States Government: *Federal Register: Rules and Regulations.* Washington DC: United States Government Printing Office; Friday 9/1/89; 54;169:36533–36546.

32.  Eisenstaedt RS, Getzen TE: **Screening blood donors for immunodeficiency virus antibody: Cost-benefit analysis.** *Am J Public Health* 1988, **78**:450–454.

33.  Stange PV, Sumner AT: **Predicting treatment costs and life expectancy for end-stage renal disease.** *N Engl J Med* 1978, **298**:372–378.

Dr Dawn Provenzale, Duke University, Department of Medicine, Division of Gastroenterology, Epidemiology Decision Analysis, Outcomes Research Group, 2200 W. Main Street, Suite A-240, Room 9, Durham, NC 27705, USA.

# Progress in tissue sampling at ERCP

## Willis G. Parsons and Douglas A. Howell

Maine Medical Center, Portland, Maine, USA

## Introduction

The importance of tissue sampling during endoscopy was recognized early in the initial development of the technique. Excellent results in sampling upper gastro-intestinal and colonic mucosal neoplasms rapidly followed and a greater than 90% yield has remained the standard for over 20 years. The technical difficulties encountered with tissue sampling at endoscopic retrograde cholangiopancreatography (ERCP) as well as the wide availability of computed tomography (CT)-guided percutaneous needle aspiration delayed the parallel development of endoscopic biopsy techniques of pancreaticobiliary strictures.

Over the last 10 years, considerable research and a growing literature have demonstrated that a variety of techniques can produce highly specific tissue diagnoses but often with disappointing yields.

Recent changes in clinical practice have placed more emphasis on endoscopic tissue sampling. This has resulted in an increasing pressure to devise convenient, safe and more sensitive endoscopic techniques for evaluating pancreaticobiliary strictures. Although percutaneous fine needle aspiration has an excellent published yield with a good safety record, in practice the technique remains hampered by the need for an adequate target, patient discomfort, and the potential for complications. In addition, since biopsy is rarely performed initially, the need for a second CT scan in the era of cost containment is undesirable. Finally, and most important, scattered reports of needle tract seeding by malignancy raise the concern that CT-guided biopsy might negatively affect curability of resectable tumours. Warshaw [1•] found a much higher incidence of free intraperitoneal malignant cells at laparotomy in those patients who had recently undergone a percutaneous fine needle aspiration. A growing consensus now supports avoiding percutaneous biopsy in potentially resectable patients.

A review of the current status and recent progress in pancreaticobiliary tissue sampling at ERCP is therefore timely and should serve to stimulate research into new devices and techniques which could be adopted in routine clinical practice.

## Bile exfoliative cytology

Although the simplest and least expensive of the available cytology techniques, direct examination of bile samples obtained during ERCP is less sensitive than other techniques for detecting carcinoma of the pancreas, bile ducts, or gallbladder. Three prospective studies [2•,3,4] showed that the sensitivity of bile exfoliative cytology for detecting malignancy was 6–26%, significantly less than brush cytology, stent cytology, or endoscopic forceps biopsy. Six other studies published since 1981 produced an overall sensitivity for exfoliative bile cytology of 38% with 100% specificity but these were retrospective analyses. Kurzawinski et al. [2•] prospectively studied 100 consecutive patients with biliary tract strictures diagnosed at ERCP or percutaneous transhepatic cholangiography (PTC). The first 47 patients were studied with bile exfoliative cytology alone while the next 46 were evaluated with a 6 F Geenen cytology brush (Wilson-Cook Medical, Inc., Winston-Salem, NC, USA) modified according to the method of Foutch et al. [5•] and then with bile exfoliative cytology. Of note, in both groups bile cytology was obtained after stricture manipulation, dilation and stent placement. Seven patients were excluded from analysis due to inadequate follow-up information. Eighty-one patients had malignant strictures and 12 had benign strictures. Bile cytology alone was less sensitive than combined bile and brush cytology (38% or 16 out of 42 versus 69% or 27 out of 39). In addition, in the combined technique group, cytologic study of brushings was more sensitive than bile analysis (69% versus 26%). The superior sensitivity and accuracy of brush cytology held true with both ERCP and PTC, with a 9% sensitivity of bile cytology in PTC. No complications relating to bile aspiration or brushing were noted. Consistent with the majority of reports in the literature, no false-positives were seen in either group, making the test specificity 100% [6].

### Abbreviations

CT—computed tomography; **ERCP**—endoscopic retrograde cholangiopancreatography; **PCR**—polymerase chain reaction; **PTC**—percutaneous transhepatic cholangiography.

The notion that dilating or otherwise traumatizing a stricture increases the yield of subsequent cytologic tests by releasing malignant cells is attractive but not proven. Mohandas *et al.* [7] studied 64 consecutive patients undergoing endoscopic biliary drainage for malignant biliary strictures. Patients with ampullary or duodenal tumours were excluded. Forty-nine of the 64 underwent guide wire placement across the stricture, dilation using a 10 F Soehendra biliary dilator (Wilson-Cook Medical, Inc.), and then bile aspiration for cytology. A control group of 15 patients with malignant strictures contained 11 whose bile was aspirated without dilation and four who failed an attempt at dilation. Of note, the stricture was caused by gallbladder carcinoma in 33 (52%), cholangiocarcinoma in 14 (22%), pancreatic carcinoma in 11 (17%) and metastases in six (9%). Bile exfoliative cytology was positive for malignancy in 27% and 63% of the patients in the control group and the dilated group, respectively. These results are remarkable as almost two-thirds of the patients who underwent dilation had positive exfoliative cytology. The relatively high sensitivity of this technique rivals the best results reported with endoscopic brush cytology, forceps biopsy, or fine needle aspiration. In the accompanying editorial to Mohandas' report, Foutch [8•] appropriately cautions us that case selection and tumour bias may explain these results. Over half of their patients had gallbladder carcinoma which is probably easier to diagnose compared with pancreas and metastatic lesions. In addition, more than 25% of their control group was composed of patients with strictures that could not be dilated, possibly skewing the results in favour of the dilated group. These patients should have been included in the dilated group as an intention-to-treat analysis.

In an effort to define more reliable cytologic indicators of malignancy, Nakajima *et al.* [9] analysed bile specimens collected from external transhepatic drains of 22 patients with malignant and 13 patients with benign strictures. The bile smears were reviewed blindly and the incidence of each cytologic feature was noted. Next, a step-wise procedure of multiple regression analysis was performed. Finally, the reliable cytologic indicators of malignancy were selected, and their occurrence was calculated for each patient with benign and malignant disease. Six cytologic features were shown to be most significantly related to malignancy: loss of honeycomb arrangement, enlarged nuclei, loss of polarity, bloody background, flat nuclei and cell-in-cell arrangement. Three or more of these criteria were observed in cases of carcinoma more often than they were in cases of benign stricture. By using these criteria, the sensitivity for diagnosing cancer was 86% and the specificity was 77%.

K-ras oncogene mutations are present in over 90% of pancreaticobiliary cancers. In a preliminary report by Lee *et al.* [10], 20 patients with biliary strictures underwent bile exfoliative cytologic and K-ras mutational analysis. Twelve patents had malignant and eight had benign strictures. Using DNA prepared from the bile sample as a template, the polymerase chain reaction (PCR) amplified a 157 base pair product surrounding a codon of the K-ras oncogene. The presence of the K-ras mutation in the PCR product was determined by restriction endonuclease mapping. Only eight (40%) of the bile samples had cellular material, and none was diagnostic for malignancy. However, of the cases in which the 157 base pair product was detected, the sensitivity of K-ras mutational analysis for malignancy was 50% while the specificity was 100%. K-ras mutational analysis may become an elegant yet expensive method of determining the aetiology of strictures that have failed other methods.

## Pancreatic juice cytology

Attempts to diagnose pancreatic adenocarcinoma by obtaining pure pancreatic juice at ERCP and analysing for malignant cells have been variably successful. Kameya *et al.* [11] compared brush cytology of malignant pancreatic duct strictures to pancreatic juice cytology after saline washing or intravenous secretin administration and reported a 51% and 63% sensitivity, respectively. The reported sensitivities of pure pancreatic juice cytology for detecting pancreatic adenocarcinoma varies significantly, with a low of 30% [12] to a high of 79% [13]. In the majority of reported studies, the sensitivity of this technique for tumours of the head of the pancreas is greater than that for tumours of the body or tail [11,13]. Nakaizumi *et al.* [14] reported a 76% sensitivity and a 100% specificity of pure pancreatic juice cytology for detecting pancreatic cancer utilizing secretin stimulation and a 15-min collection period. In that same report, they described a new technique termed endoscopic retrograde intraductal catheter aspiration cytology. The technique involves placing a 5 F aspiration cytology catheter with a radiopaque tip (Wilson-Cook Medical, Inc.) over a 0.025 inch guide wire into the pancreatic duct next to the stricture, withdrawing the guide wire, injecting secretin intravenously, and moving the catheter repeatedly back and forth a few millimetres during constant maximal aspiration. In the nine patients who underwent this technique, there were no severe complications and both the sensitivity and specificity were 100% for detecting pancreatic cancer. Of note, a correct cytologic diagnosis was difficult in specimens containing contrast medium and, as a result, the last 5-min collection period after secretin stimulation should be used.

In an interesting report, Uehara *et al.* [15] studied 14 patients with mucin-producing pancreatic tumours (11 carcinomas and three adenomas) with endoscopic ultrasonography, ERCP and pancreatic juice cytology utilizing secretin and a 17-mm diameter aspiration catheter. No pancreatic sphincterotomies were performed. They found that the sensitivities and specificities, respectively, of these tests for detecting malignancy were 82% and 90% for endoscopic ultrasound, 91% and 91% for ERCP and 91% and 100% for pancreatic juice cytology. They concluded that pancreatic juice cytology has a primary role in the evaluation of patients with suspected or known mucin-producing tumours of the pancreas.

## Stent cytology

Cytologic analysis of the biofilm and sludge removed from a biliary endoprosthesis may yield a diagnosis of cancer in 25–36% of cases [3,16,17]. However, because the stent is in place on average for several months prior to removal, this technique is impractical. Most endoscopists have placed this technique in an adjunctive role, used when tissue diagnosis is needed at a follow-up endoscopy.

## Brush cytology

The first report of endoscopic brush cytology of the pancreaticobiliary tree was made by Osnes *et al.* in 1975 [18]. The technique did not gain widespread acceptance or use for almost 15 years because the available brushes were difficult to use and because it required removal of the guide wire prior to brushing. As a result, after

obtaining brush cytology, the endoscopist was required to negotiate the stricture a second time prior to stent placement. Foutch *et al.* [5•] described a novel technique in 1989 that maintained access above an obstruction with a guide wire while brush cytology was being performed. They pierced a hole in the distal tip of a standard cytology brush sheath, passed a guide wire through the lumen of the sheath and out through the hole, and then placed this device across the stricture.

Venu *et al.* [19•] developed a new brush in 1990 that was easier to pass through complex or difficult strictures (Geenen cytology brush device; Wilson-Cook Medical, Inc.) This brush is mounted on a wire with a flexible syringe tip lead allowing easy and secure engagement of the stricture, but without the ability to maintain access above the stricture. The brush is housed within a sheath and the two are removed together after tissue sampling.

In the last 6 years, endoscopic brush cytology has become the most widely employed method for diagnosing pancreaticobiliary malignancy. It is safe, simple to use, relatively inexpensive, moderately sensitive, and highly specific. Foutch [8•] reviewed the recent literature on endoscopic brush cytology for diagnosis of malignant biliary obstruction, and Figure 1 summarizes the test characteristics. Note that the overall sensitivity of brush cytology is higher for cholangiocarcinoma (63%) than for pancreatic carcinoma (56%), with an overall sensitivity of 59% [2,12,19•,20–26]. Perhaps

| Author | Patients (n) | Technical success (%) | Sensitivity* Bile duct cancer (%) | Sensitivity* Pancreatic cancer (%) | Sensitivity* Overall (%)** |
|---|---|---|---|---|---|
| Yap *et al.*, 1995 [22] | 52 | 100 | 75 | 42 | 54 |
| Ferrari *et al.*, 1994 [21] | 74 | 100 | 20 | 66 | 56 |
| Ryan and Baldauf , 1994 [20] | 48 | 100 | 30 | 45 | 42 |
| Kurzawinski *et al.*, 1993 [2•] | 39 | 100 | 60 | 65 | 69 |
| Ryan, 1991 [12] | 69 | 90 | 44 | 30 | 44 |
| Foutch *et al.*, 1990 [23] | 34 | 100 | 100 | 60 | 60 |
| Rabinowitz *et al.*, 1990 [24]† | 65 | 100 | 62 | – | 62 |
| Scudera *et al.*, 1990 [25] | 19 | 100 | 100 | 50 | 50 |
| Venu *et al.*, 1990 [19•] | 53 | 94 | 80 | 60 | 69 |
| Sawada *et al.*, 1989 [26]‡ | 72 | 100 | – | 85 | 85 |
| Total | 525 | 98 | 63 | 56 | 59 |

*Specificity for all studies was 100% with the exception of Ryan and Baldauf [20] and Yap *et al.* [22]; both of these had a specificity of 92%. **Values may reflect results for other malignancies as well as pancreatic and bile duct cancer. †Specimens were obtained by the percutaneous route; all subjects had cholangiocarcinoma. ‡Specimens were collected from the pancreatic duct; all subjects had pancreatic cancer.

**Fig. 1.** Cumulative brush cytology results for diagnosis of malignant biliary obstruction. Published with permission [8•].

more important, the specificity for detecting malignancy was 100% in all of these series except two, where it was 92%. This means that once a positive cytology result is obtained, further diagnostic testing is unnecessary. Should the patient be a surgical candidate, then further staging evaluation (CT, endoscopic ultrasound, angiography) would be indicated.

Van der Hul et al. [27] reviewed their experience of 66 patients with proximal cholangiocarcinoma and found that ultrasonography, ERCP and PTC were helpful whereas CT, angiography and brush cytology added little additional information. However, in only four out of the 66 patients could material from endoscopic brush cytologic examination be obtained, suggesting that an endoscopic tissue diagnosis was not a primary concern.

In a study of 65 patients with biliary strictures who underwent PTC only, Rabinowitz et al. [24] demonstrated that of the 37 with cholangiocarcinoma, brush cytology correctly diagnosed 15 (40% sensitivity) with only brushing. However, almost 40% of patients with cholangiocarcinoma who were found initially negative for malignancy were discovered to have malignant cells on a second attempt. Conversely, sequential negative brush cytology results decreased the possibility of cholangiocarcinoma to 41%, 20% and 0%, respectively. These findings suggest that performing several brushings will increase the sensitivity of detecting malignancy. It is not clear, though, whether these findings can be generalized to other clinical settings such as pancreatic carcinoma or metastatic lesions found at ERCP.

Ferrari et al. at the Brigham and Women's Hospital [21] carefully reviewed their experience with 74 patients with pancreaticobiliary strictures who underwent ERCP. Fifty-two patients had malignant strictures (56% pancreatic cancer, 19% cholangiocarcinoma, 12% metastatic, 13% other) while 22 had benign strictures. The overall brush cytology sensitivity was 56% with 100% specificity using the Geenen brush system. Cytology samples were obtained from the bile duct in 55 patients and from the pancreatic duct in 19 patients without complications. Whenever possible, the cytology sheath was used as the stent inner-guide catheter after removal of the friction grip handle. This allowed for placement of a stent without the need to remove the cytology brush from its sheath. Submitting the brush itself for histologic examination did not improve the results. The authors concluded that ERCP and brush cytology should be the first diagnostic approach in cases of pancreaticobiliary malignancy, including patients with an identified mass lesion on ultrasound or CT scan.

In cases of difficult cannulation through tight biliary strictures, the endoscopist using the Geenen cytology brush system must either use the brush sheath as the stent inner-guide catheter as we described previously [28•] or remove the brush from its sheath in order to maintain access. Baron et al. [29•] studied the potential for loss of diagnostic cellular material by pulling the brush through the sheath in the canine biliary system and whether a 'salvage' technique to extract material from the sheath itself could improve the yield. In phase I of the study, 20 consecutive samples were randomly collected by pushing the brush from the end of the sheath or pulling the brush through the length of the sheath. Pulling resulted in a significant loss of cellular material, such that only 22% of samples were diagnostic, compared with 100% of the push group. In phase II, 23 consecutive samples were randomly obtained in the same fashion. However, in the pull group, the distal tip of the empty sheath was placed in saline and 5 ml was aspirated. This solution was then placed into a specimen tube with its respective brush: the 'salvage' group. Ninety-two per cent of the phase II push group specimens were diagnostic while 82% of the salvage group specimens were diagnostic, suggesting that salvage cytology can greatly increase the diagnostic sensitivity. Although it is not clear whether the normal canine biliary tree behaves the same as a diseased human system when brushed, the data is compelling and should prompt endoscopists who pull cytology brushes through the sheath to use this salvage technique. Double-lumen cytology brushes that maintain access above a stricture while allowing for removal of the brush and sheath as a unit should circumvent these concerns and are now available (Combo-cath, Microvasive or Cytomax; Wilson-Cook Medical, Inc.).

Endoscopic brush cytology of pancreatic duct strictures is being utilized more as reports of its safety and sensitivity for detecting malignancy emerge. In a preliminary report, Lee et al. [30] studied 34 consecutive patients with unexplained pancreatic duct strictures who underwent endoscopic brushing using a 5 F cytology brush (GCBH-220; Wilson-Cook Medical, Inc.). Sufficient material was obtained for analysis in 33 out of the 34 patients; 10 patients had malignant strictures and three patients developed exacerbations of pre-existing pancreatitis (one mild, two moderate) after the procedure. The sensitivity of pancreatic duct brush cytology for detecting cancer was 40% with a 100% specificity. In a subset of 16 patients who underwent both bile duct and pancreatic duct brushings, the sensitivity of pancreatic duct cytology was 50% while that of bile duct cytology was 0%.

Van Laethem et al. [31] prospectively studied 38 patients with dominant main pancreatic duct strictures by ERCP, pancreatic brush cytology and pancreatic brush K-ras mutation analysis. Twenty patients had adenocarcinoma, six had mucin-secreting tumours and 12 had chronic pancreatitis. Eleven out of the 20 patients with adenocarcinoma had positive pancreatic brush cytology while no patients with chronic pancreatitis had positive cytology (sensitivity 55%, specificity 100%). Point mutations at codon 12 of the K-ras oncogene were detected in 17 out of the 20 patients with pancreatic adenocarcinoma (sensitivity 85%), in one of the six with mucin-secreting tumours and in none of the patients with chronic pancreatitis. This preliminary report suggests that genetic analysis of pancreatic duct brushing material at ERCP is more sensitive than standard brush cytology and may have a role in the evaluation of these patients.

In an effort to determine whether flow cytometric analysis for DNA content could increase the sensitivity of detecting malignancy in brushings, Ryan and Baldauf [20] obtained 51 sets of brushings from 48 patients with pancreaticobiliary strictures at ERCP. Two tissue samples were taken from each stricture and sent randomly for either routine cytology or flow cytometry. Brushings were obtained from either the bile duct of the pancreatic duct, depending on which duct was easiest to cannulate and most affected by the disease process. Both routine cytology and flow cytometry had a 41% sensitivity for diagnosing malignancy. The specificity was 92% for routine cytology and 77% for flow cytometry, with false-positive results obtained in one patient by the former technique and in three by the latter. When the studies were combined, so that the presence of either tumour cells or abnormal DNA content was diagnostic of malignancy, the sensitivity rose to 63% but the specificity fell to 69%. Of interest, for those patients with pancreatic carcinoma, mean survival was longer in those with a diploid cell population (8.9 months) compared with those with aneuploid brushings (3 months), as revealed by flow cytometry. The high incidence of false-positive results when combining flow cytometry with routine cytology is disturbing and should limit the application of this technique to research studies only.

In a similar study, Lee *et al.* [32] obtained bile duct brushings from 28 patients with various biliary pathologies. Routine cytology and DNA content as measured by an image analyser (CAS-200; Cell Analysis System, Inc., Elmhurst, IL, USA) were determined. The sensitivity of image analysis for the diagnosis of cancer was 63%, the specificity was 75% and the positive predictive value was 50%.

## Endoscopic transpapillary biopsy

Although it is much less frequently performed than bile and brush cytology, forceps biopsy of biliary strictures at ERCP began at the birth of biliary sphincterotomy in Erlangen, Germany. Classen and Demling performed their pioneering first pull-type sphincterotomy to enable placement of a standard endoscopic biopsy forceps to sample a malignant bifurcation stricture in 1974 (personal communication). Because of the size of standard endoscopic biopsy forceps, a sphincterotomy is a necessary but not always sufficient procedure to allow fluoroscopically guided biopsies. As a result, in the subsequent 20 years, the use of endoscopic forceps biopsy has received only scattered attention in the literature and in practice. In the exhaustive review of Kurzawinski *et al.* of cytology for biliary strictures [33•], the data from four series using endobiliary biopsy between 1986 and 1991 is pooled, yielding a 68% sensitivity and a 100% specificity. The largest of these series contained only 17 patients, however [34].

Kubota *et al.* [35•] utilized a recently developed malleable forceps (FB39; Olympus, Tokyo, Japan) whose outer sheath consists of a 1.92-mm outer diameter fluorinated ethylene propylene tube to acquire transpapillary tissue in a consecutive series of 43 patients with pancreaticobiliary strictures found at ERCP. There were 19 cholangiocarcinomas, 15 pancreatic carcinomas, five benign biliary strictures and four benign pancreatic strictures. Although 14 patients underwent papillotomy prior to biopsy, the forceps biopsy could be placed into the appropriate duct selectively with free-hand technique in all patients. Tissue acquisition (four specimens per patient) was successful in 41 out of the 43 patients (95%), without complications. The overall sensitivity for detecting malignancy was 81% (89% sensitivity for cholangiocarcinoma, 71% sensitivity for pancreatic carcinoma) with a 100% specificity. The authors concluded that this was a simple, safe and convenient method that should be used as an initial diagnostic method during ERCP.

## Endoscopic needle aspiration

From this review of exfoliative and brush cytology and forceps biopsy, no consecutive large series approaches the 90% sensitivity enjoyed in endoscopic sampling of hollow organ mucosal lesions. This should not be surprising since tumours producing pancreaticobiliary strictures are greatly extrinsic malignancies arising beneath the ductal epithelium and compressing the ducts. The benign epithelium is usually well preserved, explaining the persistence of strictures rather than the development of solid tumour obstruction. Sampling well below the stricture mucosa would be necessary to increase the above reviewed modest yields.

We developed a ball-tipped catheter with a retractable 22-gauge, 7-mm long needle (Howell biliary aspiration needle; HBAN 22; Wilson-Cook Medical, Inc.) to perform endoscopic needle aspiration for cytology of biliary strictures and reported initial results in 1992 [28•].

Of the 31 consecutive patients reported in that study, carcinoma was confirmed in 26 (19 pancreatic adenocarcinoma, five cholangiocarcinoma, one gallbladder carcinoma and one metastatic colon carcinoma) while five had benign lesions. All patients underwent sphincterotomy and endoscopic needle aspiration while 29 patients also underwent brushing using the Geenen guide wire tip cytology brush. The technique of endoscopic needle aspiration is crucial to obtaining the highest possible yield. After cannulating the bile duct with the HBAN 22 device, the tip is advanced to a point just below the stricture. Next, the needle is extended into the tumour and aspirations are obtained using a 20 ml dry syringe while gently moving the needle back and forth within the tumour (Fig. 2). We generally chose three sites for biopsy, releasing the suction between each placement of the needle. After all aspirations were performed, the needle was retracted into the ball tip and the catheter was withdrawn from the endoscope. The contents of the needle were expressed using an air filled syringe and, if necessary, by running the stainless steel stylet back down the catheter. Slides were prepared and sent for analysis.

Positive endoscopic needle aspirate cytology was obtained in 16 out of the 26 patients (61.5% sensitivity) with no false-positive results or complications. Positive brushings were obtained in only two out of the 24 patients (8.3% sensitivity), perhaps due to pre-selection which favoured smaller, earlier tumours not seen or successfully biopsied at CT scanning. The sensitivity of endoscopic needle aspiration suggests that it should be utilized at the index ERCP along with brush cytology and, perhaps, endoscopic transpapillary forceps biopsy.

Recent refinement of the technique of endoscopic needle aspiration has included priming the needle with heparinized saline to avoid clogging of the needle tip and aspirating with a small amount of saline in the syringe to produce hydraulic rather than vacuum suction for greater aspiration force at the tip [36]. Cells admixed with saline will not adhere to glass slides which were already somewhat inconvenient to produce during the procedure. With this modification, the needle is flushed with Mucolexx (Lerner Labs, Pittsburgh, PA, USA) or other cytology transport media. The speci-

(a)

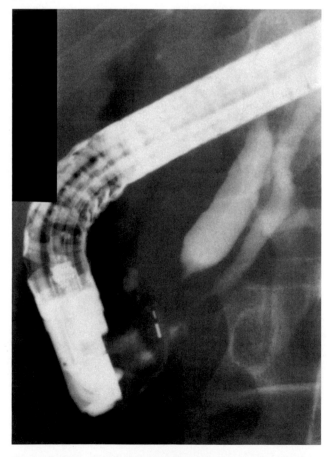

(b)

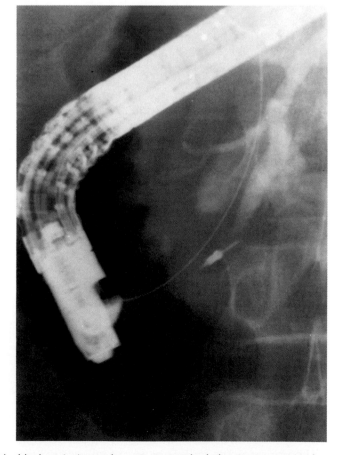

**Fig. 2.** (a) Distal common bile duct and main pancreatic duct strictures ('double duct sign') at endoscopic retrograde cholangiopancreatography in an elderly patient with adenocarcinoma of the pancreas. (b) Sampling of the main pancreatic duct stricture (same patient as in Fig. 2a) using the Howell biliary aspiration needle.

men can then be spun and the cellular pellet fixed by cell block technique producing a histologic section which can provide additional information regarding tumour differentiation. Figure 3a demonstrates a large piece of benign biliary epithelium whereas the adjoining Figure 3b reveals a moderately differentiated adenocarcinoma, obtained using the Howell biliary aspiration needle. Finally, we demonstrated no loss of sensitivity with this refinement [36].

## Combined endoscopic sampling

With the development of easier endoscopic brush cytology, endoscopic transpapillary forceps biopsy and endoscopic needle aspiration, a prospective study comparing the yields of these techniques was needed and this was provided by Sherman *et al.* [37] at Indiana University Medical Center. Between 1990 and 1994, 127 patients with biliary strictures underwent 'triple sampling' with the Geenen cytology brush (one brush), the Howell aspiration needle (two thrusts), and endobiliary

forceps biopsy (three to four bites). Strictures were ultimately judged malignant in 77 and benign in 45. High-grade dysplasia was tallied as cancer. Figure 4 displays their positive sampling frequency in the malignant strictures undergoing the three simultaneous sampling methods. Note that the overall sensitivity rate for detecting cancer was 71% when all three techniques were combined. Indeed, combining a second or a third method clearly increases the sensitivity of detecting malignancy compared with any one method alone. On the basis of these results, their conclusion that at least two tissue sampling methods be routinely employed makes sense. An excellent, up-to-date review of endoscopic tissue sampling techniques in the detection of pancreatic adenocarcinoma, including this triple sampling data, is provided by Lehman [38•]. Figure 5 summarizes the literature on the sensitivity of endoscopic biliary tissue sampling techniques in patients with strictures from pancreatic adenocarcinoma. Note that none of the three techniques is clearly superior to the others. In addition, the overall sensitivity for detecting pancreatic adenocarcinoma with each technique is

(a)

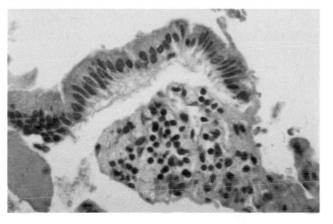

(b)

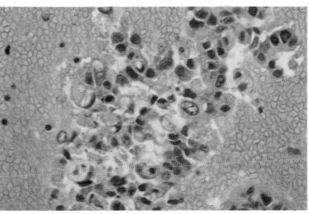

**Fig. 3.** (a) Photomicrograph of benign ductal epithelium obtained by the Howell biliary aspiration needle (HBAN 22; Wilson-Cook Medical, Inc.). (b) Photomicrograph of cell block made from a Howell needle aspirate revealing a moderately differentiated adenocarcinoma.

| | Pancreas carcinoma (%) (n = 38) | Cholangiocarcinoma (%) (n = 27) | Metastases (%) (n = 12) | All cancers (%) (n = 77) |
|---|---|---|---|---|
| Brush | 45 | 44 | 33 | 43* |
| FNA | 34 | 41 | 33 | 37* |
| Biopsy | 42 | 59 | 33 | 47† |
| Brush + FNA | 45 | 59 | 50 | 51‡ |
| Brush + biopsy | 58 | 74 | 58 | 64 |
| FNA + biopsy | 55 | 74 | 58 | 62 |
| Brush + FNA + biopsy | 63 | 81 | 75 | 71 |

*$P < 0.05$ versus brush + biopsy, fine needle aspiration (FNA) + biopsy and brush + FNA + biopsy; †$P < 0.05$ versus brush + biopsy and brush + FNA + biopsy; ‡$P < 0.05$ versus brush + FNA + biopsy.

**Fig. 4.** Positive sampling frequency in malignant strictures undergoing three simultaneous sampling methods. Published with permission [37].

| Study* | | Pancreatic adenocarcinoma | | |
|---|---|---|---|---|
| | n | Brush | FNA | Biopsy |
| Aabakken et al. [34] | 7 | – | – | 1 (14%) |
| Foutch et al. [23] | 5 | 3 (60%) | – | – |
| Howell et al. [28•] | 19 | 0 (0%) | 10 (53%) | – |
| Ferrari et al. [21] | 24 | 16 (67%) | – | – |
| Kubota et al. [35] | 14 | – | – | 10 (71%) |
| Ryan and Baldauf [20] | 22 | 10 (45%) | – | – |
| Scudera et al. [25] | 10 | 5 (50%) | – | – |
| Venu et al. [19•] | 5 | 3 (60%) | – | – |
| Sherman et al. [37] | 38 | 17 (45%) | 13 (34%) | 16 (42%) |
| Total | 144 | 54/123 (44%) | 23/57 (40%) | 27/59 (46%) |

*All studies report a specificity of 96–100%. Specimens with atypia only are considered negative for malignancy in this figure.

**Fig. 5.** Sensitivity of endoscopic biliary tissue sampling techniques in patients with malignant strictures from pancreatic adenocarcinoma. FNA = fine needle aspiration. Adapted with permission [38•].

lower than that reported for cholangiocarcinoma or metastatic disease. This likely reflects its extrinsic nature which compresses the duct epithelium without destroying it.

The need for improved cytologic yields, especially at the index ERCP when a pancreaticobiliary stricture is encountered, has sparked interest in developing disposable endoscopic devices that obtain tissue using several different techniques. In a preliminary report, Parasher et al. [39] describe the development of a wire-guided brush that allows simultaneous exfoliative cytology and submucosal ductal scrape biopsy. Brushing/biopsies were obtained using a brush made of a semi-rigid blunt ended bristles mounted over a 6 F ball-tipped nylon catheter which goes over a 0.035 inch Teflon guide wire by initiating a push-pull manoeuvre through the stricture. Prior sphincterotomy was not required. Seven patients with malignancy (four with cholangiocarcinoma, three with pancreatic cancer) were studied, although in the first three patients an earlier prototype device was used which did not permit passage of the stricture and, as a result, no tissue was obtained. All patients had positive cytology, either by brush or scrape biopsy technique. Although the presence of submucosal tissue was verified using histologic staining of muscle and collagen, no complications were noted.

Haluszka et al. [40] developed a modification of a multiple biopsy device (Triton Technologies, Salem,

Ohio, USA) to obtain samples of bile duct epithelium for conventional histology and of bile for flow cytometric analysis. The strictures were traversed with the modified dilation catheter that contains specialized side ports, and samples were obtained via suction and the Triton cutting device. Of the six patients with biliary strictures who were studied, three had malignancy. Not all samples contained fragments of tissue sufficient for histology.

To simplify the technical challenges of performing multiple techniques of tissue sampling during a single procedure, we have developed a new device (Howell biliary introducer with needle; HBIN 35; Wilson-Cook Medical, Inc.). The device is designed to permit dilation of the stricture, followed by 22-gauge fine needle aspiration, 5 F forceps biopsy and, finally, brush cytology all in rapid sequence (Fig. 6). The device consists of a introducer fashioned from a 10 F double-lumen dilating catheter with a tapered radiopaque tip, a 0.035 inch guide wire channel and a 5 F biopsy channel fitted with a 45° ramp. After placement of a guide wire, the introducer can be advanced through the papilla without sphincterotomy and the stricture is dilated. After pulling the ramp to a position just below the stricture, the preloaded metal ball-tipped 5 F catheter loaded with a retractable 22-gauge Chiba type biopsy needle is thrust at 45° deeply into the submucosal tumour (Figs 6a and 6b). The biopsy technique and sample preparation is as previously described [28•].

After withdrawal of the needle, 5 F forceps biopsies are obtained using the JB-38W forceps designed for the mother/baby duodenoscope system (Olympus, Figs 6c and 6d).

Finally, the ramp is then positioned above the top of the stricture permitting placement of the spring wire tipped Geenen cytology brush into the dilated ducts above (Figs 6e and 6f). By pulling the side-by-side introducer and brush to and fro through the stricture, the already traumatized mucosa is further abraded to produce a highly cellular specimen. The introducer with the brush left in its separate channel can then be withdrawn, leaving the guide wire in place for stent placement. The brush specimen is prepared with a push technique to avoid loss of cellular material [29•].

Preliminary results confirm that the device can be successfully introduced with rapid specimen collection. The initial combined yield of at least one positive test in 10 out of 15 patients with malignancy (67%) compares favourably with the best combined yield series in the literature. Whether the elusive goal of 90% yield can be achieved with this device must await further experience and refinement.

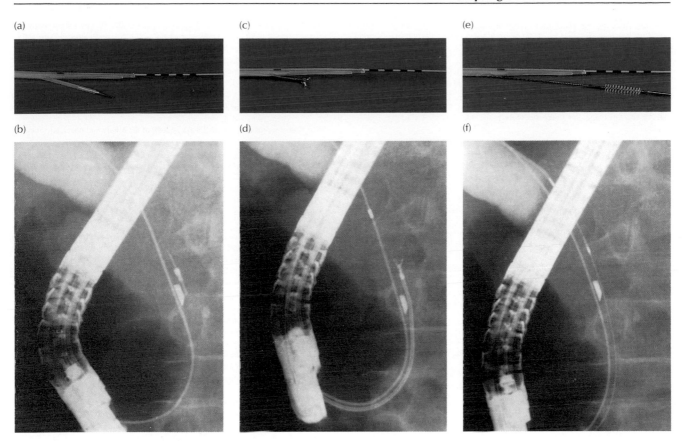

**Fig. 6.** (a) Photograph of the Howell biliary introducer with needle (HBIN 35, Wilson-Cook Medical, Inc.) with the preloaded metal ball-tipped 5 F catheter loaded with the 22-gauge biopsy needle in biopsy position. (b) A bile duct stricture secondary to a head of the pancreas carcinoma is being biopsied using the biopsy needle of the HBIN 35 device. (c) Photograph of the HBIN 35 device with the 5 F biopsy forceps (Olympus JB-38W) in biopsy position. (d) The malignant bile duct stricture is biopsied using the Olympus JB-38W forceps through the HBIN 35 device. (e) Photograph of the HBIN 35 device with the spring wire tipped Geenen cytology brush in position. (f) The malignant bile duct stricture is brushed using the Geenen cytology brush through the HBIN 35 device.

## Conclusion

Tissue sampling at ERCP provides a unique challenge in endoscopy as evidenced by this comprehensive review. Because of the extrinsic nature and multiple tumour types involved, a single technique of tissue sampling which can produce yields in excess of 90% seems unlikely at the present time. To date, the greatest yields have utilized combinations of sampling techniques and it is likely that this will remain a requirement for the future. Improved equipment and refinements are needed to standardize and simplify the sequence of procedures.

Given that the aetiology of pancreaticobiliary strictures dictates both the management and prognosis, accurate and sensitive tissue sampling at ERCP will continue to be an area of active research.

## References and recommended reading

Papers of particular interest, published within the annual period of review, have been highlighted as:

• of special interest
•• of outstanding interest

1. Warshaw AL: **Implications of peritoneal cytology for staging of early**
   • **pancreatic cancer.** *Am J Surg* 1991, **161**:26–29.
   Patients with pancreatic adenocarcinoma who underwent percutaneous fine needle aspiration had a 75% incidence of positive peritoneal cytology compared with 19% of those not undergoing this procedure.

2. Kurzawinski TR, Deery JS, Dick R, Hobbs KEF, Davidson BR: **A prospec-**
   • **tive study of biliary cytology in 100 patients with bile duct strictures.**
   *Hepatology* 1993, **18**:1399–1403.
   Prospective study of 100 patients comparing bile exfoliative cytology alone to brush and exfoliative cytology demonstrating that brush cytology was more sensitive.

3. Foutch PG, Kerr DM, Harlan JR, Kummet KD: **A prospective controlled**
   **analysis of endoscopic cytotechniques for diagnosis of malignant biliary**
   **strictures.** *Am J Gastroenterol* 1991, **86**:577–580.
   Prospective study of 30 patients with bile duct strictures revealing 36% sensitivity for stent cytology, 33% sensitivity for brush cytology and 6% sensitivity for bile cytology for detecting malignancy.

4. Chang L, French S, Hierro M, Lo SK: **A prospective study comparing**
   **endobiliary biopsy, brush and aspiration cytology during ERCP in**
   **diagnosing biliary obstructive lesions [abstract].** *Am J Gastroenterol* 1992,
   **87**:1282A

Abstract reporting that endobiliary biopsy of biliary strictures was more sensitive (64%) than either brush cytology (21%) or exfoliative bile cytology (8%) for detecting malignancy.

5. Foutch PG, Harlan JR, Kerr D, Kummet TD: **Wire-guided brush cytology:**
• **a new endoscopic method for diagnosis of bile duct cancer.** *Gastrointest Endosc* 1989, **35**:243–247.
Description of the 'Foutch' technique for performing brush cytology of biliary strictures while maintaining wire access above the stricture.

6. Davidson BR: **Progress in determining the nature of bile duct strictures.** *Gut* 1993, **34**:725–726.
Brief review of the literature on endoscopic tissue sampling of bile duct strictures.

7. Mohandas KM, Swaroop VS, Gullar SU, Dave UR, Jagannath P, DeSouza LJ: **Diagnosis of malignant obstructive jaundice by bile cytology: results improved by dilating the bile duct strictures.** *Gastrointest Endosc* 1994, **40**:150–154.
Series report showing that dilation of malignant biliary strictures to 10 F enhances the sensitivity of subsequent bile exfoliative cytology.

8. Foutch PG: **Diagnosis of cancer by cytologic methods performed during**
• **ERCP.** *Gastrointest Endosc* 1994, **40**:249–252.
Thoughtful review of endoscopic cytology techniques as well as an editorial to four accompanying articles [7,20,21,29•] in the March/April 1994 issue of *Gastrointestinal Endoscopy*.

9. Nakajima T, Tajima Y, Sugano I, Nagao K, Sakuma A, Koyama Y, *et al.*: **Multivariate statistical analysis of bile cytology.** *Acta Cytol* 1994, **38**:51–55.
Retrospective multiple regression analysis of exfoliative bile cytologic features, yielding an 86% sensitivity with a disappointing 77% specificity.

10. Lee JG, Leung JWC, Cotton PB, Mannon PJ: **K-ras oncogene mutational analysis by PCR improves the diagnostic yield from bile by ERCP [abstract].** *Gastrointest Endosc* 1994, **40**:405A.
Abstract describing the use of K-ras mutational analysis to determine the nature of biliary strictures in 20 patients.

11. Kameya S, Kuno N, Kasugai T: **The diagnosis of pancreatic cancer by pancreatic juice cytology.** *Acta Cytol* 1981, **25**:354–360.
Prospective comparison of brush cytology to pancreatic juice cytology of malignant pancreatic duct strictures, reporting 51% and 63% sensitivities, respectively.

12. Ryan M: **Cytologic brushing of ductal lesions during ERCP.** *Gastrointest Endosc* 1991, **37**:139–142.
Retrospective review of 69 patients who underwent endoscopic brush cytology of pancreaticobiliary strictures. Technical success rate was 90%, sensitivity was 44% and specificity was 100%.

13. Endo Y, Morii T, Tamura H, Okuda S: **Cytodiagnosis of pancreatic malignant tumors by aspiration under direct vision, using a duodenal fiberscope.** *Gastroenterology* 1974, **67**:944–951.
Fourteen patients with pancreatic carcinoma underwent duodenoscope-directed collection of pancreatic juice for cytology, yielding a 79% sensitivity and 100% specificity.

14. Nakaizumi A, Tatsuta M, Uehara H, Yamamoto R, Takenaka A, Kishigami Y, *et al.*: **Cytologic examination of pure pancreatic juice in the diagnosis of pancreatic carcinoma. The endoscopic retrograde intraductal catheter aspiration cytologic technique.** *Cancer* 1992, **70**:2610–2614.
Pure pancreatic juice cytology had a 76% sensitivity for detecting pancreatic carcinoma. Endoscopic retrograde intraductal catheter aspiration technique is described.

15. Uehara H, Nakaizumi A, Iishi H, Tatsuta M, Kitamra T, Okuda S, *et al.*: **Cytologic examination of pancreatic juice for differential diagnosis of benign and malignant mucin-producing tumors of the pancreas.** *Cancer* 1994, **74**:826–833.
Cytologic examination of pancreatic juice was better than endoscopic ultrasound or pancreatography for differentiating benign from malignant mucin-producing pancreatic tumours.

16. Wiersema M, Lehman G, Hawes R, Sherman S, Earle D: **Improvement of diagnostic yield of brush cytology in malignant biliary strictures by the use of supplemental tissue sampling techniques [abstract].** *Gastrointest Endosc* 1992, **38**:265A.
Abstract noting a 25% sensitivity of stent cytology in diagnosing pancreatic or bile duct carcinoma if atypia was excluded.

17. Kohler B, Kaufman V, Maier M, Riemann JF, Wegener K: **Accuracy of histological and cytological examination for malignant cells in biliary endoprostheses [abstract].** *Gastrointest Endosc* 1994, **40**:399A.
Abstract demonstrating that stent cytology had 33% sensitivity and 100% specificity in the diagnosis of various pancreaticobiliary cancers.

18. Osnes M, Serck-Hanssen A, Myren J: **Endoscopic retrograde brush cytology (ERBC) of the biliary and pancreatic ducts.** *Scand J Gastroenterol* 1975, **10**:829–831.
The first report of endoscopic brush cytology of the biliary and pancreatic ducts.

19. Venu RP, Geenen JE, Kini M, Hogan WJ, Payne M, Johnson GK, *et al.*:
• **Endoscopic retrograde brush cytology a new technique.** *Gastroenterology* 1990, **99**:1475–1479.
Description of the Geenen cytology brush device and its 94% technical success rate, 70% sensitivity and 100% specificity in the evaluation of 53 consecutive patients with pancreaticobiliary strictures.

20. Ryan ME, Baldauf MC: **Comparison of flow cytometry for DNA content and brush cytology for detection of malignancy in pancreaticobiliary strictures.** *Gastrointest Endosc* 1994, **40**:133–139.
Both routine brush cytology and flow cytometry of brush material have a 42% sensitivity for detecting malignancy. When the two are combined, the sensitivity rises to 64% but the specificity falls to 69%.

21. Ferrari AP, Lichtenstein DR, Slivka A, Chang C, Carr-Locke DL: **Brush cytology during ERCP for the diagnosis of biliary and pancreatic malignancies.** *Gastrointest Endosc* 1994, **40**:140–145.
Meticulous review of the Carr-Locke experience with brush cytology, showing a 56% sensitivity and 100% specificity for detecting malignancy. Submitting the brush for histological examination is not helpful.

22. Yap CK, ten Kate FJW, Ramsoekh B: **A retrospective analysis of brush cytology in biliary tract strictures: sensitivity, specificity, atypia and the effect of indwelling biliary stents.** *Endoscopy* 1995, in press.
Article in press that reports 42% sensitivity of brush cytology for pancreatic cancer, 75% sensitivity for cholangiocarcinoma and an overall sensitivity of 54%.

23. Foutch PG, Kerr DM, Harlan JR, Manne RK, Kummet TD, Sanowski RA: **Endoscopic retrograde wire-guided brush cytology for diagnosis of patients with malignant obstruction of the bile duct.** *Am J Gastroenterol* 1990, **85**:791–795.
A retrospective review of 34 patients with pancreaticobiliary strictures who underwent endoscopic retrograde wire guided brush cytology ('Foutch' technique), showing 60% sensitivity and 100% specificity. Sensitivities were 100% for cholangiocarcinoma, 60% for pancreatic carcinoma and 22% for metastases.

24. Rabinowitz M, Zajko AB, Hassanein T, Shetty B, Bron KM, Schade RR, *et al.*: **Diagnostic value of brush cytology in the diagnosis of bile duct carcinoma: A study in 65 patients with bile duct strictures.** *Hepatology* 1990, **12**:747–752.
Retrospective PTC study of 65 patients with biliary strictures. Repeated brushings increased yield over the initial 40% obtained with the first brush.

25. Scudera PL, Koizumi J, Jacobson IM: **Brush cytology examination of lesions encountered during ERCP.** *Gastrointest Endosc* 1990, **36**:281–284.
Retrospective review showing 60% sensitivity of brush cytology for detecting malignancy in biliary strictures. Using the Geenen cytology brush device, sensitivity was 50% with 100% specificity.

26. Sawada Y, Gonda H, Hayashida Y: **Combined use of brushing cytology and endoscopic retrograde pancreatography for the early detection of pancreatic cancer.** *Acta Cytol* 1989, **33**:870–874.
Seventy-two patients underwent pancreatic duct stricture brushing, yielding 85% sensitivity for detecting carcinoma.

27. Van Der Hul RL, Pliasier PW, Lameris JS, Veeze-Kuijpers B, Van Blankenstein M, Terpstra OT: **Proximal cholangiocarcinoma: A multidisciplinary approach.** *Eur J Surg* 1994, **160**:213–218.
Retrospective review of 66 patients with cholangiocarcinoma.

28. Howell DA, Beveridge RP, Bosco JJ, Jones M: **Endoscopic needle aspira-**
• **tion biopsy at ERCP in the diagnosis of biliary strictures.** *Gastrointest Endosc* 1992, **38**:531–535.
Our description of the Howell biliary aspiration needle and its use in 31 patients with biliary strictures at ERCP showing a 61.5% sensitivity and 100% specificity for detecting cancer.

29.    Baron TH, Lee JG, Wax TD, Schmitt CM, Cotton PB, Leung JW: **An in vitro,**
•      **randomized, prospective study to maximize cellular yield during bile**
       **duct cytology.** *Gastrointest Endosc* 1994, **40**:146–149.
*In vitro* study showing that if a brush is pulled from the sheath during bile duct brush
cytology there is a significant loss of cellular material.

30.    Lee JG, Schutz SM, Layfield L, Leung JWC, Cotton PB: **A prospective study**
       **of endoscopic pancreatic duct cytology in 34 consecutive patients [ab-**
       **stract].** *Gastrointest Endosc* 1994, **40**:407A.
Abstract showing 40% sensitivity and 100% specificity of pancreatic duct brush
cytology for detecting pancreatic carcinoma.

31.    Van Laethem JL, Vertongen P, Deviere J, Rickeart F, Cremer M, Robberecht
       P: **Detection of c-Ki-ras gene codon 12 mutations in pancreatic duct**
       **brushing samples in the diagnosis procedure of pancreatic tumors [ab-**
       **stract].** *World Congress of Gastroenterology, Los Angeles,* October 1994,
       98A.
Abstract describing a prospective study comparing pancreatic duct brush cytology
with pancreatic duct brush K-ras mutational analysis. The sensitivity of brush
cytology was 55% while that of K-ras mutational analysis was 85% for detecting
pancreatic cancer.

32.    Lee JG, Layfield L, Kerns BJ, Leung JWC, Cotton PB: **What you see is not**
       **what you get. The utility of image analysis in exfoliated bile duct cells for**
       **diagnosis of cancer [abstract].** *Gastrointest Endosc* 1994, **40**:403A.
Abstract reporting that the sensitivity of measuring the DNA content of bile duct
brushings for the diagnosis of cancer was 63% while the specificity was 75% .

33.    Kurzawinski T, Deery A, Davidson BR: **Diagnostic value of cytology for**
•      **biliary stricture.** *Br J Surg* 1993, **80**:414–421.
An excellent, exhaustive review of the history and recent progress in cytology of
pancreaticobiliary strictures.

34.    Aabakken L, Karesen R, Serck-Hanssen A, Osnes M: **Transpapillary biop-**
       **sies and brush cytology from the common bile duct.** *Endoscopy* 1986,
       **18**:49–51.
Series report of 17 patients with biliary strictures who underwent transpapillary
forceps biopsies and brush cytology.

35.    Kubota Y, Takaoka M, Tuni K, Ogura M, Kin H, Fujimura K, *et al.*:
•      **Endoscopic transpapillary biopsy for diagnosis of patients with pancrea-**
       **ticobiliary ductal strictures.** *Am J Surg* 1993, **88**:1700–1704.

Using the Olympus FB39 forceps to sample 43 consecutive patients with pancreaticobiliary strictures, the technical success rate was 95%, the sensitivity was 81% and
the specificity was 100%.

36.    Muggia RA, Bosco JJ, Jones MS, Howell DA: **Improved cytologic tech-**
       **nique for endoscopic needle aspiration (ENA) [abstract].** *Gastrointest
       Endosc* 1993, **39**:279A.
Abstract reporting that refinement of the technique of endoscopic needle aspiration
did not decrease the sensitivity for detecting cancer.

37.    Sherman S, Esher EJ, Pezzi JS, Rupp TH, Gottlieb K, Ikenberry SO, *et al.*:
       **Yield of ERCP tissue sampling of biliary strictures by brush, forceps,**
       **and needle aspiration methods [abstract].** *Gastrointest Endosc* 1995, in
       press.
Abstract in press reporting data from 127 patients with biliary strictures who underwent 'triple sampling' with the Geenen cytology brush, the Howell aspiration needle
and endobiliary forceps biopsy. The overall sensitivity for detecting cancer was 71%
when all three techniques were combined.

38.    Lehman GA: **Application of ERCP and endoscopic tissue sampling tech-**
•      **niques in the detection of pancreatic neoplasms.** *Int J Pancreatol* 1994,
       **16**:264–268.
Excellent literature summary of endoscopic tissue sampling for diagnosing pancreatic
adenocarcinoma, including the Indiana University 'triple sampling' technique data.

39.    Parasher VK, Ramsoekh B, Rauws E, Tytgat GNJ, Huibregtse K: **Wire**
       **guided simultaneous brush cytology and 'scrape' biopsy of pancreato-**
       **biliary strictures — a new technique [abstract].** *Gastrointest Endosc* 1994,
       **40**:65A.
Abstract describing preliminary results obtained with a wire-guided brush that allows
simultaneous exfoliative cytology and submucosal ductal scrape biopsy.

40.    Haluszka O, Bohorfoush AG, Arndorfer R, Komorowski R, Varma R: **A new**
       **combination dilation/biopsy catheter provides histology and flow cy-**
       **tometry of bile duct strictures [abstract].** *Gastrointest Endosc* 1994,
       **40**:382A.
Abstract describing a modified dilation catheter for sampling biliary strictures that
contains specialized side ports. Samples are obtained via suction and the Triton cutting
device.

Willis G. Parsons and Douglas A. Howell, Maine Medical Center, Portland, Maine,
USA.

# Endoscopy of the oesophagus

## David Armstrong, Subbaramiah Sridhar and Gervais Tougas

Division of Gastroenterology, McMaster University Medical Centre, Hamilton, Ontario, Canada

## Introduction

Publications dealing with the diagnosis of oesophageal disease will, as last year, be considered separately from those dealing with the therapy of oesophageal disease. Diagnostically, it is important to obtain prognostic information and there is a continuing need for appropriate and acceptable grading systems to describe disease severity, be it for candidiasis, reflux oesophagitis, Barrett's oesophagus or carcinoma. Surveillance in Barrett's oesophagus remains a vexed question as does the diagnosis of human immunodeficiency virus (HIV)-related oesophageal disease. Therapeutically, developments continue apace; effective acid antisecretory therapy has been shown clearly to decrease the need for dilation in patients with peptic oesophageal strictures and new technical approaches are being applied to the stenting of malignant strictures. However, one of the most exciting reports concerns the short- and medium-term efficacy of intrasphincteric botulinum toxin for the treatment of achalasia of the cardia.

## Diagnostic oesophageal endoscopy

Endoscopy is very safe but is not problem free; overall complication rates are of the order of 0.1% with a mortality of less than 0.005%. In the oesophagus, the most common major complication is perforation which occurs in about 0.03% of examinations, although the incidence is higher in the presence of an underlying oesophageal lesion or if a therapeutic manoeuvre is undertaken [1••]. The use of a slimmer (5.3 mm), transnasal pharyngo-oesophagogastroduodenoscope may minimize complications as it can more often be used without sedation [2•]. Furthermore, it promises to facilitate the management of tortuous or complex oesophageal strictures, either benign or malignant, which may require dilation or intubation.

## Gastro-oesophageal reflux disease

Endoscopy is the gold standard when evaluating the efficacy of medical therapy for oesophagitis in clinical trials but it does not identify all patients with gastro-oesophageal reflux disease (GORD). Thirty-four out of 36 consecutive patients with symptoms typical of GORD had increased oesophageal acid exposure on pH monitoring; however, 11 patients had no endoscopic abnormality. Furthermore, although another 11 patients had Savary–Miller grade 1 oesophagitis, the description of the grades indicates that some patients may actually have had non-erosive oesophagitis [3••]. This lack of standardization among endoscopic grading systems perpetuates the difficulty of comparing the results of many studies. With the increasing choice of medical and laparoscopic techniques to treat GORD, future studies must use standardized, objective measures to assess treatment efficacy in the short- and long-term.

## Mucosal curiosities

Oesophageal glycogenic acanthosis, described in association with GORD [4•], has also been described in three out of four patients with Cowden's disease [5•]. The pale plaques characteristic of glycogenic acanthosis are in contrast to the yellow plaques typical of ectopic sebaceous glands in the oesophagus [6•] (Fig. 1). Squamous cell papillomata are benign findings, usually incidental, which were reported in about 0.05% of 36 500 endoscopies; ranging in diameter from 2 to 11 mm, they were removed by diathermy without untoward sequelae in 15 patients [7•].

## Carcinoma/dysplasia surveillance: Barrett's oesophagus

Reports that omeprazole induces regression of Barrett's oesophagus emphasize the need for accurate assessments of the extent of metaplastic changes [8]. Conventionally, Barrett's oesophagus is diagnosed if 2–3 cm of the distal oesophagus is lined with columnar epithelium. However, a review of data from the Veterans' Affairs Gastroesophageal Reflux Study Group indicates that specialized columnar epithelium was found at only one out of two endoscopic examinations, 6 weeks apart, in 20% of patients. Furthermore, when investigations were repeated, the location of the lower oesophageal sphincter (determined manometrically)

## Abbreviations

CMV—cytomegalovirus; CT—computed tomography; EMRC—endoscopic mucosal resection with a cap-fitted endoscope; GORD—gastro-oesophageal reflux disease; HIV—human immunodeficiency virus; LOS—lower oesophageal sphincter; RDEB—recessive dystrophic epidermolysis bullosa.

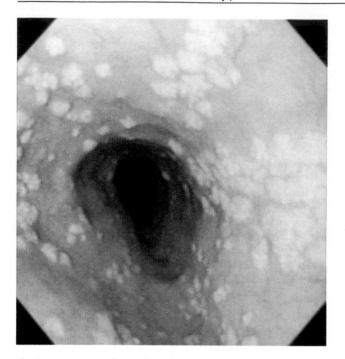

**Fig. 1.** Appearance of oesophageal ectopic sebaceous glands. Courtesy of G.N. Tytgat.

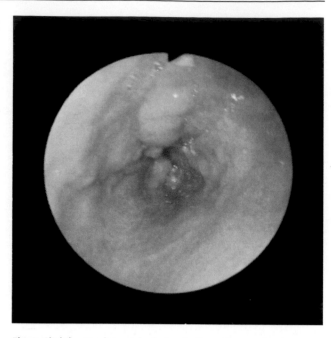

**Fig. 2.** Slightly raised, irregular lesion in Barrett's oesophagus; biopsy showed mild dysplasia. Courtesy of G.N. Tytgat.

and the most proximal level of Barrett's epithelium differed by more than 4 cm in 11% and 9% of patients, respectively [9••]. Clearly, great care is needed when monitoring the progression of Barrett's oesophagus. It is too early to decide whether combined magnification endoscopy and chromoendoscopy [10•] will permit more precise identification of areas of metaplasia or irregularity suggestive of dysplasia (Fig. 2). Practically, it should be noted that four (8.7%) out of the 46 subjects had reactions, albeit minor, to the iodine-based chromoendoscopy dye.

Debate continues regarding the need for surveillance and the endpoints of surveillance for patients with Barrett's oesophagus. Realistically, no single correct surveillance protocol will satisfy all requirements. Using a computer cohort simulation to examine 12 management strategies, Provenzale *et al.* [11••] concluded that the optimal strategy was dependent upon the desired outcome. In their model, annual surveillance produced the greatest increase in life expectancy, whereas surveillance every 2–3 years produced the greatest increase in quality-adjusted life expectancy and 5-yearly surveillance increased life expectancy with a cost–effectiveness ratio similar to that for other common medical practices. Thus, the decision as to the best surveillance strategy requires input from patients, physicians, health-care finance providers and society.

In a case–control study, 38 patients with benign Barrett's oesophagus were compared with 50 patients with Barrett's oesophagus and adenocarcinoma. Dysplasia

in the columnar epithelium and the presence of aneuploidy or G2/tetraploidy emerged as independent risk factors for the development of adenocarcinoma. If dysplasia alone was sought, biopsy had a sensitivity of 76% and a specificity of 74% for the presence of malignancy whereas, if either dysplasia, aneuploidy or G2/tetraploidy were present, the sensitivity and specificity were 98% and 55%, respectively. The authors recommend that patients with flow cytometric abnormalities should receive more frequent endoscopic screening [12•].

Barrett's oesophagus was noted in four out of 46 patients who had undergone a Heller's myotomy for achalasia [13•]. Increased oesophageal acid exposure and symptoms typical of gastro-oesophageal reflux were documented in all four patients with Barrett's oesophagus whilst the majority of subjects had normal acid exposure, no symptoms and no Barrett's oesophagus during a mean follow-up period of 13 years. Thus, surveillance should probably not be offered to all patients post-myotomy but rather to patients with severe reflux symptoms.

There is continuing concern that delayed intervention in patients with high-grade dysplasia may miss an undetected, synchronous adenocarcinoma. Recent data suggest also that short-segment Barrett's oesophagus is less benign than has been thought hitherto; a retrospective review suggests that short-segment Barrett's is a risk factor for adenocarcinoma of the cardia whilst oesophageal adenocarcinoma is associated with longer segments of Barrett's epithelium [14•].

## Squamous carcinoma of the oesophagus

A large prospective study, currently in progress, has examined the histological precursors of oesophageal squamous carcinoma in the Chinese county of Linxian where the incidence of oesophageal carcinoma is about 100–150-times higher than comparable adjusted rates for United States caucasians [15•]. Follow-up over 3.5 years in 682 patients after endoscopy and oesophageal biopsy in 1987 showed that the risk of carcinoma increased with increasing severity of dysplasia. The risk was comparable for severe dysplasia (cumulative incidence 65%) and for identified carcinoma *in situ* (cumulative incidence 69%). There was also an increased risk of malignancy in patients with basal cell hyperplasia (cumulative incidence 5%) but not in patients with oesophagitis or acanthosis [15•] (Fig. 3). The authors conclude that there is little need to differentiate between severe dysplasia and carcinoma *in situ*. These results cannot be extrapolated directly to surveillance for Barrett's oesophagus but they are consistent with reports of adenocarcinoma being discovered unexpectedly following resection of the oesophagus for high-grade dysplasia in patients with Barrett's oesophagus. Parallel follow-up of 10 066 Linxian subjects over 7.5 years after the acquisition of oesophageal balloon cytology specimens showed increases in the incidence of oesophageal and gastric cardia cancer which were correlated with increasing severity of cellular atypia. Cancers developed in 4.0% of subjects with normal cytology, and 5.1%, 10.6%, 19.3% and 26.3% of those with hyperplasia, grade 1 dysplasia, grade 2 dysplasia and 'near cancer', respectively [16•]. This provides further support for the notion that balloon cytology is a cheap and effective screening procedure which may also have a role to play in the screening and follow-up of patients with severe GORD and Barrett's oesophagus [4•].

## Dysphagia

Inspection of the cardia, with the tip of the endoscope retroflexed, is important to exclude pseudo-achalasia.

This view may also provide positive evidence to support a diagnosis of achalasia if advancing the endoscope produces 'tenting' of the cardia into the fundus of the stomach [17•]. Dysphagia and a burning sensation in the throat have been reported as a presenting feature of heterotopic gastric mucosa in the upper oesophagus. The dysphagia, attributable to the formation of a cervical oesophageal web, improved after endoscopy and dilation whilst the burning responded to omeprazole but not to ranitidine [18•]. Ectopic gastric mucosa (a developmental abnormality found in up to 10% of the population) is not usually associated with symptoms. A radiological finding of a shallow, well-defined lesion at the level of the thoracic inlet warrants a directed endoscopic examination with biopsies to confirm the diagnosis and rule out malignancy [19•].

## Chest pain

Sudden onset chest pain in a 72-year-old man led to the discovery of a polypoid lesion in the upper third of the oesophagus. Endoscopic ultrasonography showed it to be a superficial vascular lesion which was clipped and removed with a diathermy snare [20•]. Chest pain may also be a manifestation of other rare conditions; in one patient with recessive dystrophic epidermolysis bullosa (RDEB), ingestion of a hot-dog preceded an oesophageal perforation at the site of a bulla. In the gastrointestinal tract, RDEB affects only the squamous epithelium of the mouth, oesophagus and anus and the most common oesophageal presentation is dysphagia due to a bulla, web or stricture [21•]. Vomiting also can induce chest pain; subsequent dysphagia suggests the development of an oesophageal haematoma which may be detected and assessed by endoscopy, endoscopic ultrasonography or computed tomography (CT) of the chest [22•].

## Gastrointestinal haemorrhage

Recurrent painless haematemesis, due to haemorrhage from a visible vessel in the distal third of the oesophagus, was ascribed to an extragastric Dieulafoy's vascular

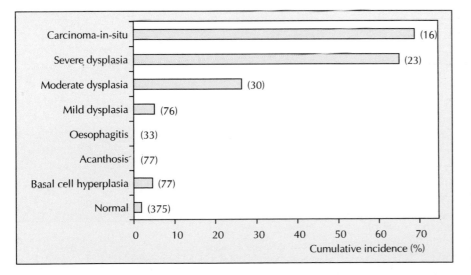

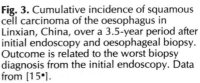

**Fig. 3.** Cumulative incidence of squamous cell carcinoma of the oesophagus in Linxian, China, over a 3.5-year period after initial endoscopy and oesophageal biopsy. Outcome is related to the worst biopsy diagnosis from the initial endoscopy. Data from [15•].

malformation in three patients. Arterial blood flow was confirmed in all cases by means of a flexible Doppler probe passed down the biopsy channel of an endoscope and the visible vessel was then injected with epinephrine. No patient had a recurrent haemorrhage during a follow-up period of 6–18 months [23•].

Oesophageal variceal haemorrhage, attributed to pseudoxanthoma elasticum and treated by endoscopic sclerotherapy, has been described in one patient although there is no indication that underlying liver disease or portal hypertension were excluded [24•]. Haematemesis was also the presenting feature of a submucosal, distal oesophageal inflammatory polyp containing abundant eosinophils [25•].

### Crohn's disease

The oesophagus is affected rarely by Crohn's disease; usually, no more than 5% of patients have oesophageal involvement [26•]. D'Haens *et al.* [27••] have reported on 14 patients with oesophageal Crohn's disease (aphthous ulcers in eight patients, 'punched out' ulcers in four patients, linear ulcers in one patient, and erosions in one patient) from a total of 38 patients with Crohn's disease who complained of dysphagia, odynophagia or heartburn. The 14 patients had a high incidence of extraintestinal disease and all had more distal disease. The oesophageal lesions healed completely in 11 patients (using corticosteroids in nine and 5-amino salicyclic acid plus antibiotics in two patients). Subsequent flares of oesophageal disease at the same site in three patients accompanied a flare of more distal disease [27••]. Omeprazole may provide symptomatic relief for oesophageal Crohn's disease without necessarily producing macroscopic healing [28•]; patients who do not respond to omeprazole may require corticosteroid therapy for symptomatic relief [29•]. An oesophago-respiratory fistula associated with a Crohn's stricture responded initially to endoscopic dilation and closure with fibrin sealant (Tissucol/Tisseel, Immuno AG, Vienna, Austria) but a subsequent recurrence necessitated surgical repair [26•].

### HIV infection

Oesophageal ulceration in HIV-infected patients may be due to *Candida albicans*, Herpes simplex or cytomegalovirus (CMV) but it may also be directly related to HIV [30•]. In one series, 70 out of 214 HIV-infected patients had oesophageal ulceration at endoscopy; most patients presented with odynophagia and the aetiology of ulceration was CMV (33 patients, 47.1%), idiopathic (30 patients, 42.9%), herpes simplex virus (three patients, 4.3%), idiopathic plus CMV (two patients, 2.9%), *Candida* (two patients, 2.9%), pill intake (one patient, 1.4%) and gastro-oesophageal reflux (one patient, 1.4%). The authors recommend that multiple biopsies be taken as there was no single feature diagnostic of an oesophageal CMV lesion [31••] (Figs 4,

5 and 6). Accurate diagnosis of HIV-associated oesophagitis is fundamental to the choice of therapy. Oral prednisone, for example, produced a complete response in 28 (77.8%) out of 36 patients with idiopathic oesophageal ulceration [32•] but it would have been expected to exacerbate candidiasis. It is not yet clear whether a recently devised endoscopic grading system for oesophageal candidiasis (Fig. 7) will be helpful in predicting a therapeutic response or relapse [33•].

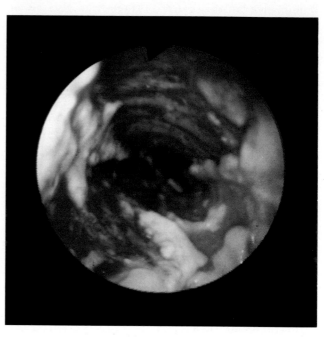

**Fig. 4.** Endoscopic photograph of sharply demarcated oesophageal ulcers in an HIV-infected patient. Cytomegalovirus is in the differential diagnosis. Courtesy of G.N. Tytgat.

| Characteristic | n (%) |
|---|---|
| **Diameter (cm)** | |
| ≤ 1.0 | 61 (43) |
| 1.1–2.0 | 41 (29) |
| 2.1–3.0 | 14 (10) |
| > 3.0 | 25 (18) |
| **Location** | |
| Proximal oesophagus | 15 (11) |
| Mid oesophagus | 81 (57) |
| Distal oesophagus | 45 (32) |
| **Depth** | |
| Shallow | 63 (46) |
| Intermediate | 38 (28) |
| Deep | 11 (8) |
| 'Heaped-up' | 16 (12) |
| Diffuse erosive | 8 (6) |
| Mass-like ulcer | 1 (1) |
| Unable to assess | 4 (2) |

**Fig. 5.** Endoscopic characteristics of 141 cytomegalovirus lesions in the oesophagus. Published with permission [31••].

(a) (b)

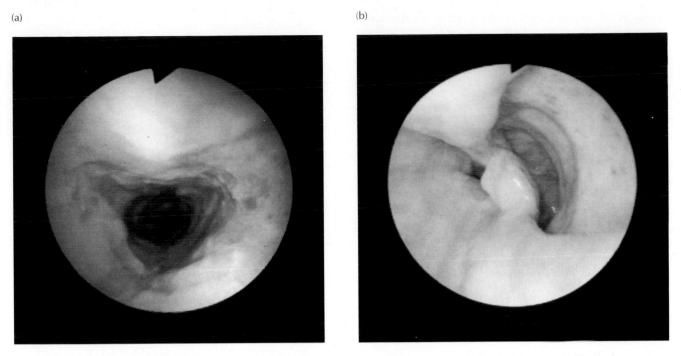

**Fig. 6.** Different endoscopic appearances of cytomegalovirus ulcers in HIV-infected patients. (a) Multiple, shallow ulcers in the distal oesophagus. (b) Mucosal bridging and residual ulceration. Courtesy of G.N. Tytgat.

Palliation of a tracheo-oesophageal fistula in an HIV-infected patient was achieved, in the short-term, with a silicon-covered, self-expanding metal stent. Such devices are worthy of consideration in the management of non-malignant fistulae in debilitated patients [34•].

## Therapeutic oesophageal endoscopy

### Haemorrhage
Under normal circumstances, modern endoscopes provide excellent images with minimal patient discomfort but the relatively narrow instrumentation channels (2.8–3.2 mm) may not permit adequate luminal aspiration or mucosal washing in the face of brisk haemorrhage. In such cases, a wide-channel endoscope with a 6.0 mm instrumentation channel would allow relatively free aspiration of the blood clot and luminal debris [35•]. However, the cost of a specialized endoscope, for use on rare occasions, may only be justifiable in tertiary-care centres.

Most Mallory–Weiss tears heal spontaneously but, occasionally, active therapy is necessary. Mallory–Weiss tears were identified in 74 (3.4%) out of 2175 consecutive patients with upper gastrointestinal bleeding but they were considered to be the cause of haemorrhage in only 50 patients. After endoscopic assessment, 13 patients were treated by injection sclerotherapy (1 : 10 000 adrenalin + 1% polidocanol) because of active bleeding (10 patients) or a visible vessel (three patients) [36•]. Complications occurred in two patients (minor rebleeding, necessitating re-injection in one patient and oesophageal perforation in the other patient) but there were no deaths in this series, regardless of the management strategy. This differs from the series reported last year [4•]. Injection sclerotherapy holds promise for the management of continuing non-variceal oesophageal haemorrhage but the precise indications have yet to be defined.

| Definition | Time to response (days; mean ± SD) |
|---|---|
| **Grade 1**<br>Scattered plaques covering < 50% of oesophageal mucosa | 7.0 ± 0.0 |
| **Grade 2**<br>Plaques covering > 50% of the oesophagus | 8.3 ± 5.1 |
| **Grade 3**<br>Confluent plaques circumferentially coating > 50% of the mucosa | 5.3 ± 1.5 |
| **Grade 4**<br>Circumferential plaques with luminal narrowing | 6.4 ± 3.2 |

**Fig. 7.** Endoscopic grading system for *Candida* oesophagitis and time to complete response to fluconazole. Published with permission [33•].

### Polyps and flat polypoid lesions
The resection of flat mucosal lesions remains a challenge, taken up by several groups. The technique of endoscopic mucosal resection with a cap-fitted endoscope (EMRC) [4•] has been modified to make it less challenging technically. The cap now has a preformed

gutter which maintains the position of the polypectomy snare while the mucosal bleb is aspirated into place [37•]. In an alternative approach, based on the Stiegmann's oesophageal varix band-ligation procedure, the lesion is aspirated into the fitted cap and an elastic ligature is applied at the base so that the newly pedunculated lesion can be resected with a polypectomy snare [38•] (Fig. 8).

The technique of strip biopsy (submucosal injection of saline to elevate a flat superficial lesion which can then be resected) has been modified to allow access to submucosal lesions. The normal overlying mucosa is removed to expose the submucosal lesion which can then be biopsied with standard biopsy forceps. Karita *et al.* [39•] report successful retrieval of diagnostic specimens in nine out of 11 patients with submucosal tumours, including one patient with a pedunculated oesophageal leiomyoma; no serious complications were reported (see Figure 13a on page 43).

### Benign strictures

Most benign oesophageal strictures are a consequence of GORD; maintenance acid antisecretory therapy is important in such patients to minimize the risk of recurrent stricturing. Two recent studies, one of 34 patients [40••] and one much larger study of 366 patients [41••], report that the incidence of redilation is lower in patients receiving prophylactic therapy with omeprazole daily than in patients receiving standard dose $H_2$-receptor antagonists.

The final analysis of a prospective comparative study in 93 patients indicates that bougie dilation is superior to balloon dilation for most benign oesophageal strictures. The use of an Eder–Puestow dilator, passed over an endoscopically placed guide wire, produced a greater increase in oesophageal diameter (2.1 versus 1.65 mm, respectively) at 12 months, a greater decrease in dysphagia at 5 months and a lower redilation rate (6 versus 18 patients, respectively) than did balloon dilation [42••].

If concomitant disease of the oropharynx or upper oesophagus prevents the antegrade passage of an endoscope, it may still be possible to dilate a stricture, if the patient has a gastrostomy. Retrograde intubation of the oesophagus allows cannulation of the oesophageal stricture with a guide wire over which appropriate dilators can then be passed in an antegrade direction [43•].

### Achalasia

A recent report suggests that the injection of botulinum toxin into the lower oesophageal sphincter (LOS) provides a viable alternative to surgical myotomy or

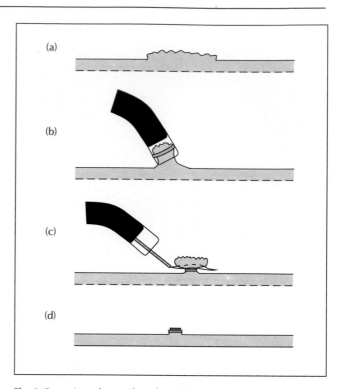

**Fig. 8.** Resection of a sessile polypoid lesion after rubber band ligation. (a) Small sessile lesion. (b) Rubber band ligature applied to base of lesion. (c) Polypectomy snare in use. (d) Rubber band remaining at the base of the resected lesion. Published with permission [38•].

endoscopic balloon dilation for the treatment of achalasia. A pilot trial in 10 patients [44••] produced complete relief of symptoms, accompanied by a significant decrease in resting LOS pressure, in seven patients. No adverse effects were noted after treatment. One patient was dissatisfied with the results of therapy and three patients required a second injection after 2 months. The remaining six patients were asymptomatic for a median period of 12 months and recurrent symptoms responded to a second injection in two patients (Fig. 9).

A retrospective comparison of Rigiflex balloon dilation and Heller's myotomy in 45 patients with achalasia was conducted by telephone interview [45•]. After an initial explanation of the expected outcomes and risks, 36 patients had previously chosen pneumatic dilation and nine had chosen surgery. The two techniques were equally effective with an excellent outcome in 88% and 89%, respectively. In another study [46•], balloon diameter, duration of dilation and number of dilations did not appear to affect the outcome. Relatively few patients were studied, however, and the lack of any observed difference may indicate a type II error. A prospective comparison of pneumatic and bougie dilation in 41 patients showed no difference in outcome with respect to symptoms, resting LOS pressure or complications [47•]. The authors concluded that neither dilator could be recommended over the other but,

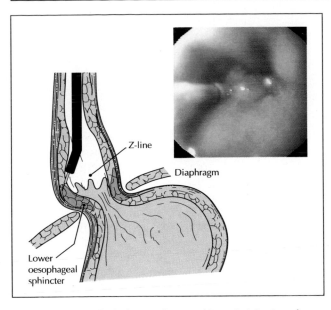

**Fig. 9.** Treatment of achalasia with intrasphincteric injection of botulinum toxin. At endoscopy, 20 U of botulinum toxin is injected into the lower oesophageal sphincter at each quadrant using a 5-mm sclerotherapy needle. Published with permission [44••].

again, there were probably too few patients to allow the detection of a difference between the techniques given the expected success rate (80–90%) and incidence of complications (5–10%).

A retrospective cohort study reported complications in 16 (9%) out of 178 patients and a perforation rate of 1.7% after 236 pneumatic dilations for achalasia or diffuse oesophageal spasm [48••]. All nine major complications were identified within 5 h of dilation; factors associated with an increased risk of complications are shown in Figure 10. Tarnasky *et al.* [49••] described oesophageal perforation in a patient with achalasia and a concomitant epiphrenic diverticulum. This complication notwithstanding, the authors contest the opinion that balloon dilation was contraindicated because the most distal oesophageal diverticulum was several centimetres proximal to the site of perforation.

Gastro-oesophageal reflux is a recognized complication of oesophagomyotomy for achalasia. Reflux-related strictures, reported in up to 3.4% of cases after surgical myotomy, can be managed safely, without reoperation, by endoscopic balloon dilation and acid antisecretory therapy [50•].

### Instrumental oesophageal perforations

The causes and management of instrumental perforations in the upper gastrointestinal tract have recently been reviewed in detail [1••]. The recommendations of the article are summarised in Figure 11. The oesophagus is the most common site of endoscopic perforation in the upper gastrointestinal tract. Perforation is often associated with a stricture or an anatomic abnormality

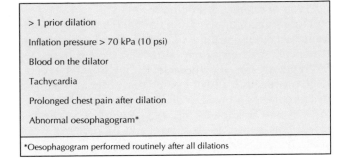

| |
|---|
| > 1 prior dilation |
| Inflation pressure > 70 kPa (10 psi) |
| Blood on the dilator |
| Tachycardia |
| Prolonged chest pain after dilation |
| Abnormal oesophagogram* |
| *Oesophagogram performed routinely after all dilations |

**Fig. 10.** Factors associated with perforation after pneumatic dilation for achalasia or diffuse oesophageal spasm. Published with permission [48••].

such as a Zenker's diverticulum even if endoscopic intubation is performed with catheter guidance [51•]. Oesophageal perforation is relatively more common at the time of dilation although perforations can also occur with overtube insertion for variceal banding. A retrospective review of chest X-rays obtained 1.5–120 h (median 6 h) after endoscopy in 15 patients who had sustained an instrumental perforation of the oesophagus identified abnormalities in 12 patients, the most common being pneumomediastinum (60%) and loss of the normal descending aortic contour at the level of the left diaphragm (33%) [52•].

### Oesophageal cancer

It has been argued that a multimodal approach to the therapy of non-resectable oesophageal squamous cell carcinoma, incorporating endoscope-based resection along with chemotherapy and radiotherapy, is preferable to a single palliative procedure [53•]. In the absence of a control group, however, it is impossible to know whether the addition of other therapeutic modes provides any benefit compared with endoscopic palliation alone. Clearly, it is preferable to have access to as many different palliative approaches as one can. Different techniques may be required for different patients, or even for the same patient at different times during the evolution of the disease [54•]. However, there is a dearth of hard data on the relative efficacies and side effects of the many different approaches.

| |
|---|
| **Prevention** |
| Avoid blind oesophageal intubation |
| Do not use endoscope as a dilator |
| Dilate strictures slowly and progressively |
| Use guide wire and fluoroscopy for complex strictures |
| |
| **Management** |
| High index of suspicion for perforation |
| Examine for crepitus |
| Plain chest X-ray and upright X-ray of abdomen |
| Gastrografin swallow if gag reflex present; barium swallow if tracheo-oesophageal fistula or if gastrografin negative |
| Consult surgeon |

**Fig. 11.** Recommendations for prevention and management of oesophageal perforation. Published with permission [1••].

*Dilation of malignant strictures*

Stricture formation, requiring bougie dilation, is a common presenting feature of oesophageal malignancy. However, stricturing may also be a consequence of radiotherapy for intrathoracic malignancy. A recent, large prospective study reported that radiation-induced strictures respond well to dilation (Savary–Gillard dilator, Wilson-Cook Inc., Winston-Salem, NC, USA) in 66% of patients with a treatment-related mortality of 1.9% and a complication rate of 10.4% [54•].

*Intubation/stenting*

Traditionally, malignant oesophageal strictures are stented with preformed, plastic-based prostheses. After dilation, the prosthesis is inserted over an endoscopically placed guide wire, often with fluoroscopic monitoring. Spinelli *et al.* [55•] report their experience using three different prostheses over a 14-year period in 76 patients from a total of 270 patients with oesophageal or gastric cardia cancers. There were no procedure-related deaths. Follow-up in 71 patients identified complications in 16 patients (22%) with perforation at the time of dilation occurring in three patients (4.2%), figures which are comparable to those in previous studies [56•]. Prosthesis migration was more common in malignancies of the distal oesophagus and cardia and the authors speculate that such patients might be better served by the insertion of a self-expanding metal stent [55•]. Warren *et al.* [57•] describe the use of a silicon Montgomery salivary bypass stent (8–20 mm external diameter; E. Benson Hood Laboratories, Pembroke, MA, USA) in 37 patients with a non-resectable carcinoma invading the oesophagus. Most procedures were performed under general anaesthetic; smaller stents (10–14 mm external diameter) were inserted using a Maloney bougie and final positioning achieved by means of a rigid oesophagoscope whilst larger (16–20 mm external diameter) stents were inserted over a flexible endoscope and advanced using a Tygon 'pusher'. There were no immediate, procedure-related deaths. Oesophageal perforation occurred in one patient (2.7%), retrograde migration occurred in four patients (10.8%) and six patients (16.2%) died in hospital of pulmonary sepsis 2–18 days after intubation.

In the last 12 months, several centres have reported their experiences with self-expanding stents whose insertion at endoscopy is considered less traumatic and technically less challenging. For the most part, these have been preliminary reports using a variety of different designs (Wallstent, Schneider Medical Inc., Lausanne, Switzerland/Schneider US Stent Division, Plymouth, Minnesota, USA [34•,58•]; Ultraflex, Microvasive, Watertown, Massachusetts, USA [59•,60•]; Gianturco-Rösch Z, Dotter Institute of Interventional Therapy, Oregon Health Sciences University, Portland, Oregon, USA [61•]). There are very few studies comparing self-expanding stents with each other, with other

prostheses or with other approaches to palliation. Furthermore, many of the reports have used assessment endpoints such as death, stent obstruction, stent migration and semiquantitative assessments of dysphagia without providing an adequate assessment of improvement in the patient's quality of life [62•].

Ell *et al.* [58•] implanted 31 self-expanding Wallstents in 23 patients after balloon dilation of the oesophageal stricture to 12–16 mm. There were no procedure-related deaths and 12 patients required no further treatment during a median follow-up period of 66 days (range 10–132 days). Since uncoated stents are potentially more susceptible to tumour infiltration, the authors have started to use silicone-rubber coated stents but they recommend that the proximal and distal 3 cm of the stent be uncoated to minimize the risk of displacement. A silicone-covered Gianturco-Rösch Z stent, incorporating anchoring hooks and a thickened rim of silicone at the cranial end of the stent, was used in 32 consecutive patients with inoperable oesophageal carcinoma. Dysphagia improved by at least two grades in 21 out of the 24 patients who had a malignant stricture, and normalization of swallowing was achieved in six out of the eight patients who had a malignant oesophago-respiratory fistula. Major stent-related complications occurred in 10 patients (31%) with a mortality of 6.2%; minor complications occurred in six patients (19%) [61•].

Raijman *et al.* [60•], using nitinol stents in 14 patients with a non-resectable oesophageal carcinoma, reported immediate improvement in dysphagia in 13 patients and a procedure-related mortality of 14%. Injection of a water-based contrast medium (diatrizoate, Hypaque 50%) at the margins of the tumour may help to confirm accurate placement of the stent at fluoroscopy [60•,63•] although it has been reported that lipiodal, an oil-based contrast medium, is preferable as it persists longer in the tissue [64•].

Patients with a malignant tracheo-oesophageal fistula present a particular problem for palliation, in part because it is difficult to occlude the fistula permanently and also because a fistula precludes continued adjuvant chemotherapy or radiotherapy. In such cases, self-expanding stents coated with silicone rubber or polyurethane have been reported to provide good palliation for patients who would not otherwise have been candidates for the use of a metallic stent [61•]. Devière *et al.* [59•] described palliation of a bronchogenic malignant broncho-oesophageal fistula with a self-expanding 'Nitinol' stent supplemented by local injection, at endoscopy, of cyanoacrylate glue to seal the fistula. This provided relief from the dysphagia and also permitted continued palliative radiotherapy.

*Alcohol injection*

There is continuing interest in endoscopic injection of ethanol as a means of providing cost-effective symptom relief for patients with inoperable oesophageal malignancy. Ethanol injection in 36 patients with inoperable cancers of the oesophagus or cardia produced significant improvements in the mean dysphagia scores, albeit delayed because of initial oedema. Mediastinitis developed in one patient and tracheo-oesophageal fistulae in two patients [65•]. In a smaller study, 95% ethanol produced good symptom relief lasting a mean of 31.5 days with no recorded complications in nine patients [66•]. Clearly, this technique should be cheaper and more widely available than laser photocoagulation. Its place in the therapeutic armamentarium will, however, remain unclear until there are more data on its efficacy, safety and cost with respect to other techniques.

## Oesophageal foreign bodies

The vast majority of oesophageal foreign bodies becomes impacted at the time of swallowing. However, Reissman *et al.* [67•] described a patient with dysphagia and chest pain which resolved following the removal, at endoscopy, of a regurgitated gastric phytobezoar. Increasingly, oesophageal foreign bodies are being removed at endoscopy although the technique of choice depends on the availability of local expertise and the nature of the foreign body. A review of the management of suspected aerodigestive foreign bodies in children suggests strongly that removal using a balloon catheter is appropriate only if the patient is co-operative and there is a smooth, inert radio-opaque object which has been present for less than 72 h. This review also emphasizes the importance of obtaining antero-posterior and lateral X-rays of the neck and chest [68•].

An alternative approach, in the case of food bolus impaction, is the administration of glucagon, an effervescent agent and water. This approach was successful, obviating the need for endoscopy, in 33 (69%) out of 48 attempts. A minor oesophageal laceration occurred in one patient but no other complications were noted [69•]. However, this protocol could not be followed in nearly half of the patients presenting with suspected food bolus impaction. Contraindications to the non-endoscopic approach included the presence of a sharp foreign body, the presence of a known malignancy, fixed stricture or oesophageal diverticulum, a history of ingestion more than 24 h previously and location of the foreign body in the upper third of the oesophagus. A prospective study in Singapore found that the majority of ingested foreign bodies were food related; only about 50% of patients with symptoms were actually found to have a foreign body. Oesophagoscopy was rarely necessary for the removal of the foreign body but, when necessary, flexible endoscopy was as effective as rigid oesophagoscopy [70•]. Oesophageal food boluses are retrieved at endoscopy using one or more of an array of instruments including baskets, rat- or alligator-toothed forceps, polypectomy snares and polyp retrievers but impacted meat boluses can be particularly stubborn as they fragment on contact. This problem was circumvented in one patient by turning the Stiegmann–Goff friction fit adaptor to yet another use; with the cap fitted to the endoscope, it was possible to aspirate the entire bolus into the cap and remove it as the endoscope was withdrawn [71•].

## Conclusion

The major points which arise from the papers published in the last year are:

- Endoscopy allows accurate diagnosis and monitoring of erosive oesophagitis but it does not identify all patients with GORD [3••].
- Endoscopic assessments of the linear extent of Barrett's oesophagus (and manometric assessments of the position of the lower oesophageal sphincter) vary considerably from one measurement to the next making it difficult to monitor the progress of the columnar metaplasia [9••].
- Cost-effectiveness for the surveillance of Barrett's oesophagus is in the eye of the beholder [11••].
- Multiple biopsies are essential to allow the accurate diagnosis and treatment of HIV-related oesophageal disease [31••].
- Effective acid antisecretory therapy decreases the incidence of recurrent stricturing after dilation of peptic oesophageal strictures [40••,41••].
- Injection of botulinum toxin into the lower oesophageal sphincter produces good short- and medium-term relief from the symptoms of achalasia of the cardia [44••] but comparative, randomized studies are needed to compare this technique with the standard approach of balloon dilation or oesophageal myotomy.
- Palliation for oesophageal carcinoma remains exceedingly difficult and no single approach is predominant.

## References and recommended reading

Papers of particular interest, published within the annual period of review, have been highlighted as:
- of special interest
•• of outstanding interest

1. Pasricha PJ, Fleischer DE, Kalloo AN: **Endoscopic perforations of the**
•• **upper digestive tract: a review of their pathogenesis, prevention, and management.** *Gastroenterology* 1994, **106**:787–802.
An excellent, comprehensive review of oesophageal perforations produced by diagnostic and therapeutic endoscopic manoeuvres.

2. Shaker R: **Unsedated trans-nasal pharyngoesophagogastroduode-**
• **noscopy (T-EGD): technique.** *Gastrointest Endosc* 1994, **40**:346–348.

A preliminary study showing that transnasal upper gastrointestinal endoscopy is feasible without sedation, albeit in healthy volunteers who are often more tolerant than patients. Formal studies of patient acceptability, diagnostic accuracy and cost–benefit ratios are necessary before widespread promulgation of this new approach.

3. Saraswat VA, Dhiman RK, Mishra A, Naik SR: **Correlation of 24-hr**
•• **esophageal pH patterns with clinical features and endoscopy in gastroesophageal reflux disease.** *Dig Dis Sci* 1994, **39**:199–205.
Prospective study in 36 consecutive patients showing that symptom severity and endoscopic abnormalities correlate with acid exposure. Patients with GORD symptoms, accompanied by increased oesophageal acid exposure, however, do not necessarily have endoscopic evidence of oesophagitis.

4. Armstrong D: **The oesophagus.** In *Annual of Gastrointestinal Endoscopy*
• edited by Cotton PB, Tytgat GNJ, Williams CB. London: Current Science Ltd; 1994:15–28.
Annual review of the role of endoscopy in the management of oesophageal disease: provides context and references for some of the developments described in the present article.

5. Hizawa K, Iida M, Matsumoto T,Kohrogi N, Suekane H, Yao T, *et al.*:
• **Gastrointestinal manifestations of Cowden's disease. Report of four cases.** *J Clin Gastroenterol* 1994, **18**:13–18.
Oesophageal lesions, found in three out of four patients with Cowden's disease (multiple hamartoma and neoplasia syndrome), were identified as glycogenic acanthosis: pale, whitish patches which could be stained using the sprayed-iodine technique. All patients had mucocutaneous and colonic lesions along with a variety of other polypoid lesions along the length of the gastrointestinal tract.

6. Marcial M, Villafaña M: **Esophageal ectopic sebaceous glands: endoscopic**
• **and histologic findings.** *Gastrointest Endosc* 1994, **40**:630–632.
Case report describing unusual, yellow oesophageal plaques equivalent to Fordyce's spots found commonly in the buccal mucosa. These lesions did not progress during a 10-year follow-up period and were not thought to be related to the patient's reflux disease.

7. Orlowska J, Jarosz D, Gugulski A, Pachlewski J, Butruk E: **Squamous cell**
• **papillomas of the esophagus: report of 20 cases and literature review.** *Am J Gastroenterol* 1994, **89**:434–437.
Case series and detailed review of a rare oesophageal lesion found incidentally at endoscopy in 20 patients over a 12-year period. After removal of the lesions in 15 patients, recurrence was observed only once, 8 years later. There was no indication of malignant change or other untoward sequelae.

8. Gore S, Healey CJ, Sutton R, Eyre-Brook I, Gear MWL, Shepherd WA, *et al.*: **Regression of columnar lined (Barrett's) oesophagus with continuous omeprazole therapy.** *Aliment Pharmacol Ther* 1993, **7**:623–628.
Convincing data to show that Barrett's epithelium can revert to squamous epithelium and that this can be achieved with omeprazole therapy over a period of 2 years.

9. Kim SL, Waring JP, Spechler SJ, Sampliner RE, Doos WG, Krol WF, *et al.*:
•• **Diagnostic inconsistencies in Barrett's esophagus.** *Gastroenterology* 1994, **107**:945–949.
Repeated tests, 6 weeks apart, in 192 patients with complicated GORD showed that manometric estimation of lower oesophageal sphincter location and endoscopic estimation of the proximal extent of Barrett's oesophagus changed by more than 4 cm in 10% of patients. Data on the progression of Barrett's oesophagus must be interpreted with care as specialized columnar epithelium and Barrett's oesophagus was diagnosed at both endoscopies in only 80% and 90% of patients, respectively.

10. Stevens PD, Lightdale CJ, Green PHR, Siegel LM, Garcia-Carrasquillo RJ,
• Rotterdam H: **Combined magnification endoscopy with chromendoscopy for the evaluation of Barrett's esophagus.** *Gastrointest Endosc* 1994, **40**:747–749.
Instillation of Lugol's iodine to identify non-staining areas suggestive of Barrett's epithelium, followed by indigo carmine spray with magnification (10× to 35×) endoscopy identified one area of dysplasia and 13 out of 46 patients with Barrett's oesophagus (10 short and three long segment). Comparative validation studies are needed.

11. Provenzale D, Kemp JA, Arora S, Wong JB: **A guide for surveillance of**
•• **patients with Barrett's esophagus.** *Am J Gastroenterol* 1994, **89**:670–680.
Markov model examining the expected outcomes for 12 management strategies applied to a hypothetical cohort of 10 000 55-year-old men with Barrett's oesophagus. The 'optimal' interval between surveillance endoscopies (1–5 years) depended upon which outcome criterion (life expectancy, quality-adjusted life expectancy or cost-effectiveness) was considered to be most important.

12. Menke-Pluymers MBE, Mulder AH, Hop WCJ, van Blankenstein M, Tilanus
• HW, The Rotterdam Oesophageal Tumour Study Group: **Dysplasia and aneuploidy as markers of malignant degeneration in Barrett's oesophagus.** *Gut* 1994, **35**:1348–1351.
Case–control study in 88 patients with Barrett's oesophagus, 50 of whom also had adenocarcinoma. Dysplasia and aneuploidy emerged from multivariate logistic regression analysis as independent risk factors for the presence of malignancy. The cost-effectiveness of adding flow cytometry to routine histology needs further investigation before widespread adoption of a new surveillance technique.

13. Jaakkola A, Reinikainen P, Ovaska J, Isolauri J: **Barrett's esophagus after**
• **cardiomyotomy for esophageal achalasia.** *Am J Gastroenterol* 1994, **89**:165–169.
Barrett's epithelium noted 6–23 years after Heller's myotomy in four out of 46 patients who had undergone surgery for achalasia. Symptoms of reflux seem to be a good marker of oesophageal acid exposure and the risk of columnar metaplasia. Thus, for the present, endoscopic surveillance probably needs to be offered only to symptomatic patients.

14. Clark GW, Smyrk TC, Burdiles P, Hoeft SF, Peters JH, Kiyabu M, *et al.*: **Is**
• **Barrett's metaplasia the source of adenocarcinomas of the cardia?** *Arch Surg* 1994, **129**:609–614.
Retrospective review of surgical specimens from 100 patients who had undergone oesophagogastrectomy for adenocarcinoma. Specialized intestinal metaplasia was found in association with 5%, 42% and 79% of subcardiac, cardiac and oesophageal tumours, respectively. The cardiac tumours were associated with short-segment Barrett's oesophagus which was undetected in seven out of 13 cardiac tumours.

15. Dawsey SM, Lewin KJ, Wang GQ, Liu F-S, Nieberg RK, Yu Y, *et al.*:
• **Squamous esophageal histology and subsequent risk of squamous cell carcinoma of the esophagus. A prospective follow-up study from Linxian, China.** *Cancer* 1994, **74**:1686–1692.
Endoscopic biopsy findings of moderate dysplasia, severe dysplasia and carcinoma *in situ* were associated with relative risks of 15.8, 72.6 and 62.5 for the development of oesophageal squamous cell carcinoma over the following 3.5 years.

16. Liu SF, Shen Q, Dawsey SM, Wang GQ, Nieberg RK, Wang ZY, *et al.*:
• **Esophageal balloon cytology and subsequent risk of esophageal and gastric-cardia cancer in a high-risk Chinese population.** *Int J Cancer* 1994, **57**:775–780.
Prospective 7.5-year follow-up of 10 066 Chinese subjects after oesophageal balloon cytology. The risk of developing oesophageal squamous cell carcinoma increased in proportion to the degree of cellular atypia. Further support for the notion that oesophageal balloon cytology may provide a low-cost, effective alternative to endoscopic surveillance in patients with Barrett's oesophagus.

17. Levine ML: **Endoscopic appearance of the lower esophageal sphincter in**
• **achalasia: a diagnostic sign [letter].** *Gastrointest Endosc* 1994, **40**:124–125.
Advancing the endoscope whilst inspecting the cardia, with the tip of the endoscope retroflexed, may show a 'tented' appearance highly suggestive of achalasia.

18. Jerome-Zapadka KM, Clarke MR, Sekas G: **Recurrent upper esophageal**
• **webs in association with heterotopic gastric mucosa: case report and literature review.** *Am J Gastroenterol* 1994, **89**:421–424.
Acid secreting heterotopic gastric mucosa in the upper oesophagus may produce acid-related symptoms amenable to acid antisecretory therapy; it may also produce local inflammation, web formation and dysphagia necessitating dilation.

19. Ueno J, Davis SW, Tanakami A, Seo K, Yoshida S, Nishitani H, *et al.*:
• **Ectopic gastric mucosa in the upper esophagus: detection and radiographic findings.** *Radiology* 1994, **191**:751–753.
Radiological demonstration of a shallow, discrete mucosal depression in the upper oesophagus is highly suggestive of ectopic gastric mucosa. Single lesions should be inspected endoscopically and biopsied to confirm the diagnosis.

20. Cantero D, Yoshida T, Ito T, Suzumi M, Tada M, Okita K: **Esophageal**
• **hemangioma: endoscopic diagnosis and treatment.** *Endoscopy* 1994, **26**:250–253.
Case report describing the presentation and treatment of a vascular oesophageal polyp. Snare polypectomy was preceded by the application of a metal, haemostatic clip to minimize the risk of haemorrhage.

21. Horan TA, Urschel JD, MacEachern NA, Shulman B, Crowson AN, Magro
• C: **Esophageal perforation in recessive dystrophic epidermolysis bullosa.** *Ann Thorac Surg* 1994, **57**:1027–1029.
Chest pain in a patient with epidermolysis bullosa should raise the spectre of severe oesophageal trauma. Normal management strategies may be inappropriate.

22. Mion F, Bernard G, Valette P-J, Lambert R: **Spontaneous esophageal**
 • **haematoma: diagnostic contribution of echoendoscopy.** *Gastrointest Endosc* 1994, **40**:503–505.
Oesophageal haematomata are part of the spectrum of oesophageal injuries induced by vomiting. They may mimic either Mallory–Weiss or Boerhaave's syndromes with haematemesis, dysphagia, odynophagia and chest pain. Various diagnostic modalities, including radiology, CT scan, endoscopy and echoendoscopy may be necessary to determine the exact cause of the symptoms.

23. Jaspersen D, Körner T, Schorr W, Brennenstuhl M, Hammar C-H: **Extra-**
 • **gastric Dieulafoy's disease as unusual source of intestinal bleeding. Esophageal visible vessel.** *Dig Dis Sci* 1994, **39**:2558–2560.
Report of three patients (0.6% of patients with upper gastrointestinal bleeding over a 3-year period) who had a protuberant visible vessel in the distal oesophagus. Arterial blood flow was identified using a transendoscopic Doppler ultrasound probe and the lesions were injected with adrenalin (1 : 10000).

24. Fruhwirth H, Rabl L, Hauser H, Schmid C, Beham A, Klein GE: **Endoscopic**
 • **findings of pseudoxanthoma elasticum.** *Endoscopy* 1994, **26**:507.
Case report of oesophageal haemorrhage as a complication of a systemic disease. Recurrent haemorrhage was treated by endoscopic sclerotherapy.

25. Bosch O, González Campos C, Jurado A, Guijo I, Miro C, Renedo G, *et al.*:
 • **Esophageal inflammatory fibroid polyp. Endoscopic and radiologic features.** *Dig Dis Sci* 1994, **39**:2561–2566.
Case report of a rare benign, submucosal lesion, known also as an eosinophilic granuloma, which developed in the distal oesophagus and presented with haematemesis and melaena.

26. Mathis G, Sutterlutti G, Dirschmid K, Feurstein M, Zimmermann G: **Crohn's**
 • **disease of the esophagus — dilation of stricture and fibrin sealing of fistulas.** *Endoscopy* 1994, **26**:508.
Case report of an oesophageal Crohn's stricture and fistula which responded, albeit temporarily, to dilation and injection of fibrin into the fistula.

27. D'Haens G, Rutgeerts P, Geboes K, Vantrappen G: **The natural history of**
 •• **esophageal Crohn's disease: three patterns of evolution.** *Gastrointest Endosc* 1994, **40**:296–300.
Case series of 14 patients; oesophageal Crohn's disease responded rapidly to therapy in the majority of patients and did not recur. In some patients, oesophageal disease settled with therapy but recurred when distal disease flared and, in a few patients, the oesophageal disease did not resolve.

28. Przemioslo RT, Mee AS: **Omeprazole in possible esophageal Crohn's**
 • **disease [letter].** *Dig Dis Sci* 1994, **39**.1594–1595.
Two patients with oesophageal Crohn's disease whose symptoms improved with omeprazole therapy although there was no resolution of the underlying Crohn's oesophagitis.

29. Beck PL, Blustein PK, Andersen MA: **Aphthous esophageal ulceration: a**
 • **novel presentation of Crohn's disease?** *Can J Gastroenterol* 1994, **8**:101–104.
Presentation of patient with odynophagia with subsequent discovery of more distal Crohn's disease. In contrast to other reports [27••], the oesophageal symptoms did not respond to omeprazole although they settled with corticosteroid therapy.

30. Chawla SK, Ramani K, Chawla K, LoPresti P, Mahadevia P: **Giant esopha-**
 • **geal ulcers of AIDS: ultrastructural study.** *Am J Gastroenterol* 1994, **89**:411–415.
Report of three HIV-infected patients with giant oesophageal ulcers (5–15 cm); electron microscopic studies showed features consistent with, but not diagnostic of, a direct HIV aetiology for the ulcers.

31. Wilcox CM, Straub RF, Schwartz DA: **Prospective characterization of**
 •• **cytomegalovirus esophagitis in AIDS.** *Gastrointest Endosc* 1994, **40**:481–484.
Clear delineation of the protean manifestations of cytomegalovirus oesophagitis in HIV-infected patients. In the absence of a characteristics appearance, all oesophageal lesions should be biopsied to obtain a definitive diagnosis.

32. Wilcox CM, Schwartz DA: **Comparison of two corticosteroid regimens**
 • **for the treatment of HIV-associated idiopathic esophageal ulcer.** *Am J Gastroenterol* 1994, **89**:2163–2167.
Idiopathic, HIV-associated oesophageal ulcers respond well to oral corticosteroids but relapse is frequent and, perhaps, more rapid after a 2-week than after a 4-week course.

33. Wilcox CM: **Short report: time course of clinical response with flucona-**
 • **zole for** *Candida* **oesophagitis in patients with AIDS.** *Aliment Pharmacol Ther* 1994, **8**:347–350.
Proposed system for grading severity of oesophageal candidiasis in patients with AIDS. The system describes the extent of disease but the prognostic importance of the grading has not yet been established.

34. Nelson DB, Silvis SE, Ansel HJ: **Management of a tracheoesophageal**
 • **fistula with a silicone-covered self-expanding metal stent.** *Gastrointest Endosc* 1994, **40**:497–499.
Palliation of tracheo-oesophageal fistula, presumed to be due to *Mycobacterium avium-intracellulare* infection, was achieved with a silicone-covered 'Wallstent'. The patient's cough and tracheal aspiration were prevented.

35. Hintze RE, Binmoeller KF, Adler A, Veltzke W, Thonke F, Soehendra N:
 • **Improved endoscopic management of severe upper gastrointestinal haemorrhage using a new wide-channel endoscope.** *Endoscopy* 1994, **26**:613–616.
Initial experiences with a prototype wide-channel fibreoptic endoscope with a 6.0-mm instrumentation channel.

36. Bataller R, Llach J, Salmerón JM, Elizalde JI, Mas A, Piqué JM, *et al.*:
 • **Endoscopic sclerotherapy in upper gastrointestinal bleeding due to Mallory–Weiss syndrome.** *Am J Gastroenterol* 1994, **89**:2147–2150.
Injection sclerotherapy with polidocanol following a Mallory–Weiss tear was followed by cessation of bleeding in 12 out of 13 patients. The precise criteria for choosing sclerotherapy over conservative therapy have not yet been defined.

37. Inoue H, Noguchi O, Saito N, Takeshita K, Endo M: **Endoscopic mucosec-**
 • **tomy for early cancer using a pre-looped plastic cap [letter].** *Gastrointest Endosc* 1994, **40**:263–264.
Modification of the cap fitted to the endoscope tip allows a polypectomy snare wire to be maintained securely in position whilst the mucosa is aspirated into the cap prior to resection.

38. Chaves DM, Sakai P, Mester M, Spinosa SR, Tomishige T, Ishioka S: **A new**
 • **endoscopic technique for the resection of flat polypoid lesions.** *Gastrointest Endosc* 1994, **40**:224–226.
Aspiration of a flat mucosal lesion, forming a raised bleb which can be banded, produces an intermediate, stable 'pedunculated' lesion which is more easily resected using a polypectomy snare.

39. Karita M, Tada M: **Endoscopic and histologic diagnosis of submucosal**
 • **tumors of the gastrointestinal tract using combined strip biopsy and bite biopsy.** *Gastrointest Endosc* 1994, **40**:749–753.
Extension of the strip biopsy technique. Removal of normal overlying mucosa allows access to submucosal tumour with standard biopsy forceps. The authors retrieved diagnostic specimens in nine out of 11 patients.

40. Marks RD, Richter JE, Koehler RE, Spenney JG, Mills TP, Champion G:
 •• **Omeprazole versus $H_2$-receptor antagonists in treating patients with peptic stricture and esophagitis.** *Gastroenterology* 1994, **106**:907–915.
A 6-month study in which 34 patients were randomized to omeprazole (20–40 mg) or an $H_2$-receptor antagonist after initial stricture dilation. Relief from dysphagia was greater and the need for dilation less if medical therapy healed the oesophagitis. Omeprazole produced greater healing (100% versus 53%) and dysphagia relief (94% versus 40%) and a trend to less frequent dilation. Omeprazole was more cost-effective.

41. Smith PM, Kerr GD, Cockel R, Ross BA, Bate CM, Brown P, *et al.*: **A**
 •• **comparison of omeprazole and ranitidine in the prevention of recurrence of benign esophageal stricture.** *Gastroenterology* 1994, **107**:1312–1318.
A 12-month study in which 366 patients were randomized to omeprazole (20 mg) or ranitidine after initial stricture dilation. Omeprazole produced greater healing of erosions (80% versus 43%) and dysphagia relief (76% versus 64%) and a lower rate of re-dilation (30% versus 46% by 12 months).

42. Cox JGC, Winter RK, Maslin SC, Dakkak M, Jones R, Buckton GK, *et al.*:
 •• **Balloon or bougie for dilatation of benign esophageal stricture?** *Dig Dis Sci* 1994, **39**:776–781.
A 1-year, prospective comparison of two dilation techniques showed that bougie dilation produced lower dysphagia scores at 5 months and a greater increase in stricture diameter at all times. In addition, fewer patients needed redilation after initial bougie dilation. The effect of oesophagitis severity on the outcome is not known. Furthermore, one might now expect the redilation rate to be reduced by maintenance therapy with an $H^+$–$K^+$ ATPase inhibitor.

43. Leong S, Kortan P, Gray R, Marcon N, Haber G: **Transgastric eso-**
 • **phagoscopy with antegrade dilation [case report].** *Endoscopy* 1994, **26**:622–624.

A feeding gastrostomy, placed radiologically, allowed retrograde oesophagoscopy and cannulation of a high oesophageal stricture which could not be intubated in an antegrade direction. A novel and opportunistic approach to complete dysphagia.

44. Pasricha PJ, Ravich WJ, Hendrix TR, Sostre S, Jones B, Kalloo AN:
•• **Treatment of achalasia with intrasphincteric injection of botulinum toxin. A pilot trial.** *Ann Intern Med* 1994, **121**:590–591.
Encouraging preliminary results following the use of botulinum toxin in 10 patients. Of nine patients who responded initially, three needed re-injection at 2 months and the remaining six were free of symptoms for a median period of 12 months. This approach promises to minimize the risks of perforation and postoperative gastro-oesophageal reflux inherent in dilation and surgery, respectively.

45. Abid S, Champion G, Richter JE, McElvein R, Slaughter RL, Koehler RE:
• **Treatment of achalasia: the best of both worlds [see comments].** *Am J Gastroenterol* 1994, **89**:979–985.
Retrospective review of symptomatic response to either balloon dilation or myotomy in 45 patients who were free to select their treatment of preference. Symptomatic response rates were comparable in the two groups (≈90% good/excellent). Suggests that patient preference and local expertise should be the major determinants of treatment choice.

46. Kim CH, Cameron AJ, Hsu JJ, Talley NJ, Trastek VF, Pairolero PC, *et al.*:
• **Achalasia: prospective evaluation of relationship between lower esophageal sphincter pressure, esophageal transit, and esophageal diameter and symptoms in response to pneumatic dilation.** *Mayo Clin Proc* 1993, **68**:1067–1073.
The conclusions — that the size of the dilator, the frequency of balloon inflations and the duration of inflation do not affect the symptomatic response — need to be validated prospectively in a larger number of patients.

47. Mearin F, Armengol JR, Chicharro L, Papo M, Balboa A, Malagelada JR:
• **Forceful dilatation under endoscopic control in the treatment of achalasia: a randomised trial of pneumatic versus metallic dilator.** *Gut* 1994, **35**:1360–1362.
Another study suggesting that there is little to choose between methods currently available for the treatment of achalasia. In this study, however, as in other studies, there were too few subjects to permit the confident detection of a difference between techniques.

48. Nair LA, Reynolds JC, Parkman HP, Ouyang A, Strom BL, Rosato EF, *et al.*:
•• **Complications during pneumatic dilation for achalasia or diffuse esophageal spasm. Analysis of risk factors, early clinical characteristics, and outcome.** *Dig Dis Sci* 1993, **38**:1893–1904.
Retrospective study of the complications ensuing from 236 balloon dilations for achalasia or diffuse oesophageal spasm in 178 patients. The procedure was safe with a perforation rate < 2%. Factors predictive of complication include high intraballoon pressure, previous dilation, prolonged chest pain, blood on the dilator and tachycardia.

49. Tarnasky PR, Brazer SR, Leung JWC: **Esophageal perforation during**
• **achalasia dilation complicated by esophageal diverticula.** *Am J Gastroenterol* 1994, **89**:1583–1585.
Case report suggesting that the presence of an oesophageal diverticulum was not causally related to the oesophageal perforation at dilation. Previous reports notwithstanding, the authors argue that an oesophageal diverticulum is not a contraindication to balloon dilation for achalasia.

50. Parkman HP, Ogorek CP, Harris AD, Cohen S: **Nonoperative management**
• **of esophageal strictures following esophagomyotomy for achalasia.** *Dig Dis Sci* 1994, **39**:2102–2108.
Gastro-oesophageal reflux occurs in about 10–20% of patients after a Heller's myotomy leading, in some patients, to postoperative peptic strictures. In this series, six patients were treated successfully with through-the-scope balloon dilation (mean 3.6 dilations per patient over a mean period of 3.8 years) and acid antisecretory therapy without need for further surgery.

51. Tsang T-K, Chodash HB: **Perforation after catheter-guided endoscopic**
• **intubation [letter].** *Gastrointest Endosc* 1994, **40**:780–781.
The 'CAGEIN' (Catheter-Guided Endoscopic Intubation) technique has been presented as a simple and safe approach to oesophageal intubation in subjects with anatomic abnormalities. The authors report the occurrence of a perforation in a Zenker's diverticulum despite the use of their 'CAGEIN' technique. Clearly, no technique is totally without risk.

52. Panzini L, Burrell MI, Traube M: **Instrumental esophageal perforation —**
• **chest film findings.** *Am J Gastroenterol* 1994, **89**:367–370.
Retrospective review of chest X-ray findings in 15 patients with known instrumental oesophageal perforation occurring over a 5-year period. Radiographic changes suggestive of perforation (pneumomediastinum, obscured left cardiophrenic angle) were

identified in 12 patients (80%); the remaining three had evidence of contrast leakage at a subsequent oesophagogram.

53. Sibille A, Lambert R, Lapeyre B, Souquet J-C, Descos F, Ponchon T:
• **Survival following non-surgical multimodal treatment for oesophageal squamous cell carcinoma.** *Eur J Gastroenterol Hepatol* 1994, **6**:287–292.
Patients unfit for surgery were entered into a multimodal protocol including options for endoscopic therapy (laser photoablation, dilation and stenting), radiotherapy and chemotherapy. The aims were to provide maximal palliation and a cure, if possible. Survival rates were dependent on the disease stage and overall survival rates were 42%, 22% and 9% at 1, 2 and 5 years. There was, however, no comparison with other modes of therapy and it is therefore difficult to quantify what additional benefit, if any, was conferred by chemotherapy and radiotherapy.

54. Swaroop VS, Desai D, Mohandas KM, Dhir V, Dave UR, Gulla RI, *et al.*:
• **Dilation of esophageal strictures induced by radiation therapy for cancer of the esophagus.** *Gastrointest Endosc* 1994, **40**:311–315.
Prospective study of dilation under endoscopic and/or fluoroscopic guidance in 103 patients with dysphagia secondary to radiotherapy and/or recurrent tumour; 66% of patients obtained good symptomatic relief with a morbidity rate of 10.4% and a mortality rate of 1.9%.

55. Spinelli P, Cerrai FG, Ciuffi M, Ignomirelli O, Meroni E, Pizzetti P: **En-**
• **doscopic stent placement for cancer of the lower esophagus and gastric cardia.** *Gastrointest Endosc* 1994, **40**:455–457.
Retrospective assessment of stent placement in 76 patients; 56% of these patients could swallow solids or semi-solids compared with 84–88% of patients who had tumours in the upper/middle third of the oesophagus. Procedure-related complications (early or late) occurred in 22% and there was no procedure-related mortality.

56. Bennett JR, Dakkak M: **An improved method for oesophageal intubation**
• **[letter; comment].** *Ann R Coll Surg Engl* 1993, **75**:449–450.
Summary of perforation and mortality rates following oesophageal intubation in the context of a comment on a modified technique described by Bramhall *et al.* for palliative tube introduction.

57. Warren WH, Smith C, Faber LP: **Clinical experience with Montgomery**
• **salivary bypass stents in the esophagus.** *Ann Thorac Surg* 1994, **57**:1102–1106; discussion 1106–1107.
Attempted insertion of a silicon stent, usually under general anaesthetic, in 37 patients, 19 of whom had an oesophago-respiratory fistula. Possible procedure-related complications included oesophageal perforation (2.7%), stent migration (10.8%), death from pulmonary sepsis (16.2%) and death from haemorrhage (5.4%). In the absence of randomized comparative trials, recommendations on the relative merits of most stent types remain speculative.

58. Ell C, Hochberger J, May A, Fleig WE, Hahn EG: **Coated and uncoated**
• **self-expanding metal stents for malignant stenosis in the upper GI tract: preliminary clinical experiences with Wallstents.** *Am J Gastroenterol* 1994, **89**:1496–1500.
Report on a series of 23 patients with obstructing carcinomata of the oesophagus or cardia. Major complications included stent migration in three patients (13%) and stent obstruction by food or tumour (35%). There were no perforations and no procedure-related deaths; dysphagia was relieved completely in 39%.

59. Devière J, Quarre JP, Love J, Cremer M: **Self-expandable stent and injec-**
• **tion of tissure adhesive for malignant bronchoesophageal fistula.** *Gastrointest Endosc* 1994, **40**:508–510.
Case report describing failure of cuffed oesophageal tube. Injection of cyanoacrylate glue after placement of an expandable Nitinol stent relieved dysphagia and allowed the patient to complete his chemotherapy regimen.

60. Raijman I, Walden D, Kortan P, Haber GB, Fuchs E, Siemans M, *et al.*:
• **Expandable esophageal stents: initial experience with a new nitinol stent.** *Gastrointest Endosc* 1994, **40**:614–621.
Report on a series of 14 patients with non-resectable oesophageal carcinoma. Major complications included deaths from gastric aspiration (7%) and myocardial infarction at 6 days (7%). There were no perforations; after stent insertion, 10 patients (71%) were able to swallow most solids and three (21%) could swallow semi-solids.

61. Wu WC, Katon RM, Saxon RR, Barton RE, Uchida BT, Keller FS, *et al.*:
• **Silicone-covered self-expanding metallic stents for the palliation of malignant esophageal obstruction and esophagorespiratory fistulas: experience in 32 patients and a review of the literature.** *Gastrointest Endosc* 1994, **40**:22–33.
Report on a series of 32 patients with inoperable oesophageal malignancy; a silicone covering was used to minimize tumour ingrowth. Major complications (31%) included stent dislocation (12.5%), tumour ingrowth or overgrowth (6%) and death from pressure necrosis of the tumour (6%). After stent insertion, 21 (88%) out of the

24 patients with dysphagia were able to swallow most solids and six (75%) of those with a fistula could eat all solids and liquids.

62.  Gelfand GAJ, Finley RJ: **Quality of life with carcinoma of the esophagus.**
•    *World J Surg* 1994, **18**:399–405.
A proposal that patients' quality-of-life be given greater consideration when evaluating palliative therapy for oesophageal carcinoma and that appropriate scales be developed to assess quality-of-life in these patients.

63.  Raijman I, Kortan P, Haber GB, Marcon NE: **Contrast injection to identify**
•    **tumor margins during esophageal stent placement.** *Gastrointest Endosc* 1994, **40**:222–224.
Accurate delineation of tumour extent is critical for correct placement of self-expandable metal stents; injection of contrast material at the upper and lower margins of the oesophageal tumour avoids some of the inaccuracy inherent in the use of external markers.

64.  Chan ACW, Leong HT, Chung SSC, Li AKC: **Lipiodal as a reliable marker**
•    **for stenting in malignant esophageal stricture [letter].** *Gastrointest Endosc* 1994, **40**:520–521.
An oil-based contrast material is cleared more slowly than a water-based marker. Better visualization is claimed during the insertion procedure and slower clearance should facilitate assessment of the stent's position postoperatively.

65.  Chung SCS, Leong HT, Leung JWC, Li AKC: **Palliation of malignant**
•    **oesophageal obstruction by endoscopic alcohol injection.** *Endoscopy* 1994, **26**:275–277.
Report on a series of 36 patients with inoperable oesophageal malignancy; local injection of ethanol led to tolerance of most solids in 14 patients (39%). Major complications included mediastinitis (2.8%) and oesophago-respiratory fistula formation (5.6%). In general, relief of dysphagia is perhaps slower and less complete than that seen after stent insertion.

66.  Moreira LS, Coelho RCL, Sadala RU, Dani R: **The use of ethanol injection**
•    **under endoscopic control to palliate dysphagia caused by esophagogastric cancer.** *Endoscopy* 1994, **26**:311–314.
A small series of nine patients with inoperable oesophageal malignancy. Local injection of ethanol led to tolerance of most solids in seven of these patients (78%). No major complications were noted.

67.  Reissman P, Fich A, Eid A, Rivkind A: **Esophageal phytobezoar causing**
•    **acute dysphagia: a rare complication of gastric bezoar.** *J Clin Gastroenterol* 1994, **18**:159–160.
Endoscopic removal of a phytobezoar impacted acutely in the oesophagus produced complete relief of dysphagia.

68.  Papsin BC, Friedberg J: **Aerodigestive-tract foreign bodies in children:**
•    **pitfalls in management.** *J Otolaryngol* 1994, **23**:102–108.
A useful retrospective chart review highlighting the problems which have arisen from suboptimal management of foreign bodies swallowed or inhaled by children. Many of the prinicples apply equally to the management of foreign bodies in adults.

69.  Robbins MI, Shortsleeve MJ: **Treatment of acute esophageal food impaction with glucagon, an effervescent agent, and water.** *AJR Am J*
•    *Roentgenol* 1994, **162**:325–328.
Prospective study of a non-endoscopic approach to the impacted oesophageal foreign body; the obstruction was cleared in 33 (69%) out of 48 attempts. However, this approach was indicated in only about 50% of patients with an oesophageal foreign body. Further studies will be necessary to study the cost-effectiveness of selection criteria and the appropriate management algorithms of these patients.

70.  Lim CT, Quah RF, Loh LE: **A prospective study of ingested foreign bodies**
•    **in Singapore.** *Arch Otolaryngol Head Neck Surg* 1994, **120**:96–101.
No foreign body was found in nearly half of the patients who presented with typical symptoms; the majority of foreign bodies were retrieved from the oropharynx. Relatively few patients (15%) needed endoscopy. Flexible and rigid oesophagoscopy were comparably effective.

71.  Pezzi JS, Shiau Y-F: **A method for removing meat impactions from the**
•    **esophagus.** *Gastrointest Endosc* 1994, **40**:634–636.
Successful removal of a meat bolus impacted 19 h previously at the level of cricopharyngeus; the Stiegmann–Goff friction fit adaptor was used to aspirate the bolus as there was insufficient room to manoeuvre a snare or polyp retriever.

David Armstrong, Division of Gastroenterology, McMaster University Medical Centre, 1200 Main Street West, Hamilton, Ontario L8N 3Z5, Canada.

# Endoscopy of the stomach

## Guido N.J. Tytgat and Jamie G. Ignacio

Academic Medical Center, Department of Gastroenterology-Hepatology,
Amsterdam, the Netherlands

## General considerations

Strong evidence for the continuation of open-access endoscopy available to general practitioners and specialists was presented in a prospective study evaluating the diagnostic outcome of upper gastrointestinal endoscopy [1•]. Patient age was used as a determining factor and significant endoscopic findings were subsequently noted to be less likely among younger patients (less than 45 years of age). Although general practitioners tended to refer younger patients than did specialists, the diagnostic yield did not differ significantly between referrals from general practitioners and specialists (Fig. 1). Noteworthy here is the reassurance provided by negative endoscopic findings in younger patients fearful of malignancy. Another study evaluating the value of prompt endoscopy against initial empirical H2-receptor treatment showed better cost effectiveness for early endoscopy, citing that the case selection for eventual endoscopy (if symptoms did not subside or if they recurred) was not improved by prior empirical treatment [2•]. Moreover, 40% of the expected ulcer cases remained undiagnosed.

An important audit on the appropriate use of endoscopy was published by British endoscopists. Eleven per cent of endoscopies were classified as inappropriate by the British panel compared to 31% when assessed by the American Rand criteria. This difference occurred largely because in the USA it is recommended that one month's anti-ulcer treatment be tried before considering endoscopy for dyspepsia. No important abnormalities were discovered in the 'British' inappropriate cases. The percentage of doctors who would request endoscopy in various situations is summarized in Figure 2 [3•].

Upper gastrointestinal endoscopy has frequently been included in the diagnostic protocol among patients with occult blood-positive stools but with negative colonoscopy findings. This practice was retrospectively examined involving 211 consecutive patients in a recent study [4•]. Overall, 42% turned out to have abnormal findings, corresponding to 35% of the symptomatic patients, and 45% of those with severe anaemia. There were many more lesions in patients who were 60 years of age or older. All of the observed abnormal findings in all patients were benign lesions and only 12% overall were amenable to specific treatment, yet 53% of identified lesions among patients with severe anaemia had a specific treatment. The presence of symptoms among patients with severe anaemia did not increase the likelihood of finding a lesion. Furthermore, it was not particularly clear whether the lesions observed were at all responsible for occult bleeding. Still, it was suggested that since iron-deficiency anaemia is a potentially serious clinical problem, affected patients should be endoscopically evaluated since almost half of them in the study presented with upper tract lesions. More reliable information, however, may be obtained from prospective studies as to the cost-effectiveness and practicality of this approach.

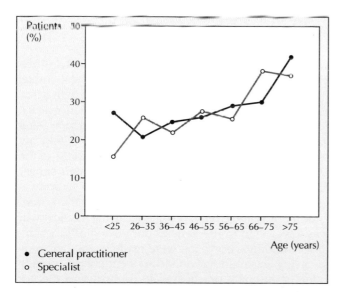

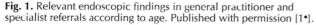

**Fig. 1.** Relevant endoscopic findings in general practitioner and specialist referrals according to age. Published with permission [1•].

---

## Abbreviations

**ELISA**—enzyme linked immunosorbent assay; **ERCP**—endoscopic retrograde cholangiopancreatography; **Ig**—immunoglobulin; **MALT**—mucosa-associated lymphoid tissue; **MMC**—migrating motor complex; **NSAID**—non-steroidal anti-inflammatory drug; **PCR**—polymerase chain reaction; **PEG**—percutaneous endoscopic gastrostomy; **PEJ**—percutaneous endoscopic jejunostomy.

---

| 1 | Asymptomatic sliding hiatus hernia seen on barium meal | 4.5% |
|---|---|---|
| 2 | Patient < 40 years of age, untreated dyspepsia for 6 weeks (asymptomatic at time of interview) | 5.0% |
| 3 | Patient < 40 years of age with a single episode of dyspepsia lasting 2 weeks | 5.0% |
| 4 | Uncomplicated heartburn responding to treatment | 7.9% |
| 5 | Uncomplicated duodenal ulcer shown on barium studies which is responding to $H_2$ antagonists | 11.2% |
| 6 | Duodenal scarring shown on barium studies; responding to $H_2$ antagonists | 13.8% |
| 7 | Patients < 40 years of age with dyspepsia who had had a negative endoscopy within 2 years | 22.0% |
| 8 | Follow-up endoscopy after gastrectomy; patient is asymptomatic | 23.3% |
| 9 | Patient < 40 years of age with mild-to-moderate symptoms of gastro-oesophageal reflux only | 28.6% |
| 10 | Follow-up to previous endoscopic findings of non-ulcer dyspepsia; patient is symptomatic | 29.5% |
| 11 | Metastatic adenocarcinoma of unknown primary site | 39.0% |
| 12 | Patient < 40 years of age with dyspepsia; has had a negative barium meal within 2 years | 50.6% |
| 13 | Evaluation of occult blood in stool, before lower gastrointestinal work-up performed | 57.7% |
| 14 | Patient < 40 years of age, with a 2–6 month history of untreated dyspepsia | 61.0% |
| 15 | Patient with chronic, non-progressive dyspepsia; probably functional in origin | 63.8% |
| 16 | Patient > 60 years of age with anorexia, early satiety or weight loss; barium meal normal | 71.1% |
| 17 | Patient > 40 years of age, with a 2–6 month history of untreated dyspepsia | 87.2% |
| 18 | Patient with anaemia (haemoglobin < 10 g) on long-term, non-steroidal anti-inflammatory drugs for chronic arthritis | 88.9% |
| 19 | Patient with dyspepsia and large-volume vomiting | 92.8% |
| 20 | Patient > 60 years of age with anorexia, early satiety or weight loss; barium meal not performed | 95.0% |
| 21 | Heartburn which failed to respond adequately to maximal medical therapy | 96.0% |
| 22 | Patient with dyspepsia who continued to have symptoms despite $H_2$ antagonists, who has not had any investigations of the upper gastrointestinal tract | 96.8% |
| 23 | Patient with progressive dysphagia | 97.0% |
| 24 | Follow-up to double-contrast barium meal showing a gastric ulcer | 97.6% |
| 25 | Patient with haematemesis | 99.0% |

Fig. 2. Percentages of doctors who would request endoscopy in different circumstances. Published with permission [3•].

Upper gastrointestinal endoscopy is a safe procedure, and risk to the patient is generally considered small. There are, however, certain clinical situations where performing endoscopy may have some potential to produce certain unique risks. Its use among 20 women in various stages of pregnancy was evaluated in a multicentre study over a period of 7.5 years, giving emphasis on the risk–benefit ratio and follow-up of foetal outcome [5•]. It was successful in the diagnosis of offending lesions in 14 patients and identifying the source in all nine bleeding patients with no deleterious effect on maternal vital signs nor inadvertent induction of labour. Likewise, no evidence of foetal distress or congenital malformations was noted in any patients. The main attraction of endoscopic haemostasis is obvious in pregnant patients with upper gastrointestinal bleeding, but this was not addressed in the study since only one patient received thermocoagulation. It is hoped that further future studies on this aspect will be undertaken.

## Helicobacter pylori

More epidemiologic data are available to determine the prevalence as well as the risk factors for infection with *H. pylori*. The Eurogast study group evaluated more than 3000 asymptomatic subjects from Europe, North America, North Africa and Japan using serologic testing. Infection prevalence was noted to be higher in older (62.4%) than in younger (34.9%) age groups, and a low educational level was shown to be a consistent determinant of high infection prevalence [6••]. In contrast, strikingly low infection prevalence rates were reported in north-eastern Malaysia on serologic testing of almost 500 blood donors (4.2%) and more than 900 subjects attending health screening clinics (4.8%) and even among subjects with duodenal ulcers (50%, 17 out of 34), gastric ulcers (5%, one out of 22) and non-ulcer dyspepsia (9%, 15 out of 159) [7•].

Whether endoscopists are at a special risk for acquiring *H. pylori* infection is somewhat controversial. Initial studies suggested that endoscopy was indeed an occupational hazard. Later studies were less confirmatory. Seroprevalence was also examined among practising gastroenterologists in Austria, showing no significant difference from age-matched controls, regardless of the number of endoscopies performed [8•]. Rather similar data were published from Poland. Although seroprevalence was higher amongst endoscopists than non-endoscopists, the overall prevalence in the medical staff was lower than in the general population [9•]. Contradictory findings, however, were made in another study involving gastroendoscopists and endoscopy nurses, citing endoscopic practice as an occupational risk for acquiring *H. pylori* [10•]. Undoubtedly increasing the use of gloves and more adequate disinfection procedures have decreased the infection risk.

Most prevalence studies are, however, cross-sectional surveys and few studies have been made about the mode of acquisition of the infection. A study by Cullen *et al.* conducted in Australia [11•] examined the pattern of *H. pylori* acquisition by detection of *H. pylori* antibodies using enzyme linked immunosorbent assay (ELISA) in serum samples of 141 adults stored serially in 1969, 1978 and 1990 for other purposes. While the prevalence of *H. pylori* antibodies did not change significantly at the three points in time (34–40%), of the 86 subjects who were seronegative in 1969 only six (7%) were noted to be seropositive in 1990. This suggests that *H. pylori* infection occurs early in life and persists later in life as a result of a cohort effect. It was further implied that recurrence of infection after initial eradication treatment would seem unlikely. This assumption is further supported by the findings of Borody *et al.* [12••] that the effective reinfection rate after eradication treatment was found to be 0.36% per patient-year among patients with cured duodenal ulcers. The duration of follow-up was almost 6 years. In that study, the importance of recrudescence is discussed. Recrudescence is a well-known phenomenon that occurs mostly within the first 4 weeks after the cessation of non-eradicating therapy, but never later than 1 year.

Recrudescence is explained by the fact that after treatment bacteria may still be present but may escape detection because of low colonization rates or because of their presence in 'sanctuary sites' in atrophic or metaplastic mucosa or perhaps by their presence in intercellular or intracellular sites.

Development of assays of salivary anti-*H. pylori* immunoglobulin (IgG showed sensitivity similar to that of serum IgG and better than salivary IgA. This test proved important in the examination of dyspeptic patients under the age of 45 years being screened for peptic ulcers, saving on 39% of endoscopies in salivary IgG-negative patients [13•].

More evidence for the essential role of *H. pylori* in gastric ulcers was reported. Serum IgG antibody to *H. pylori* was detectable in sera stored for more than 20 years, showing positive results in 93% of 150 patients with gastric ulcers and 92% of those 65 with duodenal ulcers [14•]; the respective odds ratios were 3.2 and 4.0. In another study, after a 1-year follow up of a total of 50 patients with healed gastric ulcers, recurrence rates were significantly lower among subjects whose ulcers were healed by eradication therapy (3.1%) as compared with those healed without bacterial eradication [15•].

Labenz and Börsch in another study [16••] showed that recurrence of peptic ulcer bleeding was considerably reduced after bacterial eradication. It has been proposed that eradication treatment be considered in patients with conservatively managed bleeding from *H.*

*pylori*-positive ulcers. This is an important observation, confirming previous observations that healing of the gastroduodenal mucosa through cure of the infection eliminates any further risk of recurrent ulcer bleeding. It should be pointed out that this protection does not extend to drug-associated mucosal damage, as illustrated in Figure 3.

Because of all the above compelling reasons it is readily understood why a National Institutes of Health consensus working party came to the conclusion that attempts at *H. pylori* eradication should be carried out for all patients with *H. pylori*-associated duodenal and gastric ulcers, whether at first presentation or at recurrence [17••].

Endoscopic visual predictors of gastric ulcer recurrence were presented in a study by Sakaki *et al.* [18•]. Using a standard endoscope, well-demarcated ulcer scars were found to be indicative of penetration of the muscularis propriae after histologic correlation of resected specimens. By examining the scarring pattern with the use of a magnifying endoscope, the presence of a coarse regenerating mucosal pattern was associated more with muscularis propria penetration and insufficient mucosal regeneration and was found to be predictive of a significantly higher ulcer relapse rate. Ulcer scar pattern evaluation was even more closely related to recurrence than *H. pylori* positivity after multivariate analysis (Fig. 4).

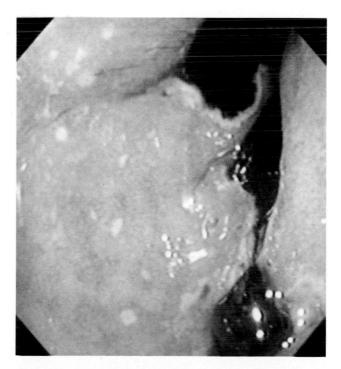

**Fig. 3.** Multiple non-steroidal anti-inflammatory drug-induced bleeding ulcers in the duodenal bulb.

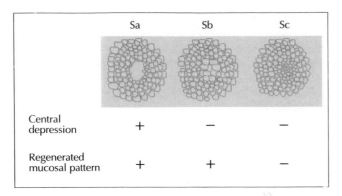

|  | Sa | Sb | Sc |
|---|---|---|---|
| Central depression | + | – | – |
| Regenerated mucosal pattern | + | + | – |

**Fig. 4.** Endoscopic classification of scar patterns of peptic ulcer from the viewpoint of magnifying endoscopy. Sa = depression without regenerating mucosal pattern is shown in the centre; Sb = a course regenerating mucosal pattern is shown up to the centre; Sc = a fine pattern similar to that in the surroundings is exhibited. Published with permission [18•].

The link between *H. pylori* infection and gastric carcinogenesis was recently examined in a study showing a high incidence of bacterial colonization in early gastric carcinoma [19••] (Fig. 5). In this study, *H. pylori* positivity was noted in up to 72% in early glandular carcinoma and 100% in early diffuse carcinoma. A drop in the incidence of infection among cases of advanced diffuse carcinoma to 71% suggests a process that seems to be independent of oxyntic gland atrophy and intestinal metaplasia, since the latter two are seen less in advanced diffuse carcinoma. The study also stressed the importance of chronic atrophic gastritis and intestinal metaplasia, particularly type III metaplasia, in the pathogenesis of gastric cancer. Two distinct pathways

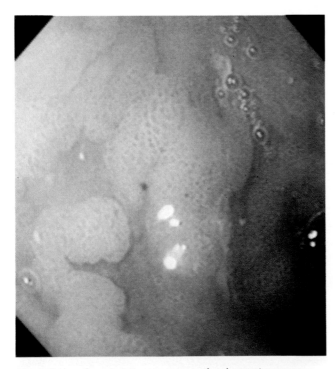

**Fig. 5.** Rather characteristic appearance of early gastric cancer; elevated/depressed type as seen in a patient with severe *H. pylori* gastritis.

of gastric carcinogenesis may operate, both starting with chronic active *H. pylori*-associated gastritis and one passing through a sequence of atrophic gastritis, intestinal metaplasia (especially type III) and dysplasia to end preferentially in glandular (intestinal-type) cancer. The other pathology, presumably starting earlier in life, moves more directly and quicker from chronic gastritis to cancer, preferentially the diffuse type, without apparent interposition of metaplastic–dysplastic change. Such high frequencies of *H. pylori* association and early gastric cancer were not obtained in a study from the Netherlands [20••]. *H. pylori* was found in 61% of intestinal-type early gastric cancer and in 55% of diffuse-type early gastric cancer. Age-adjusted prevalence of intestinal metaplasia was significantly higher in patients with early gastric cancer compared to controls.

New data on the possible positive association between *H. pylori* colonization and the development of gastric non-Hodgkin's lymphoma have surfaced. Parsonnet *et al.* [21••] in a case–control study involving two large cohort groups showed a higher risk of gastric lymphoma among *H. pylori*-positive subjects as well as the presence of the micro-organism before the development of lymphoma, which occurred a median of 14 years after serum collection. Earlier reports have shown regression of mucosa-associated lymphoid tissue (MALT) variants of B-cell lymphoma after *H. pylori* eradication [22••] as well as proliferation of B-cells from MALT tumours after exposure to *H. pylori* antigens [23•]. The final step to prove an actual causative role, that of demonstrating a decrease in the risk of lymphoma development with eradication of *H. pylori*, as is the case in peptic ulcer disease, is expected in the near future.

Definite proof of the potentiating effect of *H. pylori* on the ulcerogenic properties of non-steroidal anti-inflammatory drugs (NSAIDs) is still controversial. Goggin *et al.* [24•], using a modified Lanza score (Fig. 6), found no increase in gastric damage scores in *H. pylori*-positive patients receiving NSAIDs compared with those who were *H. pylori* negative, although the dyspeptic symptoms were greater among *H. pylori*-positive patients on NSAIDs. This is in contrast to earlier suggestions to the contrary [25].

The role of the endoscopist is vital both for primary diagnosis and for monitoring therapy in *H. pylori* infection. Endoscopic mucosal alterations have been put forward to suggest *H. pylori* infection such as chronic antral erosions, antral fine nodularity (Fig. 7), antral spotty erythema or patchy erythema alternating with pale areas. Whether these criteria are truly useful in clinical practice needs further evaluation. Graham *et al.* [26•] recommend obtaining antrum and corpus biopsy specimens for histology, culture and rapid

| Grade | Endoscopic appearance |
|-------|----------------------|
| 0 | No evidence of erosions or submucosal haemorrhages |
| 1 | Single erosion or submucosal haemorrhage |
| 2a | More than one, but not numerous, erosions or submucosal haemorrhages |
| 2b | Oedema with two or more erosions or submucosal haemorrhages |
| 3 | Numerous areas of erosions or submucosal haemorrhages |
| 4 | Invasive ulcer or large areas of erosions or submucosal haemorrhages with active bleeding |

**Fig. 6.** Modified Lanza system for scoring mucosal damage in the stomach and duodenum. Adapted with permission [24•].

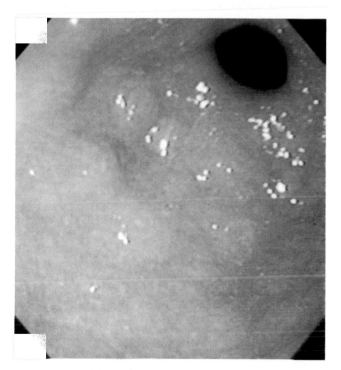

**Fig. 7.** Antral nodularity in *H. pylori*-associated gastritis.

urease testing with large calibre forceps. The specimens for culture should be taken first so as not to risk contamination of the specimens with formalin. The endoscopist must provide the pathologist with adequate material. As a rule, the larger the specimen the better. Large specimens provide a sufficient surface area to examine and are relatively easy for a technician to properly orientate.

Various *H. pylori* eradication treatment regimens have been assessed and compared. A randomized comparison between 2 weeks and 1 week of quadruple therapy (triple therapy while continuing the usual dose of an $H_2$-receptor antagonist) was made in an effort to assess the compliance of patients to treatment as well as eradication rates [27•]. Better compliance and eradication rates similar to the 2-week quadruple treatment were observed in patients receiving the 1-week regimen. Problems with metronidazole resistance have been consistently observed in some areas, and an open trial from the Netherlands suggested substituting metronidazole with clarithromycin as part of a triple-therapy regimen. Although the eradication rate with the clarithromycin-containing regimen was slightly below that of triple therapy using metronidazole (72% versus 95%, respectively), such rates may prove to be acceptable in regions with a high rate of metronidazole resistance [28•]. Another study compared eradication rates using omeprazole and amoxycillin with that employing triple therapy (bismuth subsalicylate, metronidazole and tetracycline) plus ranitidine and showed no statistical difference (79% versus 84%, respectively) [29•].

Treatments that impact favourably upon the eradication of *H. pylori* and ulcer recurrence have been summarized [30•]. On long-term follow-up of post-eradication patients, 95% were observed to have had a one-grade fall in serum IgG titres against *H. pylori*, and 94% seroconverted 12 months after eradication treatment. This prompted the investigators to recommend serum IgG level determinations after 8 months instead of endoscopy to judge the success of eradication therapy [31•]. Ashorn *et al.* [32•], however, noted a decrease in antibody levels in almost half of the subjects where *H. pylori* persisted. Since symptoms were similar between patients who had their infection eradicated and those who did not, endoscopy was still regarded as necessary in the follow-up of post-eradication therapy patients.

Iatrogenic transmission of *H. pylori* through infected endoscopes still remains a problem. Roosendaal *et al.* [33•] showed that *H. pylori*-negative gastric biopsy specimens (by culturing, histological, as well as serologic testing) still turned out to contain *H. pylori* DNA by polymerase chain reaction (PCR). Despite routine manual and machine washing and disinfection, it was suggested that PCR positivity was a result of specimen contamination by infected endoscope channels. A more extensive machine disinfection procedure was described using an enzymatic soap solution aimed at digestion of mucus and tissue parts in the biopsy channel. Endoscopes undergoing this disinfection procedure yielded no *H. pylori* DNA on PCR after flushing their biopsy channels [33•]. These findings and recommendations are particularly important to consider in future *H. pylori* studies regarding eradication and re-infection rates or patient–patient transmission.

Although the use of *H. pylori* eradication therapy on patients with dyspepsia is still not recommended, a group from Denmark observed normalization of interdigestive intestinal motility patterns, specifically phases I and II of the migrating motor complex (MMC), together with disappearance of symptoms in patients with *H. pylori*-positive dyspepsia after bacterial eradication [34•]. This may imply a limited but specific subset of dyspepsia patients who may benefit from bacterial eradication. However, in another trial, symptom resolution was not observed among dyspeptic children after eradication treatment [35•]. No difference in gastric emptying was observed between *H. pylori*-positive and -negative patients, and orocaecal transit time was even faster among patients harbouring the micro-organism [36•].

## Rugal hyperplastic gastritis — hypertrophic gastritis

The endoscopic and radiologic findings of enlarged gastric folds have always been a source of difficulty in terms of diagnosis. It is well known that forceps biopsy of such lesions have been inadequate in most cases and full thickness biopsy obtained by surgical means have been reported to be a major problem in the destination from initis plastica and gastric lymphoma. The use of endoscopic ultrasonography has recently been assessed as a less invasive and more accurate method for diagnostic evaluation of large gastric folds in 28 patients [37•]. In that study, gastric wall thickening involving layers three and four revealed primary gastric adenocarcinoma (linitis plastica) after laparotomy in three patients despite non-malignant findings on large cup forceps biopsy. Wall thickening limited to layer two was more indicative of benign disease after a mean follow-up period of 35 months. Endosonography was therefore considered an accurate predictor whether forceps biopsy of large gastric folds would be diagnostic. It was further successful in detecting gastric varices, thereby avoiding a potentially catastrophic forceps biopsy of the area.

Although the exact pathogenic mechanism has not yet been established, the recent association of enlarged fold gastritis with *H. pylori* infection has stimulated major interest. Effects of bacterial eradication in cases of enlarged fold gastritis were observed by a group from Japan [38•]. Two groups were studied: one with severe fold enlargement and another with moderate changes. Larger folds were associated with more severe mucosal inflammation, while elevated fasting serum gastrin levels were a feature common to both groups. Abnormally low pre-treatment basal and stimulated acid outputs were observed among subjects in both groups, the decrease being more pronounced in patients with more severe fold enlargement. Eradication treatment resulted in normalization of acid secretion, the change being more pronounced in the severe group than in the moderate group. Post-treatment reduction

of fold width, inflammatory infiltrates and fasting serum gastrin levels were further observed in both groups. This study highlights the association between bacterial inflammation and fold enlargement and further raises the issue of the possible role of *H. pylori* mucosal inflammation in gastric carcinogenesis through abnormally elevated serum gastrin levels seen in patients with enlarged fold gastritis.

Also, Ménétrier's disease is associated in the majority of cases with *H. pylori*. Elimination of the infection may cause disappearance of the enlarged folds and arrest of the excessive protein loss [39•].

## Gastric neoplasias

Prognostication of gastric cancer has so far been accomplished with the use of currently existing staging systems. The tumour node metastasis classification by the American Joint Committee on Cancer which is used primarily in Western countries and the system described by the Japanese Research Society for Gastric Cancer have been the standards for staging. Although both systems satisfactorily predict treatment results and survival and provide accurate pathological assessment, they are quite complicated and difficult to memorize. In an effort to provide an easy to use system that can be universally utilized in different centres, a group from Japan applied the Dukes' classification of colon and rectum cancer for use in gastric cancer [40•]. Close to 500 patients were staged according to the Japanese system, Dukes' classification, and the Astler–Coller modification of Dukes' system. A definite step-wise relationship between stage and survival was observed in both Dukes' classification and the Japanese system. Among Dukes' C patients, further prognostic importance was given to the number and anatomical level of positive lymph nodes, but not the depth of wall invasion (Fig. 8).

A large study on gastric polyps focusing on the frequency, location, age and sex distribution [41••] recently shed light on conflicting, currently available information. Clinical and pathological data from more than 5000 gastric polyps involving more than 4800 patients were collected. Fundic gland cysts accounted for 47% followed by hyperplasminogenous polyps (28.3%), tubular adenoma (9%) and adenocarcinoma (7.2%) (Figs 9 and 10). Fundic gland cysts (Fig. 11) were mostly found in the older age groups, while Peutz–Jeghers polyps, juvenile polyps and pancreatic heterotopia were found in younger individuals. Glandular cysts, hyperplasminogenous polyps, inflammatory fibroid polyps and carcinoid tumours were noted to be more common in women. Polyps located in the corpus were likely to be glandular cysts and

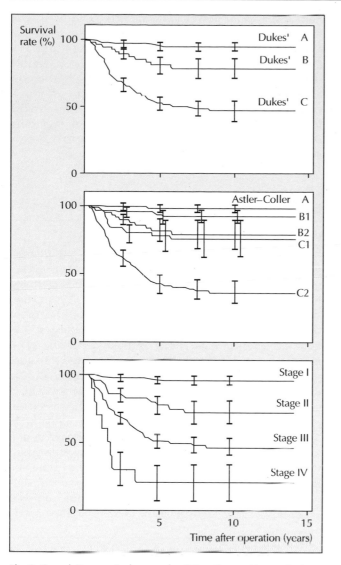

**Fig. 8.** Cumulative survival curves for 476 patients with curatively treated gastric cancer according to the criteria of Dukes' (top), Astler–Coller's (middle) and Japanese (bottom) classifications. Vertical bars represent 95% confidence intervals. Published with permission [40•].

| | Polyps | % of polyps | % without glandular cysts |
|---|---|---|---|
| **Tumour-like lesions** | | | |
| *Total* | 3928 | 81.0 | 64.0 |
| Glandular cysts | 2281 | 47.0 | – |
| Hyperplasiogenous polyps | 1373 | 28.3 | 53.4 |
| Inflammatory fibroid polyps | 151 | 3.1 | 5.9 |
| Brunner's gland heterotopia | 58 | 1.2 | 2.3 |
| Pancreatic heterotopia | 41 | 0.8 | 1.6 |
| Peutz–Jegher's polyps | 16 | 0.3 | 0.6 |
| Cronkhite–Canada polyps | 1 | 0.1 | 0.1 |
| Juvenile polyps | 7 | 0.1 | 0.3 |
| **Neoplasias** | | | |
| *Total* | 924 | 19.0 | 36.0 |
| 1. Epithelial | | | |
| 　Benign | 495 | 10.2 | 19.3 |
| 　　Tubular adenomas | 438 | 10.2 | 19.3 |
| 　　Tubulopapillary adenomas | 48 | 1.0 | 1.9 |
| 　　Papillary adenomas | 5 | 0.1 | 0.2 |
| 　　Pyloric gland adenoma | 4 | 0.1 | 0.2 |
| 　Malignant | | | |
| 　　Adenocarcinomas | 348 | 7.2 | 13.5 |
| 2. Endocrine | | | |
| 　Carcinoid tumours | 81 | 1.7 | 3.2 |

**Fig. 9.** Frequency distribution of gastric polyps (in 4852 patients) with and without inclusion of glandular cysts. Adapted with permission [41••].

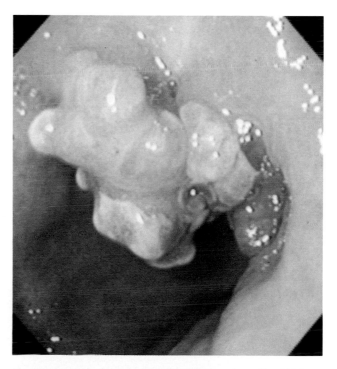

**Fig. 10.** Irregularly shaped antral hyperplastic polyp with whitish areas corresponding to granulation tissue.

carcinoid tumours, while antral polyps could most likely be either pancreatic heterotopia, Brunner's gland heterotopias, or inflammatory fibroid polyps. This study offers the endoscopists additional guidelines on how to approach gastric polyps other than endoscopic polypectomy or forceps biopsy (Fig. 12). Potential for malignancy of individual forms of gastric polyps is the subject of an ongoing evaluation.

Diagnosis of submucosal tumours has remained a challenge to the endoscopist and various techniques of biopsy have been described. Recently, using a two-channel endoscope, Karita *et al.* [42•] described a technique combining mucosal resection of the overlying normal mucosa of 11 such tumours and later performed a forceps bite biopsy of the now exposed submucosal tumours, nine of which were in the stom-

ach. Nine out of 11 submucosal lesions were successfully diagnosed with this procedure, two being unsuccessful because of the tough consistency of the tu-

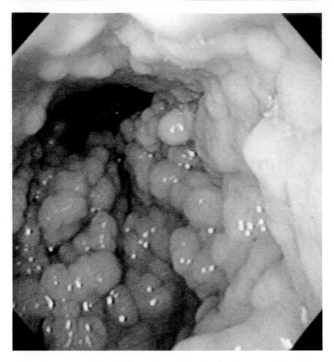

**Fig. 11.** Gastric polyposis because of fundic gland cysts in familial adenomatous polyposis

mours. No significant complications were reported but the mucosal defects were treated with endoscopic application of liquid thrombin and administration of $H_2$-receptor antagonists (Fig. 13).

Progress in the design of endoscopic biopsy forceps has been evaluated in a prospective randomized com-

parison between newer generation disposable biopsy forceps and reusable ones with respect to specimen volume and histologic depth [43••] (Figs 14 and 15). Specimen volumes were similar between comparably sized forceps, but newer standard cup disposable forceps yielded tissue comparable in depth to those obtained by using large calibre ('jumbo') reusable forceps. Various issues have been raised regarding disposable equipment, due understandably to concerns about possible infectious disease transmission.

## Enteral feeding

### Percutaneous endoscopic gastrostomy

Increasing experience with percutaneous endoscopic gastrostomy (PEG) has resulted in its use in non-specialized settings. Indications and outcomes have been noted to be similar in the general hospital setting [44•] compared with the teaching hospitals. New models of PEG tubes designed for prolonged use and better ambulatory patient acceptance have been evaluated. In the past, insertion of a gastrostomy button necessitated a mature gastrocutaneous tract made by a previously inserted PEG tube. A recent report describes an experience with a one-stage gastrostomy button that does not need an existing mature gastrocutaneous tract in 24 patients [45•]. The main innovation of this system is the inclusion of a tapered introducer which precedes the gastrostomy button, both being inserted over a guide wire using the standard pull technique. Complications were comparable to those of standard PEG tubes. Encountered problems were leakage of gastric contents to the outside

| | Frequency (%) | Mean diameter (mm) | Gross form | Surface eroded | Average age (years) | M : F | Location (%) Cardia/ fundus/ corpus | Antrum/ pylorus | Multiple polyps (%) | Polyposis (%) |
|---|---|---|---|---|---|---|---|---|---|---|
| **Tumour-like lesions** | | | | | | | | | | |
| Gastric galndular cysts | 47.0 | 4 | Hemispherical, shiny | – | 57 | 1.9:1.0 | 100.0 | – | 13.7 | 48.9 |
| Hyperplastic polyps | 28.3 | 11 | Polyp, broad-based or wasted | +++ 91.6% | 72 | 2.4:1.0 | 56.3 | 43.9 | 26.0 | 8.0 |
| Inflammatory fibroid polyps | 3.1 | 10 | Polyp, broad-based | + 30% | 64 | 1.7:1.0 | 18.6 | 81.3 | 10.0 | 0.4 |
| **Neoplasias** | | | | | | | | | | |
| Tubular adenoma | 9.0 | 8 | Flat, elevated | – | 70 | 1:1 | 54.7 | 45.3 | 14.4 | – |
| Tubular papillary adenoma | 1.0 | 16 | Polyp, broad-based | – | 70 | 1:1 | 63.2 | 36.7 | – | – |
| Adenocarcinoma | 7.2 | 17 | Polyp or elevated | + | 69 | 0.9:1.0 | 54.0 | 45.2 | 13.2 | – |
| Carcinoid tumour | 1.7 | 8 | Flat, papular | – | 64 | 2.2:1.0 | 96.1 | 3.9 | 21.0 | 30.0 |

**Fig. 12.** Gastric polyps: criteria for endoscopic diagnosis. M = male; F = female. Adapted with permission [41••].

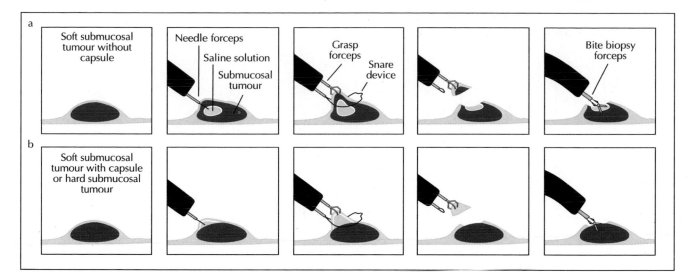

**Fig. 13.** Method for histologic diagnosis using combined strip biopsy and bite biopsy. The same procedure is used for strip biopsy of a soft, non-capsulated mucosal tumour (a) and a hard, encapsulated mucosal tumour or submucosal tumour (b). The mucosa overlying the submucosal tumour is punctured with needle forceps, and 2–3 ml normal saline solution is injected into the submucosal tumour itself or into the tissue above the submucosal tumour. The snare device is placed around the elevated tissue, which is held in the grasping forceps, and then tightened in preparation for resection. A portion of the elevated tissue is resected using a blend of cutting and coagulation current. Bite biopsy forceps are inserted through the mucosal defect created by strip biopsy, and a tissue specimen is obtained from the exposed surface of the submucosal tumour. Published with permission [42•].

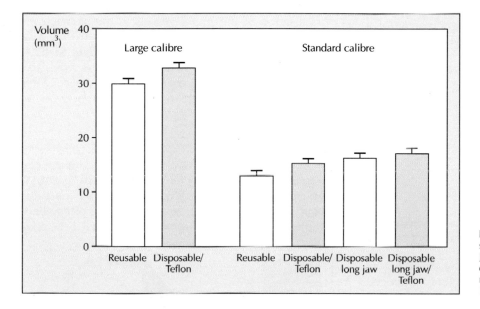

**Fig. 14.** Mean volumes of biopsy specimens obtained with each forceps. Jumbo forceps yielded biopsy specimens double the size of those obtained with regular forceps. Published with permission [43••].

through the shaft lumen as the button was opened during feeding (two patients), occlusion with inspissated feeding solution (two patients), tube migration to the transverse colon (one patient) and mushroom tip migration out of the stomach resulting in a fistula between the stomach and the tube tip (one patient). Prophylactic antibiotics were used and no cases of peristomal wound infection were observed. A second look gastroscopy was advised to make sure of proper positioning of the mushroom tip within the stomach.

## Percutaneous endoscopic jejunostomy

Percutaneous endoscopic jejunostomy (PEJ) has been associated with a high rate of failure primarily due to the difficult insertion procedure and catheter failure of small-calibre tubes. Initial experience on a novel over-the-wire technique for insertion of a large-calibre (12 F) PEJ tube through a pre-existing PEG has been described in 18 patients [46•]. In the past, PEJs were difficult to position in the jejunum and eventually ended up positioned in the duodenal bulb, making it prone to dislodgement and eventual aspiration of gastric contents. Use of a standard endoscopic retrograde cholangiopancreatography (ERCP) guide wire facilitated positioning of the PEJ in the fourth part of the duodenum or jejunum under direct endoscopic guidance. Furthermore, gastric suctioning and decompression was subsequently possible while feeding through the jejunostomy tube. The success rate was 89% and a larger multicentre trial is currently being undertaken.

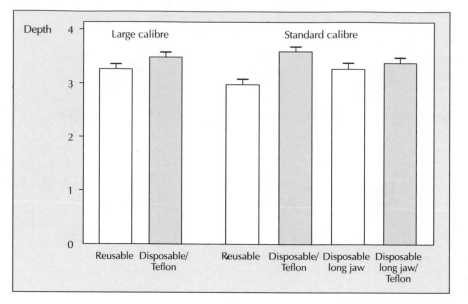

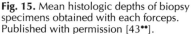

**Fig. 15.** Mean histologic depths of biopsy specimens obtained with each forceps. Published with permission [43••].

## Gastric outlet obstruction

Recent experience on endoscopic balloon dilatation of ulcer-induced gastric outlet obstruction was reported [47•]. Thirty patients symptomatic for an average of 6 months prior to treatment were dilated to an average of 15 mm. Eighty per cent experienced sustained symptom relief after a mean follow-up period of 15 months. Failure to dilate was noted in 13% and was attributed to long strictures. Perforation was reported in two patients with uneventful postoperative courses. Such high success rates of endoscopic therapy definitely merit good comparative trials with existing surgical procedures.

## Congestive gastropathy and vascular disorders

The clinical profile of congestive gastropathy was presented by a group from India [48•]. The objectives of the study were to determine which factors influenced its development, as well as to correlate it with findings of gastritis and *H. pylori* infection. Endoscopically, congestive gastropathy was described as mild, that is discrete areas of erythema with or without mosaic pattern (small elevated erythematous areas outlined by a subtle yellowish network), or severe, with the presence of cherry red spots. It was observed to be present in 60% of patients with portal hypertension, the incidence being aggravated by severe liver disease, a past history of haematemesis, and the presence of gastric or oesophageal varices. The severity was associated with the presence of large oesophageal varices and also with gastric varices. Although portal hypertension is essential for the development of congestive gastropathy, its severity was noted to be independent of the level of portal venous pressure. Similarly, the presence of *H. pylori* infection, degree of capillary dilatation, or his-

tologic gastritis were not found to influence the severity of congestive gastropathy.

Visualization of the mural vessels in the stomach remains a fascinating challenge [49•] (Fig. 16). *In vivo* spectrophotometry shows that infrared light at 620–820 nm penetrates the abdominal and gastric wall, and can be picked up by the charge-coupled device. After injecting indocyanine green the venous network is visualized.

A new entity has been described; diffuse haemorrhagic gastroenteropathy, characterized by profuse gastrointestinal bleeding, caused by diffuse friable haemorrhagic mucosa. Mucosal capillaries and postcapillary venules contain fibrin thrombi. Endothelial cells con-

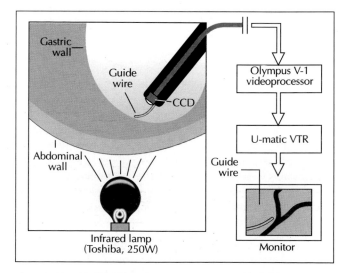

**Fig. 16.** Infrared electronic endoscopy system. CCD = charge-coupled device; VTR = video tape recorder. Published with permission [49•].

tain elongated intermediate filaments and reduplicated basement membrane. Presumably the bleeding is due to mucosal ischaemia secondary to capillary endothelial damage [50•].

## References and recommended reading

Papers of particular interest, published within the annual period of review, have been highlighted as:

- of special interest
- • of outstanding interest

1. Adang RP, Vismans JFJFE, Talmon JL, Hasman A, Ambergen AW, Stock-
• brugger RW: **The diagnostic outcome of upper gastrointestinal endoscopy: are referral sources and patient age determining factors?** *Eur J Gastroenterol Hepatol* 1994, **6**:329–335.
A study supporting the current practice of free-access endoscopic service for general practitioners as well as specialists. The diagnostic yield of endoscopy for referrals from both groups of physicians was similar, despite the generally younger referrals from general practitioners.

2. Bytzer P, Moller Hansen J, Schaffalitzky de Muckadell OB: **Empirical H₂**
• **blocker therapy or prompt endoscopy in management of dyspepsia.** *Lancet* 1994, **343**:811–816.
Endoscopy upon initial presentation of patients complaining of dyspepsia was assessed to be more cost-effective than initial empirical H₂-receptor antagonist therapy.

3. Quine MA, Bell GD, McCloy RF, Devlin HB, Hopkins A: **Appropriate use**
• **of upper gastrointestinal endoscopy. A prospective audit. The Steering Group of the Upper Gastrointestinal Endoscopy Audit Committee.** *Gut* 1994, **35**:1209–1214.
Careful study of the indications for endoscopy, indicating substantial geographical differences and major discrepancy from the American Rand criteria. This paper should be read by all endoscopists.

4. Chen YK, Gladden DR, Kestenbaum DJ, Collen MJ: **Is there a role for**
• **gastrointestinal endoscopy in the evaluation of patients with occult blood-positive stool and negative colonoscopy?** *Am J Gastroenterol* 1993, **88**:2026–2029.
Forty-five per cent of patients with severe anaemia and negative colonoscopy findings were found to have abnormal upper gastrointestinal endoscopy findings. However, the presence of upper gastrointestinal symptoms did not increase the likelihood of significant gastroscopy findings among severely anaemic patients.

5. Cappell MS, Sidhom O: **A multicenter, multiyear study of the safety and**
• **clinical utility of esophago-gastroduodenoscopy in 20 consecutive pregnant females with follow-up of fetal outcome.** *Am J Gastroenterol* 1993, **88**:1900–1905.
Oesophagogastroduodenoscopy was found to be safe in 20 pregnant patients. Labour was not induced and no foetal distress nor malformations were noted as consequences.

6. The EUROGAST Study Group: **Epidemiology of, and risk factors for,**
•• *Helicobacter pylori* **infection among 3194 asymptomatic subjects in 17 populations.** *Gut* 1993, **34**:1672–1676.
A large epidemiologic survey of the prevalence of *H. pylori* on four continents. Advanced age and low educational level were noted to predispose to higher infection prevalence.

7. Uyub AM, Raj SM, Visvanathan R, Nazim M, Aiyar S, Anuar AK: ***Helico-***
• ***bacter pylori* infection in north-eastern peninsular Malaysia: evidence for an unusually low prevalence.** *Scand J Gastroenterol* 1994, **29**:209–213.
A surprisingly low prevalence rate of *H. pylori* infection was noted in the region, both among blood donors as well as peptic ulcer patients. The low incidence of peptic ulcer was further attributed to the low H. pylori infection rate.

8. Pristautz H, Eherer A, Brezinschik R, Truschnig-Wilders M, Petritsch W,
• Schreiber F, *et al.*: **Prevalence of *Helicobacter pylori* antibodies in the serum of gastroenterologists in Austria.** *Endoscopy* 1994, **26**:690–696.
The practice of gastrointestinal endoscopy was not found to predispose one to infection with *H. pylori* as observed in this serologic survey among gastroenterologists. This was noted regardless of the number of endoscopic procedures alone.

9. Matysiak-Budnik T, Gosciniak G, Brugmann D, Lubczynska-Kowalska W,
• Poniewierka E, Knapik Z, *et al.*: **Seroprevalence of *Helicobacter pylori***

infection in medical staff in Poland. *Eur J Gastroenterol Hepatol* 1994, **6**:309–311.
*H. pylori* seroprevalence was higher among nurses than among physicians and among endoscopists than among non-endoscopists. However, medical staff had a lower seroprevalence than the general population.

10. Chong J, Marshall BJ, Barkin JS, McCallum RW, Reiner DK, Hoffman SR,
• *et al.*: **Occupational exposure to *Helicobacter pylori* for the endoscopy professional: a sera epidemiological study.** *Am J Gastroenterol* 1994, **89**:1987–1992.
American gastroendoscopists and endoscopy nursing personnel were observed to have high occupational risks of acquiring *H. pylori* infection. The infection rates were observed to be higher among Caucasian as well as foreign-born subjects.

11. Cullen DJE, Collins BJ, Christiansen KJ, Epis J, Warren JR, Surveyor I, *et*
• *al.*: **When is *Helicobacter pylori* infection acquired?** *Gut* 1993, **34**:1681–1682.
An important study tracing the status of serum samples stored for 25 years regarding positivity for anti-*H. pylori* antibodies. Very few antibody-negative sera became antibody-positive in the involved time span, implying that the persistence of infection is the result of a cohort effect.

12. Borody TJ, Andrews P, Mancuso H, McCauley D, Jankiewicz E, Ferch N, *et*
•• *al.*: ***Helicobacter pylori* reinfection rate, in patients with cured duodenal ulcer.** *Am J Gastroenterol* 1994, **89**:529–532.
Subsequent reinfection by *H. pylori* was observed to be a very unusual phenomenon in this study from Australia among patients with duodenal ulcers cured by bacterial eradication. An important study highlighting the utility of eradication treatment for peptic ulcers.

13. Patel P, Mendall MA, Khulusi S, Molineaux N, Levy J, Maxwell JD, *et al.*:
• **Salivary antibodies to *Helicobacter pylori*: screening dyspeptic patients before endoscopy.** *Lancet* 1994, **344**:511–512.
Determination of salivary anti-*H. pylori* IgG exhibited high sensitivity. Thirty-nine per cent of endoscopies were saved following detection of peptic ulcers using the assay in the treatment protocol described.

14. Nomura A, Stemmermann GN, Chyou PH, Perez-Perez GI, Blaser MJ:
• *Helicobacter pylori* **infection and the risk for duodenal and gastric ulceration.** *Ann Intern Med* 1994, **120**:977–981.
Pre-existing *H. pylori* infection increases the risk for gastric and duodenal ulcer, as observed in this nested case–control study on a cohort of more than 5000 Japanese–American men.

15. Labenz J, Börsch G: **Evidence for the essential role of *Helicobacter pylori***
• **in gastric ulcer disease.** *Gut* 1994, **35**:19–22.
Data concerning patients with gastric ulcers showed an ulcer recurrence rate of 3.1% after a 1-year follow-up after bacterial eradication therapy against *H. pylori*.

16. Labenz J, Borsch G: **Role of *Helicobacter pylori* eradication in the preven-**
•• **tion of peptic ulcer bleeding relapse.** *Digestion* 1994, **55**:19–23.
Further evidence of the prevention of bleeding relapse as well as ulcer relapse after eradication of *H. pylori* is presented. The authors recommend that eradication be considered in all patients with conservatively managed bleeding from *H. pylori*-positive ulcers.

17. NIH Consensus Development panel: ***Helicobacter pylori* in peptic ulcer**
•• **disease.** *JAMA* 1994, **272**:65–69.
All *H. pylori*-associated ulcers, both primary or recurrent, should be treated with antibiotics to eradicate the organism.

18. Sakaki N, Takemoto T: **The relationship between endoscopic findings of**
• **gastric ulcer scar and ulcer relapse.** *J Clin Gastroenterol* 1993, **17** (suppl 1):S64–S69.
An interesting study making use of a magnifying endoscope and histologic correlation of gastric ulcer healing patterns. Coarse regenerating mucosal patterns and well-delineated scars were associated with higher ulcer gastric ulcer recurrence rates more closely than *H. pylori* infection.

19. Fiocca R, Luinetti O, Villani L, Chiaravalli A, Cornaggia M, Stella G, *et al.*:
•• **High incidence of *Helicobacter pylori* colonization in early gastric cancer and the possible relationship to carcinogenesis.** *Eur J Gastroenterol Hepatol* 1993, **5** (suppl 2):S2–S8.
*H. pylori* was found in all cases of early diffuse gastric carcinoma and 72% of early glandular carcinoma. The sequence of *H. pylori* infection to chronic active gastritis to intestinal metaplasia was suggested for glandular cancer, and that involving infection–gastritis-dysplasia in diffuse cancer were suggested.

20. Craanen ME, Blok P, Dekker W, Tytgat GNJ: *Helicobacter pylori* **and early**
•• **gastric cancer.** *Gut* 1994, **35**:1372–1374.
Atrophic changes and intestinal metaplasia were significantly more common in intestinal-type early gastric cancer compared with diffuse-type early cancer. *H. pylori* was found in 61% of intestinal-type early gastric cancer and in 55% of diffuse-type early cancer.

21. Parsonnet J, Hansen S, Rodriguez L, Gelb AB, Warnke RA, Jellum E, *et*
•• *al.*: *Helicobacter* **infection and gastric lymphoma.** *N Engl J Med* 1994, **18**:1267–1271.
The presence of *H. pylori* results in a higher risk of development of gastric non-Hodgkin's lymphoma as concluded in this case–control study. However, the exact evidence for a definite causative role is still unproven.

22. Wotherspoon AC, Dogliono C, Diss TC, Pan L, Moschini A, de Boni M, *et*
•• *al.*: **Regression of primary low-grade B-cell gastric lymphoma of mucosa-associated lymphoid tissue type after eradication of** *Helicobacter pylori.* *Lancet* 1993, **342**:575–577.
An important study showing *H. pylori* eradication treatment as specific management for gastric lymphoma of the MALT type.

23. Hussell T, Isaacson PG, Crabtree JE, Spencer J: **The response of cells from**
• **low-grade B-cell gastric lymphomas of mucosa-associated lymphoid tissue to** *Helicobacter pylori.* *Lancet* 1993, **342**:571–574.
*H. pylori* antigens resulted in the proliferation of B-cells into lymphoma of the MALT variety through mechanisms involving T-cells *in vitro*.

24. Goggin PM, Collins DA, Jazrawi RP, Jackson PA, Corbishley CM, Bourke
• BE, *et al.*: **Prevalence of** *Helicobacter pylori* **infection and its effects on symptoms and non-steroidal anti-inflammatory drug induced gastrointestinal damage in patients with rheumatoid arthritis.** *Gut* 1993, **34**:1677–1680.
*H. pylori* infection was not found to potentiate NSAID-induced gastropathy, but was associated with increased dyspeptic symptoms.

25. Heresbach D, Raoul JL, Bretagne JF, Minet J, Donnio PY, Ramee MP, *et al.*: *Helicobacter pylori*: **risk and severity factor of non-steroidal anti-inflammatory drug induced gastropathy.** *Gut* 1992, **33**:1608–1611.

26. Graham DY, Karttunen TJ, Genta RM: **The evaluation of treatment of** *H.*
• *pylori* **infections: strategies for the design of clinical trials.** *Jpn J Endoscopy* 1994, **8**:991–1002.
Useful information is given on the role of endoscopy and large calibre biopsy specimens in the diagnosis of *H. pylori* infection.

57. De Boer WA, Driessen WMM, Potters VPJ, Tytgat GNJ: **Randomized study**
• **comparing 1 with 2 weeks of quadruple therapy for eradicating** *Helicobacter pylori.* *Am J Gastroenterol* 1994, **89**:1993–1997.
A 1-week course of quadruple treatment (colloid bismuth subcitrate, tetracycline, metronidazole, among patients taking $H_2$ blockers) resulted in better patient compliance and similar *H. pylori* eradication rates compared to the 2-week regimen.

28. Thijs JC, Van Zwet AA, Molenaar W, Oom JAJ, De Korte H, Runhaar EA:
• **Short report: clarithromycin, an alternative to metronidazole in the triple therapy of** *Helicobacter pylori* **infection.** *Aliment Pharmacol Ther* 1994, **8**:131–134.
Although associated with a slightly lower eradication rate, clarithromycin could be used as a substitute for metronidazole in areas where metronidazole resistance is significant.

29. Labenz J, Ruhl GH, Bertrams J, Borsch G: **Clinical course of duodenal ulcer**
• **disease one year after omeprazole plus amoxycillin or triple therapy plus ranitidine for cure of** *Helicobacter pylori* **infection.** *Eur J Gastroenterol Hepatol* 1994, **6**:293–297.
Omeprazole plus amoxycillin was observed to be equally as effective as triple therapy plus ranitidine in *H. pylori eradication.*

30. Tytgat GNJ: **Treatments that impact favorably upon the eradication of**
• *Helicobacter pylori* **and ulcer recurrence.** *Aliment Pharmacol Ther* 1994, **8**:359–368.
Overview of all current antimicrobial regimens aimed at eradication of the infection. Successful eradication of the organism almost eliminates ulcer recurrence.

31. Wang WM, Chen CY, Jan CM, Chen LT, Perng DS, Lin SR, *et al.*:
• **Long-term follow-up and serological study after triple therapy of** *Helicobacter pylori***-associated duodenal ulcer.** *Am J Gastroenterol* 1994, **89**:1793–1796.
Serum anti-*H. pylori* antibody status was followed up for 1 year after eradication therapy. Complete eradication was signalled by seroconversion usually after 1 year

from eradication. Antibody status determination was further suggested as a substitute for endoscopy as an indicator for success of eradication.

32. Ashorn M, Ruuska T, Karikoszki R, Miettinen A, Maki M: *Helicobacter*
• *pylori* **gastritis in dyspeptic children. A long-term follow-up after treatment with colloidal bismuth subcitrate and tinidazole.** *Scand J Gastroenterol* 1994, **29**:203–208.
*H. pylori*-associated dyspepsia improves after successful eradication.

33. Roosendaal R, Kuipers EJ, Van den Brule AJC, Pena AS, Uyterlinde AM,
• Walboomers JMM, *et al.*: **Importance of the fiberoptic cleaning procedure for detection of** *Helicobacter pylori* **in gastric biopsy specimens for PCR.** *J Clin Microbiol* 1994, **4**:1123–1126.
An important study suggesting evidence of persistence of *H. pylori* in biopsy channels of endoscopes despite standard manual and machine disinfection procedures.

34. Qvist N, Rasmussen L, Axelsson CK: *Helicobacter pylori*-**associated gas-**
• **tritis and dyspepsia. The influence on migrating motor complexes.** *Scand J Gastroenterol* 1994, **29**:133–137.
Phases I and II of the MMC were noted to be abnormal in patients with dyspepsia. Normalization was observed after a course of eradication therapy, along with symptom involvement.

35. Trespi E, Broglia F, Villani L, Luinetti O, Fiocca R, Solcia E: **Distinct**
• **profiles of gastritis in dyspepsia subgroups. Their different clinical responses to gastritis healing after** *Helicobacter pylori* **eradication.** *Scand J Gastroenterol* 1994, **29**:884–888.
Eradication therapy resulted in reduced dyspeptic symptoms in patients with ulcer-like dyspepsia, but not in dysmotility-like and reflux-like dyspepsias.

36. Minocha A, Mokshagundam S, Gallo SH, Rahal PR: **Alterations in upper**
• **gastrointestinal motility in** *Helicobacter pylori*-**positive nonulcer dyspepsia.** *Am J Gastroenterol* 1994, **89**:1797–1800.
Gastric emptying is similar in non-ulcer dyspepsia patients regardless of *H. pylori* status. Orocaecal transit time was noted to be significantly faster among *H. pylori* non-ulcer dyspepsia patients, but its significance is still unclear.

37. Mendis RE, Gerdes H, Lightdale CJ, Botet JF: **Large gastric folds: a**
• **diagnostic approach using endoscopic ultrasonography.** *Gastrointest Endosc* 1994, **4**:437–441.
It was possible to predict malignant disease by endoscopic ultrasonography by determining which layer was involved. Deeper layer involvement was associated more with malignancy than was superficial layer involvement.

38. Yasunaga Y, Shinomura Y, Kanyama S, Yabu M, Nakanishi T, Miyazaki Y,
• *et al.*: **Improved fold width and increased acid secretion after eradication of the organism in** *Helicobacter pylori*-**associated enlarged fold gastritis.** *Gut* 1994, **35**:1571–1574.
*H. pylori* infection was suggested as the reason for enlarged fold gastritis in the series and was associated with decreased acid secretion. Eradication resulted in decreased fold size and normalization of acid secretion.

39. Bayerdörffer E, Ritter MM, Hatz R, Brooks W, Ruckdeschel G, Stolte M:
• **Healing of protein losing hypertrophic gastropathy by eradication of** *Helicobacter pylori.* **Is** *Helicobacter pylori* **a pathogenic factor in Ménétrier's disease.** *Gut* 1994, **35**:701–704.
A patient with protein losing hypertrophic gastropathy was cured by eradication of *H. pylori.*

40. Adachi Y, Mori M, Maehara Y, Sugimachi K: **Dukes' classification: a valid**
• **prognostic indicator for gastric cancer.** *Gut* 1994, **35**:1368–1471.
Dukes' classification of colorectal cancer was adapted for use in gastric cancer for its simplicity. Analysis shows it to be as accurate a predictor of survival as the Japanese system of classification.

41. Stolte M, Sticht T, Eidt S, Ebert D, Finkenzeller G: **Frequency, location,**
•• **and age and sex distribution of various types of gastric polyps.** *Endoscopy* 1994, **26**:659–665.
A large retrospective analysis of gastric polyps, examining the clinical and histopathological aspects.

42. Karita M, Tada M: **Endoscopic and histologic diagnosis of submucosal**
• **tumors of the gastrointestinal tract using combined strip biopsy and bite biopsy.** *Gastrointest Endosc* 1994, **6**:749–753.
Initial experience in a procedure where exposure of submucosal tumours prior to forceps bite biopsy was accomplished by prior snare resection of the overlying normal mucosa.

43. Yang R, Naaritoku W, Laine L: **Prospective randomized comparison of**
•• **disposable and reusable biopsy forceps in gastrointestinal endoscopy.** *Gastrointest Endosc* 1994, **40**:671–674.
New generation disposable biopsy forceps are compared with reusable ones, showing comparable specimen volumes and histologic depth.

44. Panos MZ, Reilly H, Moran A, Wallis PJW, Wears R, Chesner IM: **Percu-**
• **taneous endoscopic gastrostomy in a general hospital: prospective evalu-ation of indications, outcome, and randomized comparison of two tube designs.** *Gut* 1994, **35**:1551–1556.
PEG is shown to be applicable and effective in a general hospital setting, as shown in this study. Experience between a 9 F and a 12 F PEG tube was also described.

45. Marion MT, Zweng TN, Strodel WE: **One-stage gastrostomy button: an**
• **assessment.** *Endoscopy* 1994, **26**:666–670.
Preliminary experience with a new PEG button design where a pre-existing PEG tract is not required.

46. Duckworth PF Jr, Kirby DF, McHenry L, DeLegge MH, Foxx-Orenstein A:
• **Percutaneous endoscopic gastrojejunostomy made easy: a new over-the-wire technique.** *Gastrointest Endosc* 1994, **3**:350–353.
A procedure of PEJ insertion through a pre-existing PEG making use of a standard ERCP guide wire to pass the PEJ into the jejunum.

47. DiSaario JA, Fennerty MB, Tietze CC, Hutson WR, Burt RW: **Endoscopic**
• **balloon dilation for ulcer-induced gastric outlet obstruction.** *Am J Gas-troenterol* 1994, **89**:868–871.

Balloon dilation of gastric outlet obstruction caused by peptic ulcers was noted to be safe and effective.

48. Parikh SS, Desai SB, Prabhu SR, Trivedi MH, Shankaran K, Bhukanwala
• FA, *et al.*: **Congestive gastropathy: factors influencing development, endoscopic features,** *Helicobacter pylori* **infection and microvessel dis-ease.** *Am J Gastroenterol* 1994, **89**:1036–1042.
The severity of congestive gastropathy was not observed to be dependent on portal venous pressure, capillary dilation, *H. pylori*, or histologic gastritis. Severe congestive gastropathy was, however, observed in patients with large oesophageal and gastric varices.

49. Hayashi N, Kawano S, Tsuji S, Tokai Y, Nagano K, Fusamoto H, *et al.*:
• **Identification and diameter assessment of gastric submucosal vessels using infrared electronic endoscopy.** *Endoscopy* 1994, **26**:686–689.
Using infrared light the venous gastric wall system can be visualized.

50. Fishbein VA, Rosen AM, Lack EE, Montgomery EA, Fleischer D: **Diffuse**
• **hemorrhagic gastroenteropathy: report of a new entity.** *Gastroenterology* 1994, **106**:500–505.
Diffuse mucosal bleeding may be caused by a small vessel vasculopathy.

Guido N.J. Tytgat and Jamie G. Ignacio*, Academic Medical Center, Department of Gastroenterology-Hepatology, Meibergdreef 9, 1005 AZ Amsterdam Zuidoost, the Netherlands and *Department of Medicine, Mary Mediatrix Medical Center, J.P. Laurel Highway, Mataas NA, Lupa, Lipa City 4217, Batangas, Philippines.

# Endoscopy of the small bowel: PEG and PEJ

## Leonard J. Ram and Jamie S. Barkin

University of Miami, School of Medicine/Mount Sinai Medical Center Divisions of
Gastroenterology, Miami Beach, Florida, USA

## Introduction

Over the past year there has been a steady growth of information regarding the indications, benefits and risks of enteroscopy, percutaneous endoscopic gastrostomy (PEG) and percutaneous endoscopic jejunostomy (PEJ). In enteroscopy, the application of video technology and overtube use has enabled a far greater diagnostic and therapeutic benefit to patients with disease occurring deeper in the reaches of the small intestine, 'the final frontier' for gastrointestinal endoscopy. Further refinements in the techniques of PEG and PEJ and timely reviews on risks, benefits and outcomes have enabled us to better understand the appropriate application of these procedures. Thus, although no breakthrough information appeared in 1994, the increasing comfort that endoscopists have with these three procedures indicates that they are becoming a permanent part of our armamentarium in digestive disease.

## Enteroscopy

There is no doubt that the use of 'push' enteroscopy is a preferred method for visualizing the small intestine. The major indications for enteroscopy are to search for a source of occult gastrointestinal bleeding and to evaluate suspected small intestinal mucosal disease. The push method, compared with Sonde enteroscopy, offers the advantage of visualizing better the circumference of the mucosa and an increased capability of biopsy and therapy of potential or actively bleeding lesions. In addition, the procedure time is markedly less. The main disadvantage of the push method is the inability to visualize the more distal small intestine. This is becoming less of an issue as longer and longer push enteroscopes are being designed and put into use. Familiarity with the use of an overtube has prevented gastric looping, which markedly prevented distal advancement.

Barkin et al. [1••,2••] published two papers detailing their experience with push enteroscopy using the longer video enteroscopes. The SIF-100 (length 2500 mm), SIF-10.5L (length 2495 mm) and SIF-3000 (length 2995 mm), all produced by Olympus (Lake Success, NY, USA), are passed in a similar manner as standard upper endoscopes. Their increased length, and the use of an overtube, require minimal further training for endoscopists already skilled in upper endoscopy. These endoscopes all use video technology. All have four-directional tip deflection and a working channel of 2.8 mm, and may have adapted accessory equipment, for example, biopsy forceps, BICAP and heater probe. A 65-cm polyurethane overtube is used to allow straightening of the endoscope in the stomach and duodenum. The examination is performed under fluoroscopic guidance.

A total of 95 patients underwent the procedure [1••,2••]. The quality of small bowel visualization, ease of tube insertion, and the tip deflection at maximum insertion were rated excellent in all patients. Tolerance to the procedure was rated good (similar to gastroscopy) in all patients. Average procedure time was 1 h. Mean length of insertion past the ligament of Treitz without the overtube was 11 cm compared with 108 cm with the overtube (SIF-100), 90 cm (SIF-10.5L) and 113 cm (SIF-3000).

Seventy-five patients underwent evaluation for occult gastrointestinal bleeding. All had undergone multiple negative diagnostic procedures. Surprisingly, 31 patients (41%) had findings proximal to the ligament of Treitz. A significant percentage of these would have been within the reach of a standard gastroscope. The authors recommend that standard oesophagogastroduodenoscopy be repeated prior to enteroscopic evaluation. Twenty patients (27%) had lesions distal to the ligament, which included five with arteriovenous malformations, and one with 'prominent vessels'. Three of these patients were treated with BICAP cautery to good effect. In addition, six patients were found to have malignant jejunal tumours that were unsuspected on radiologic contrast studies. In all, 68% of patients were found to have potential bleeding lesions. Long-term follow-up was not available.

---

**Abbreviations**

ERCP—endoscopic retrograde cholangiopancreatography; **FAP**— familial adenomatous polyposis; **HIV**—human immunodeficiency virus; **PEG**—percutaneous endoscopic gastrostomy; **PEJ**—percutaneous endoscopic jejunostomy.

Enteroscopy should be used early in the workup of patients with significant occult bleeding who have had colonoscopy and upper endoscopy that did not reveal a lesion.

In the evaluation of suspected small bowel pathology, 14 out of 20 patients (70%) had findings on enteroscopy. These findings included sprue in five patients, Crohn's disease in two and one with metastatic melanoma. The authors explained a high diagnostic rate of sprue on enteroscopy but not upper endoscopy because of the potential patchy distribution of the disease, which may be limited to the jejunum.

Only one complication occurred: a pharyngeal tear that was treated medically with good outcome. The authors feel that the complication rate of enteroscopy should not differ from standard upper endoscopy.

In other articles related to enteroscopy, Bertoni et al. [3•] found a high incidence (eight out of 16 patients; 50%) of jejunal polyps in patients with documented familial adenomatous polyposis (FAP) syndromes. Using a gastroscope, paediatric colonoscope, or enteroscope, without an overtube or fluoroscopy, the authors passed the scope on average 30 cm beyond the ligament of Treitz. They found the majority of polyps were in the proximal 20 cm of jejunum, and were often associated with gastric and duodenal polyps. As upper gastrointestinal tract cancer is the most common cause of death in FAP patients once their colon is removed, the authors recommend a regular surveillance endoscopy programme with visualization through the proximal jejunum in these patients.

Maurino et al. [4•] found that out of 100 patients referred for small bowel biopsy, 36 had severe villous atrophy by histology, and 34 out of these 36 (94%) had endoscopic findings in the second portion of the duodenum suggestive of these histologic findings. Reduction in number or loss of Kerking's folds was the most sensitive and specific finding suggestive of microscopic disease. Other findings including mosaic pattern, scalloped folds and visibility of underlying blood vessels were progressively less helpful. It is our opinion that all patients with suspected small intestinal mucosal disease, whether manifested by iron deficiency anaemia, malabsorption, or abnormal radiologic findings, regardless of endoscopic findings, undergo random small bowel biopsies. The macroscopic appearance of the small bowel may guide the endoscopist to the area likely to give the highest histologic yield. Conflicting data persist on whether visualization and biopsy of the jejunal mucosa, in the absence of duodenal findings, is necessary to exclude mucosal disease as the cause of malabsorption. However, if the histologic diagnosis is

secure on duodenal biopsy, there is probably no need for jejunal biopsy.

Zwas et al. [5] point out the importance of ileal intubation and biopsy in patients with suspected inflammatory bowel disease and negative colon findings. Seven cases in which ileal disease was not suspected on small bowel series, but was found on ileoscopy (six macroscopic, one microscopic) were reported. Smedh et al. [6••] found intraoperative enteroscopy useful for guiding surgical management in patients undergoing laparotomy for Crohn's disease. They found that, in 33 patients, the mucosal inflammation was more extensive than serositis (76%) and fat wrapping (48%), and less extensive than mural thickness (67%). In patients with fistula or abscess, or who had undergone previous resection, serosal disease was more extensive. Intraoperative enteroscopy influenced surgical decisions in 20 of these patients, more often reducing the extent of resection, or allowing stricturoplasty instead of resection. As patients with Crohn's disease often require re-operation, preserving the bowel is of the utmost importance. If intraoperative enteroscopy facilitates limitation of bowel loss, it should be used on a regular basis.

Studying intraoperative enteroscopy in patients with bleeding, Hoffman et al. [7] reported five patients who had Sonde enteroscopy passed directly by the surgeon through the bowel. They found that this technique led to less diagnostic uncertainty than standard endoscopes, which traumatize the bowel wall and may create a suction artefact. As the surgeon may manipulate the tip of the Sonde scope, the entire mucosa may be visualized. This is not possible with standard Sonde enteroscopy passed per os.

In summary, enteroscopy plays a vital diagnostic and therapeutic role in patients with suspected small bowel disease.

## PEG/PEJ

The indications, techniques, complications and outcomes continue to be defined for placement of feeding and decompression tubes into the gastrointestinal tract. In a retrospective study of PEG placement in 14 human immunodeficiency virus (HIV)-seropositive patients with corresponding age- and sex-matched controls [8•], Cappell and Godil found that the minor complication rate was similar between groups. However, as expected, the major complication rate was greater in the HIV group, although these were easily treated and rapidly resolved. Interestingly, the HIV group benefited substantially from PEG feeding with a 7.4% weight gain in 3–8 weeks. Nine of the HIV patients were able to be discharged after PEG placement. As HIV-positive patients are living longer, and more disease complications are being successfully treated, their malnutrition is becoming a common source of morbidity. In patients with a 'reasonable' life expectancy who are able to utilize their gastrointestinal tract as a nutritional source, PEG is a reasonable option to decrease the malnutrition.

Marin *et al.* [9•] found that PEG placement in children was safe and effective, providing that multi-organ failure was absent as this substantially increased the complication rate. In particular, children with congenital heart disease and cystic fibrosis derived the most benefit from supplemental PEG feeding (85% and 80% with weight gain compared with baseline, respectively). Therefore, PEG placement and enteral feeding should be considered early in the course of these patients to reduce the morbidity associated with chronic malnutrition.

Kuemmerle and Kirby [10•] presented a patient who had complete pharyngeal obstruction from malignancy whose PEG stoma was dilated and used as the port of entry for endoscopy of the upper gastrointestinal tract. Using through-the-scope balloons, the stoma was sequentially dilated to 10 mm, allowing passage of a paediatric gastroscope. The stomach, duodenum and oesophagus (retrograde) were examined and a 1 cm antral ulcer was found. Theoretical risks of this technique include separation of the stomach from the abdominal wall during passage of the dilators or the endoscope, but this should only occur if the tract is not mature. Limitations of this technique include an inability to visualize the entire upper gastrointestinal mucosa, or to pass the pylorus, because of sharp angulation from the stoma to the pyloric channel. We have used a wire guide during dilation, either with balloons or Savarys that allow us to re-enter the stomach even with oedema of the orifice.

PEJ placement is often difficult using the standard technique of tube grasping by a biopsy forceps as the tube is usually drawn back into the stomach or proximal duodenum during withdrawal of the endoscope. Duckworth *et al.* [11•] described a method for PEJ placement in 18 patients admitted for PEG placement. A standard endoscopic retrograde cholangiopancreatography (ERCP) guide wire was grasped externally with a biopsy forceps through the 28 F PEG stoma and brought into the distal duodenum. The 12 F jejunostomy tube was then guided over the taut wire into the distal duodenum under direct vision. The endoscope was removed, followed by the wire. The procedure was successful in 15 patients and, in 13, the tube reached to or beyond the ligament of Treitz. In one patient, it migrated back to the duodenal bulb, and this was the only patient who

had tube feeding reflux back into the stomach. The authors feel that placement of the tube beyond the third portion of the duodenum theoretically anchors it there and prevents migration. Unfortunately, no long-term follow-up information is provided. However, this technique seems to provide an improvement for PEJ placement. In a similar fashion, Ginsberg *et al.* [12] described a technique in which the PEJ feeding tube is anchored to the jejunal mucosa using a mucosal clip. The procedure was successful in five out of six patients, and proximal migration did not occur in any of these during the procedure. As with the above technique, long-term follow-up is not available, and the risk of using anchoring clips in the jejunum remains to be determined. However, both of these techniques should improve our ability for placement of PEJ.

Vargo *et al.* [13•] described the use of transabdominal ultrasound to aid in placing a decompression PEG in a woman with ovarian cancer and malignant small bowel obstruction. During insertion into the stomach, ultrasound was used to guide the placement of the tube away from the fluid-filled loops of the small bowel and into the stomach. After successful placement, the patient was discharged without a nasogastric tube.

As commercial replacement kits for PEG are expensive, Kadakia *et al.* [14•] studied the use of a modified Foley catheter for replacement use. In a prospective, randomized manner, a 20 F silicone Foley catheter with a retention disk and 3 mm ring were compared with a 20 F standard PEG replacement tube, also modified with a retention ring. Complications, be they balloon deflation, tube cracking, or tube clogging, were similar in both groups. There was no distal tube migration in either group, probably secondary to the use of the retention disk and ring. The authors made the salient points of placing a disk and ring on each replacement tube. Although the complication of balloon deflation would not occur with a mushroom- or button-type replacement, the authors state that the use of this type of replacement tube should be limited as these are even more expensive than balloon replacements. We feel that balloon deflation occurs frequently enough to justify the use of non-balloon replacements. The major problem is eventual tube clogging, which will exist with any of these methods. Fortunately, with continued initial placement of externally removable tubes, the need for endoscopy for tube replacement will become less frequent.

Coben *et al.* [15•] performed an elegant study to evaluate gastro-oesophageal reflux disease using lower oesophageal sphincter manometry in 10 patients with PEG. They found, as expected, that PEG itself did not change lower oesophageal sphincter pressures; however, the method of feeding did indeed alter the lower oesophageal sphincter pressure. Rapid bolus feeding of 350 cm³ reduced lower oesophageal sphincter pressure from 16 mm to 2 mm and led to scintigraphically proven reflux to the sternal notch in one patient. Conversely, continuous feeding at 80 cm³/h did not lead to these findings. In patients at risk for aspiration, continuous feeding should be the preferred method. In addition to the known complications of PEG, we must now add neoplastic seeding from a known upper aerodigestive tract cancer. Schiano et al. [16•] placed a PEG in a man with pharyngeal squamous cell carcinoma and, 4 months later, found that he had the same tumour protruding from the PEG stoma. While this rare complication should not sway us from appropriate placement of PEG, it is something to be aware of.

The role of PEGs in nursing home patients was evaluated by Kaw and Sekas [17••]. They reviewed the outcome of PEG placement in 46 nursing home patients followed over an 18-month period. In 91% of these patients there was a neurological indication for PEG placement, predominantly dementia and cerebrovascular accident. In none of the cases did PEG feeding enable a patient to be discharged from the nursing home, nor did PEG alter the albumin or cholesterol levels, or the weight of the patient. Thirty-four complications requiring hospital admission or an emergency room visit were noted, predominantly tube obstruction, but also aspiration pneumonia (20% of patients). The latter was far more common in patients who were obtunded rather than awake. Eight per cent of deaths were attributable to aspiration of gastric contents.

We can conclude from these studies that certain groups, such as children, may benefit from PEG. Others, such as the nursing home patients with advanced neurological disease, may not. It is important for all of us to carefully decide if PEG is indicated on an individual basis, and to be aware of the fact that some patients may be hurt more than they are helped. Unfortunately, it may not be possible to withhold PEG placement in patients without contraindications to its placement, and laws regarding placement of feeding tubes in these types of patients vary and are in constant flux.

## Conclusion

The role of these 'recent' arrivals to the endoscopic frontier will become further defined as our understanding of the risks and benefits becomes clearer. Enteroscopy allows us to diagnose jejunal disease and apply therapy to certain lesions. As equipment and techniques are further refined, we should be able to progress even further into the small intestine. The grasping of scopes passed from each end into the ileum may not be far off. PEG and PEJ continue to provide options for long-term enteral feeding at a fraction of the overall cost of surgical placement. Further analysis of outcomes will help define which patient groups benefit most from this form of therapy.

## References and recommended reading

Papers of particular interest, published within the annual period of review, have been highlighted as:

- •        of special interest
- ••      of outstanding interest

1.    Barkin JS, Chong J, Reiner DK: **First generation video enteroscope-fourth**
••    **generation push-type small bowel enteroscopy utilizing overtube.** Gastrointest Endosc 1994, **40**:743–747.
Twenty-nine patients underwent push enteroscopy for evaluation of occult gastrointestinal bleeding and suspected small bowel pathology using a 2500 mm video enteroscope. Findings and therapeutic interventions are discussed. This paper shows the usefulness of video push enteroscopy, its safety, ease of use and lack of patient discomfort.

2.    Chong J, Tagle M, Barkin JS, Reiner DK: **Small bowel push-type fiberoptic**
••    **enteroscopy for patients with occult gastrointestinal bleeding or suspected small bowel pathology.** Am J Gastroenterol 1994, **89**:2143–2146.
Sixty-six patients were evaluated with push enteroscopy. Findings included small bowel arteriovenous malformations, cancers, sprue, and Crohn's disease. The diagnostic yield was above 50%. This paper presents data verifying the place of enteroscopy in the armamentarium of endoscopists.

3.    Bertoni G, Sassatelli R, Tansimi P, Ricci E, Conigilano R, Bedogni G:
•    **Jejunal polyps in familial adenomatous polyposis assessed by push type endoscopy.** J Clin Gastroenterol 1993, **17**:343–348.
Fifty per cent of patients with FAP have proximal jejunal polyps. These patients should undergo endoscopic surveillance including visualization of the jejunum.

4.    Maurino E, Capizzano H, Niveloni S, Kogan Z, Valero J, Boerr L, et al.:
•    **Value of endoscopic markers in celiac disease.** Dig Dis Sci 1993, **38**:2028–2033.
Ninety-four percent of patients with biopsy-proven mucosal atrophy have endoscopic abnormalities. Absence of these findings should not dissuade biopsy, but their finding may direct it.

5.    Zwas FR, Bonheim NA, Berken CA, Gray S, et al.: **Ileoscopy as an important tool for the diagnosis of Crohn's disease: a report of seven cases.** Gastrointest Endosc 1993, **40**:89–91.
Seven patients without colonic findings were found to have Crohn's disease on ileoscopy.

6.    Smedh K, Olaison G, Nystrom PO, Sjodahl R: **Intraoperative enteroscopy**
••    **in Crohn's disease.** Br J Surg 1993, **80**:897–900.
Thirty-three patients with Crohn's disease underwent intraoperative endoscopy. Findings altered the surgical management in 20 of these. This paper shows the importance of this technique to minimize surgical bowel loss in patients with Crohn's disease.

7.    Hoffman JS, Cave DR, Birkett D: **Intraoperative enteroscopy with a sonde intestinal fiberscope.** Gastrointest Endosc 1994, **40**:229–230.
Sonde enteroscopy minimizes trauma during intraoperative endoscopy and leads to less diagnostic confusion.

8.    Cappell MS, Godil A: **A multicenter case controlled study of percutaneous**
•    **endoscopic gastrostomy in HIV seropositive patients.** Am J Gastroenterol 1993, **88**:2059–2066.
PEG is safe and has clinical benefit in patients who are malnourished with HIV.

9.    Marin OE, Glassman MS, Schoen BT, Caplan DB: **Safety and efficacy of**
•    **percutaneous endoscopic gastrostomy in children.** Am J Gastroenterol 1994, **89**:357–361.
PEG is safe and has clinical benefit in children without multi-organ failure. It most benefited children with congenital heart disease and cystic fibrosis.

10.    Kuemmerle JF, Kirby DF: **Diagnostic endoscopy via gastrostomy or PEG**
•    **stoma.** Am J Gastroenterol 1993, **88**:1445–1446.
Dilation of a PEG stoma allows upper gastrointestinal endoscopic examination. This technique is useful in patients whose proximal tract is obstructed.

11. Duckworth PF Jr, Kirby DF, McHenry L, DeLegge MH, Foxx-Orenstein A:
• **Percutaneous endoscopic gastrojejunostomy made easy: a new over the wire technique.** *Gastrointest Endosc* 1994, **40**:350–353.
Use of an ERCP guide wire enabled distal placement of a jejunostomy tube. Long-term lack of migration is not evident.

12. Ginsberg GG, Lipman TO, Fleischer DE: **Endoscopic clip assisted placement of enteral feeding tubes.** *Gastrointest Endosc* 1994, **40**:220–222.
A mucosal clip fastens a jejunostomy tube to the jejunal mucosa.

13. Vargo JJ, Germain MM, Swenson JA, Harrison CR: **Ultrasound assisted**
• **percutaneous endoscopic gastrostomy in a patient with advanced ovarian carcinoma and recurrent intestinal obstruction.** *Am J Gastroenterol* 1993, **88**:1946–1948.
Transabdominal ultrasound assisted in safe placement of a PEG for decompression. This technique may be helpful in patients with relative contraindications to PEG placement such as bowel obstruction.

14. Kadakia SC, Cassaday M, Shaffer RT: **Comparison of Foley catheter as a**
• **replacement gastrostomy tube with commercial replacement gastrostomy tube: a prospective randomized trial.** *Gastrointest Endosc* 1994, **40**:188–193.
A modified Foley catheter is just as efficacious as a commercial replacement tube for PEG replacement, and considerably less expensive. Both tubes still clog frequently.

15. Coben RM, Weintraub A, DiMarino AJ Jr, Cohen S: **Gastroesophageal**
• **reflux during gastrostomy feeding.** *Gastroenterology* 1994, **106**:13–18.
Decreased lower oesophageal sphincter pressure and scintigraphic reflux was much more common with bolus feeding than with continuous feeding.

16. Schiano TD, Pfister D, Harrison L, Shike M: **Neoplastic seeding as a**
• **complication of percutaneous endoscopic gastrostomy.** *Am J Gastroenterol* 1994, **89**:131–133.
The PEG stoma was seeded with a squamous cell carcinoma in a patient with the same tumour in the pharynx. This is the first report of this type of PEG complication.

17. Kaw M, Sekas G: **Long term follow up of consequences of percutaneous**
•• **endoscopic gastrostomy tubes in nursing home patients.** *Dig Dis Sci* 1994, **39**:738–743.
Nursing home patients with neurologic indications for PEG placement generally did not derive any benefit from these tubes. Tube feedings contributed to death from aspiration in 8% of patients. This paper points out the limitations of PEG in this patient population.

Dr Leonard J. Ram and Dr Jamie S. Barkin, Division of Gastroenterology, Mount Sinai Medical Center, 4300 Alton Road, Miami Beach, FL 33140, USA.

# Endoscopy of upper gastrointestinal bleeding

## James Y.W. Lau and S.C. Sydney Chung

Department of Surgery, The Chinese University of Hong Kong, Prince of Wales Hospital, Shatin, Hong Kong

## Introduction

Therapeutic endoscopy has emerged as the primary treatment modality in the management of upper gastrointestinal bleeding. In the past year, there were reports confirming the efficacy of endoscopic haemostasis and on the refinements of various endoscopic techniques. In addition, the fundamental issue of the place of therapeutic endoscopy in the overall management of gastrointestinal bleeding was re-examined.

## Peptic ulcer bleeding

### An overview

In a didactic and extensive review of the literature, Laine and Peterson [1••] provided a thorough account on all aspects of bleeding peptic ulcer disease. Evidence from recent meta-analyses indicates that endoscopic therapy reduces both the operation rate and overall mortality. Endoscopic treatment should now be the primary intervention. Both clinical factors and endoscopic features are important in predicting further bleeding. Endoscopic signs in particular allow clinicians to formulate management strategies and stratify care. High-risk stigmata require prophylactic endoscopic treatment and intensive observation whilst patients with low-risk stigmata can be discharged early. Injection therapy and thermal contact devices are comparable in safety and efficacy. The use of laser therapy is limited by the cost of the laser unit and difficulty in its transportation. In a compiled series of 1684 patients, the risks of the two major complications of endoscopic therapy, induction of bleeding requiring surgery (0.3%) and perforation (0.5%), were small. Surgery should be performed if endoscopic treatment fails or is not available. The prospect of bleeding peptic ulcer disease lies with its prevention. *Helicobacter pylori* eradication appears promising in reducing ulcer rebleeding while the role of elective surgery is diminishing.

## The impact of therapeutic endoscopy

The introduction of therapeutic endoscopy has led to the reduction in emergency operation for bleeding peptic ulcers. Whether therapeutic endoscopy has decreased the overall mortality remains controversial. Some surgeons held the view that endoscopic treatment delayed surgery in those who required it and adversely affected their outcome. Williams *et al.* [2] compared the results of their current practice with endoscopic treatment as the primary intervention with two historical series from the pretherapeutic endoscopy era. They concluded that both the incidence of operation and the overall mortality had decreased. On the other hand, impressive results in the management of peptic ulcer bleeding could be achieved without therapeutic endoscopy. By strict adherence to the criteria of operating on patients with shock upon admission, resuscitation requirements > 4 units of blood, age older than 65 years, ulcer size larger than 2 cm or with stigmata of recent haemorrhage and previous admission for ulcer complication, Benders *et al.* [3] operated on 66 patients with no hospital mortality in a 5-year period. The operative rate, however, was not apparent from the report. Mueller *et al.* [4] adopted a similar strategy with early surgery according to a well-defined protocol; spurting haemorrhage, non bleeding visible vessel on the posterior wall of the duodenum, blood transfusion > 6 units in the first 24 h and haemodynamic instability and signs of rebleeding in the first 48 h. In a consecutive series of 157 patients, the mortality at 30 days was 7%; only one death was related to surgery.

At the other extreme, Qvist *et al.* [5] adopted a policy of persistent endoscopic treatment even in rebleeding patients and restrictive use of surgery in the management of their patients. A low overall mortality rate of 6.4% was achieved. In their report, it was apparent that increasing mortality was associated with rebleeding and further attempts at therapeutic endoscopy. Vigilance, early intervention within a well-defined protocol and skilled endoscopists and surgeons in close cooperation are essential ingredients common to all success stories in the management of peptic ulcer bleeding. There has

---

**Abbreviations**

ETH—ethanolamine oleate; **Nd:YAG**—neodymium yttrium aluminium garnet; **SRH**—stigmata of recent haemorrhage; **STD**—sodium tetradecyl sulphate; **TIPS**—transjugular intrahepatic portosystemic stent-stunt.

yet to be a randomized trial comparing early surgery and therapeutic endoscopy as the primary treatment of bleeding ulcers. Therapeutic endoscopy and surgery should be complementary to each other with endoscopic treatment as the primary intervention. The early promise of *H. pylori* eradication in the prevention of ulcer relapses and recurrent bleeding has given rise to a more conservative attitude in referring patients for surgery. Early surgery is indicated if endoscopic treatment fails. How long one should persist with endoscopic treatment in rebleeding cases without compromising the patient remains uncertain.

## Predicting rebleeding
### Stigmata of recent haemorrhage
The lack of uniformity in the interpretation of these endoscopic signs was highlighted by a report from Laine *et al.* [6•]. At the American College of Gastroenterology Postgraduate Course, 202 endoscopists of variable experience were shown slides of stigmata of recent haemorrhage (SRH). Endoscopists disagreed more than a quarter of the time. This disagreement was related to the experience of the endoscopists and could be improved with a brief session of teaching. The consensus over colour was particularly poor. The findings of the report explained in part the discrepancy in the reported prevalence and rebleeding risks of SRH in the literature. It also raised concerns over the validity of past reports on SRH and, in particular, when one generalizes findings from one report to another. The value of refinements of visible vessels by colour has become dubious in light of its poor interobserver agreement (Fig. 1).

### Sequential studies of endoscopic signs of peptic ulcer bleeding
A sequential endoscopic study of the evolutionary changes of SRH [7] in 144 patients revealed that the fading time of a visible vessel (4.1 ± 2.1 days) was significantly longer than that of an adherent clot (2.4 ± 0.8 days) or an old stigma (2.4 ± 1.3 days). Following the disappearance of SRH, the risk of bleeding became negligible. The fading time was independent of factors such as age, sex, ulcer location and, surprisingly, the severity of bleeding and endoscopic local therapy. Stigmata of haemorrhage represent different phases of an evolutionary scheme with healing and there is transition from a visible vessel, an adherent clot, a flat pigmentation to, eventually, a clean base ulcer. In this study, some visible vessels disappeared without going through the transition phases. This could be explained by the 2-day interval between endoscopic examinations. It is apparent that there is heterogeneity within each subgroup. Some visible vessels disappeared faster. A limitation of the study lies in the arbitrary distinction between a vessel and an adherent clot. The entity of a clot covering a vessel should be recognized. In our own experience, uncovering of clots on day one certainly revealed a number of vessels (Fig. 2).

### Objective assessment of the ulcer base
Endoscopic signs in peptic ulcer bleeding are far from perfect in the quantitation of rebleeding risks and prognosis. Critical variables determining rebleeding such as size, depth and state of vessels, cannot be inferred from inspection of the ulcer base alone. Kohler

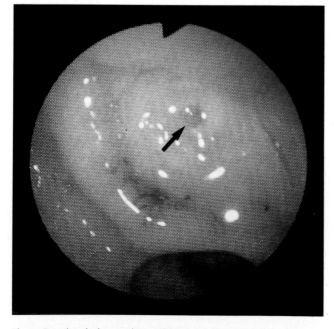

**Fig. 1.** Duodenal ulcer with a visible vessel. Courtesy of G.N. Tytgat.

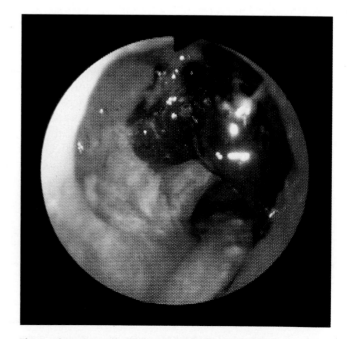

**Fig. 2.** Ulceration with adherent coagulation. Courtesy of G.N. Tytgat.

and Rieman [8] suggested that a pulsed Doppler probe might be more accurate than the endoscopic appearance in predicting rebleeding. The authors used a pulsed endoscopic Doppler in 140 patients with Forrest II and III ulcer bleeding. The agreement between endoscopic findings and ultrasonographic findings was only 59%. Injection therapy was guided by positive Doppler signs. Recurrent haemorrhage occurred in 9% of their treated patients. No rebleeding occurred in Doppler-negative ulcers.

### Clinical parameters

Clinical parameters have been used over the years to identify high-risk patients. In a retrospective review of 2217 consecutive patients with non-variceal upper gastrointestinal bleeding [9•], death occurred in 189 (8.5%) patients and rebleeding in 243 (11%). Logistic regression analyses showed that death was significantly associated with rebleeding, age greater then 60 years and the finding of fresh blood at endoscopy. Rebleeding was, in turn, associated with endoscopic stigmata of active bleeding, shock and the identification of gastric or duodenal ulcers.

In another multivariate analysis of 204 patients from Taiwan [10•], hypovolaemic shock, a non-bleeding visible vessel and an adherent clot on the ulcer base were found to be significant, independent risk factors for rebleeding. Repeat endoscopy in 19 rebleeding patients revealed persistence of stigmata of bleeding.

## Refining endoscopic treatment

### Comparative trials in injection therapy

More reports confirming the efficacy of endoscopic therapy in controlling peptic ulcer bleeding appeared in 1994. Carter and Anderson [11] randomized 49 patients with ulcer bleeding to receive adrenaline injection (21 patients) and laser photocoagulation (23 patients). Five patients proceeded directly to surgery. No difference was demonstrated in the two subgroups.

In another report [12•], 107 patients with peptic ulcer haemorrhage, all of whom had major stigmata of haemorrhage, were randomized to receive adrenaline alone or adrenaline plus 5% ethanolamine oleate (ETH). The rebleeding rate was similar in both groups (eight out of 55 in the adrenaline alone group and seven out of 52 in the sclerosant group). The transfusion requirement, hospital stay and operation rate were also similar in both groups. The finding confirms that adding a sclerosant confers no advantage.

In an interesting study from Taiwan [13•], 52 patients with Forrest Ia or Ib bleeding ulcers were randomized to receive injection with adrenaline (27 patients) or pure water (25 patients). No statistical difference was noted in the rate of initial (92.5% versus 88%) or permanent (81.5% versus 76%) haemostasis, operation rate (11% versus 16%) or mortality (3.7% versus 4%). It was suggested that injection therapy worked by the effect of local tamponade from tissue swelling. In practice, there is really little to choose as the systemic effect following the local injection of adrenaline is clinically insignificant.

In an uncontrolled retrospective series, Herold *et al.* [14] reviewed the use of fibrin injection in 452 patients with Forrest I and II bleeding. Injection of fibrin sealant was performed with or without hypertonic saline plus adrenaline. The haemostatic effect could not be entirely attributed to fibrin in some patients as other agents were used as well. The authors also suggested that fibrin sealant promoted healing.

Berg *et al.* [15] conducted a prospective randomized trial comparing injection with fibrin glue to polidocanol in 79 (38 versus 41) patients with Forrest I and II bleeding. Repeat endoscopies were performed on days 1, 3 and 5. Rebleeding as defined endoscopically following fibrin glue injection (13%) was less than that in the polidocanol group (24%).

### The value of second-look endoscopy

Some endoscopists hold the view that early repeat endoscopy after successful initial haemostasis may identify early rebleeding or persistence of high-risk stigmata. Prophylactic injection may then be useful in aborting rebleeding. Villanueva *et al.* [16•] conducted a prospective randomized trial in which 104 patients with peptic ulcer bleeding were assigned to two groups; with or without elective second-look endoscopy following successful initial endoscopic haemostasis. These patients were either actively bleeding during initial endoscopy or had non-bleeding visible vessels in the floor of their ulcers. Those assigned to second-look endoscopy were re-injected if indicated. Patients who received repeat endoscopy did marginally better with less rebleeding (21% versus 29%), less need for surgery (8% versus 15%), a smaller transfusion requirement, a shorter hospital stay and lower mortality (2% versus 4%). The difference did not reach statistical significance after enrollment of 52 patients in each group. The authors concluded that this difference was unlikely to be large and routine second-look endoscopy could not be justified.

### The efficacy of therapeutic endoscopy in anticoagulated patients

In a series of 52 patients on warfarin with signs of upper gastrointestinal haemorrhage [17], 25 were bleeding from peptic ulcers, six from gastric erosions, four from Mallory–Weiss tears and eight from other causes. Nine (17%) were bleeding from unknown causes. Twenty-three patients with peptic ulcer bleeding underwent endoscopic treatment with adrenaline injection or heat probe. Endoscopic haemostasis was equally effective in achieving haemostasis when compared with 50 closely matched control subjects presenting with gastrointestinal haemorrhage not on warfarin. Rebleeding was similar in both groups. Patients on anticoagulant with upper gastrointestinal bleeding should be managed in the same manner as others not on anticoagulant. Endoscopic treatment should be offered when indicated.

### Complication of injection therapy: intramural haematoma

Reported systemic and local complications with endoscopic injection have been few. In a prospective study of 227 patients, Rohler et al. [18] reported five patients with intramural haematoma following injection therapy for bleeding peptic ulcers. All patients had concomitant severe medical illnesses and coagulation disturbance. In three patients, acute pancreatitis developed concurrently with duodenal haematoma. Two patients required gastrectomy; one for the complication of posterior stomach wall necrosis and the other for recurrent bleeding. Both patients died subsequently.

### The prevention of rebleeding in peptic ulcer disease

In a prospective randomized trial, Jensen et al. [19**] demonstrated that the use of maintenance ranitidine significantly reduced the risk of recurrent bleeding in duodenal ulcer disease unrelated to non-steroidal anti-inflammatory agents. In the study, 65 patients with endoscopically proven, bleeding duodenal ulcers were randomly assigned to receive maintenance ranitidine (150 mg at bedtime; n = 32) or placebo (n = 33). After a mean follow-up of 61 weeks, rebleeding rates were 9% and 36%, respectively. Symptomatic recurrences without bleeding were seen in an additional 12% and 21%, respectively. The protection against rebleeding with a maintenance $H_2$-antagonist, however, was incomplete. In a small report, Graham et al. [20•] compared the use of H. pylori eradication with a course of ranitidine without maintenance medication in treating duodenal ulcer bleeding. No rebleeding was noted in the H. pylori eradication group (17 patients) while 28.6% (four out of 14 patients) treated with an $H_2$-antagonist rebled. H. pylori eradication prevented recurrent bleeding. Labenz and Borsch [21] prospectively studied two groups of patients (42 versus 24) and came to the same conclusion: H. pylori eradication led to significantly fewer ulcer recurrences (2.4% versus 62.5%) and bleeding relapses (0 versus 37.5%). If the promise of these studies holds true, eradication of H. pylori will have a major impact on the epidemiology of ulcer bleeding.

## Variceal bleeding

### Sclerotherapy versus sham therapy

The efficacy of sclerotherapy was confirmed in a prospective randomized trial by the Veterans Affairs Cooperative Variceal Sclerotherapy Group involving 12 medical centres [22•]. Over a period of 5 years, 253 male alcoholic patients who were either actively bleeding at presentation or had a previous history of bleeding were enrolled. They were assigned to receive sclerotherapy with 1.5% sodium tetradecyl sulphate (STD; 122 patients) or placebo (131 patients). The sham-therapy group experienced significantly more bleeding episodes (112 versus 52) and the rate of recurrent bleeding was higher (rate ratio 1.54). The mean transfusion requirement and the need for shunt surgery were also higher in the sham-therapy group. Long-term survival was not different between the groups.

### Prophylactic treatment of oesophageal varices

Approximately one-third of the patients with the diagnosis of oesophageal varices will bleed from them and most of the bleeding episodes occur within the first year of diagnosis. The mortality associated with the index bleed ranges from 40% to 60%. The overall mortality risk for the initial 6 months following a bleed is similar. Because of this high early mortality, prophylactic treatment in order to prevent first bleeding is attractive. The prophylactic treatment should ideally be efficacious, safe and inexpensive. The options include endoscopic sclerotherapy, drug treatment and surgery. Greig et al. [23•] reviewed the literature extensively and concluded that prophylaxis with β-blockade seemed to be the best therapeutic option with six previous randomized controlled trials showing benefits in preventing first bleed. Controlled randomized trials of the use of prophylactic sclerotherapy had yielded conflicting results. Its use was limited by the associated complications and occasional deaths. The only favourable report on the use of surgical prophylaxis came from the Japanese with shunting procedures. In selected Child's A and B patients, clear benefits were shown both in terms of bleeding rate and 5-year survival. None of the Western trials were comparable.

### Predicting the first variceal bleeding

Siringo et al. [24] prospectively followed up 87 cirrhotic patients with oesophageal varices but without previous haemorrhage for a mean of 24 months. Variceal bleeding occurred in 22 patients (25.3%), nine of them within the first 6 months. Cox regression analysis identified variceal size, cherry-red spots (Fig. 3), serum bilirubin and congestion index (the ratio of cross-sectional area of the portal vein and blood flow velocity on Doppler flowmetry) as independent predictors of variceal bleeding. The addition of Doppler ultrasound flowmetry to clinical, biochemical and endoscopic parameters im-

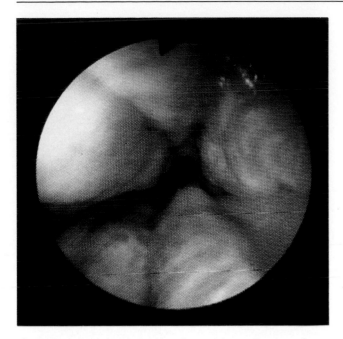

**Fig. 3.** Oesophageal varices with a cherry red spot. Courtesy of G.N. Tytgat.

proved the prediction of patients with bleeding in the first 6 months.

A study from Japan [25] utilized electronic video endoscopy and colorimetric analysis of oesophageal varices in predicting variceal rupture. A small group of 30 patients (15 with and 15 without previous variceal bleeding) was studied. The ratio of red colour tone was lower in bleeders than non-bleeders and the area ratio of red colour sign was significantly higher in the former. Endoscopic findings according to rules by the Japanese Research Society for Portal Hypertension did not differ in the two groups. Image processing may be more effective for predicting oesophageal variceal bleeding than the traditional rules.

### On demand sclerotherapy

Little controversy exists in offering patients sclerotherapy when they present with their first variceal haemorrhage. Moreto et al. [26•], in a prospective randomized trial, investigated whether these patients should continue to be treated until eradication of varices. Patients successfully treated with sclerotherapy in their first episodes of variceal bleeding were randomly assigned to two treatment groups; the combined sclerotherapy group with 50 patients who continued to have planned injections and the short-term sclerotherapy group with 56 patients who were injected only in recurrent bleeding. Varices were grouped into junctional (upper gastric and cardia) and oesophageal. Combined sclerotherapy was more effective in preventing bleeding from the oesophageal varices but not those from the junctional source. No survival difference was observed between the groups. It was concluded

that patients with oesophageal varices after their first episode of variceal bleeding should be injected electively.

McKee et al. [27] conducted a similar prospective randomized trial in poor risk cirrhotic patients who belonged to Child's class C or were older than 65 years. Forty patients who survived their first endoscopically proven variceal bleeding were randomly assigned to planned injections at 3-weekly intervals or on-demand injections when they rebled. In this small group of patients, planned injection reduced the episodes of rebleeding but did not improve survival.

### Sclerotherapy: which agent to use?

In a double-blinded, prospective, randomized trial, Chan et al. [28•] compared the use of 3% STD and 5% ETH in 95 patients with acute variceal bleeding. The technique of intravariceal injection was employed with injections of 2 ml aliquots, up to 20 ml at each session. Treatment was repeated at weekly intervals until eradication. Primary control of bleeding was comparable in the STD (n = 48) and ETH groups (n = 47) (87.5% versus 87.2%, respectively). STD appeared to obliterate varices in significantly fewer sessions compared with ETH (3.3 ±1.3 versus 4.5 ±1.9). Postinjection pyrexia was more common with STD. No difference was noted in the rate of oesophageal ulceration and subsequent stricture formation. Perforation occurred in one patient in the STD group.

### Endoscopic sclerotherapy, band ligation or cyanoacrylate glue

The saga over the choice of sclerotherapy and band ligation continued into 1994. Five independent review articles [29••,30••,31•,32••,33] examined the issue in light of published randomized trials. Mounting evidence indicates that variceal ligation has fewer complications than sclerotherapy. Ligation also obliterates varices in fewer sessions. In the original trial from Denver, survival benefit was observed in the variceal ligation group. In terms of primary control of acute variceal bleeding, the two modalities were shown to be comparable. In a review article, Schapiro [33] raised the question whether band ligation with its lesser incidence of complication could be used in the prophylactic therapy of varices that had not bled. Complications arising from variceal ligation have, however, been increasingly reported. They included over-tube pinch injury and massive haemorrhage from postligation ulcerations. Sakai et al. [34] reported early mortality in a small group of Child's C patients from massive rebleeding and questioned the use of ligation in these patients. Approaches using combinations of variceal ligation and sclerotherapy have also been described in short communications in the literature; they have yet to be substantiated by larger trials. Cyanoacrylate injection has been popular in the control of variceal bleeding in certain parts of Europe with success. Binmoeller *et al.* [29••] cited experiences from Europe and Egypt, and suggested that tissue adhesives were highly effective in achieving immediate haemostasis, and, more importantly, the incidence of rebleeding following its injection was less compared with other agents. Pulmonary and portal vein embolism are significant complications of tissue adhesive injection. A randomized trial comparing tissue adhesives with either band ligation or sclerotherapy is long overdue.

## Octreotide versus sclerotherapy

Planas *et al.* [35•] randomized 70 consecutive patients with oesophageal variceal bleeding to receive either somatostatin (an initial bolus of 250 g followed by an infusion of 250 g/h for 48 h plus additional 6-hourly boluses of 250 g for the first 24 h) or sclerotherapy. The two groups were well matched with regard to sex, age, aetiology of cirrhosis and severity of liver failure. There was no difference between the two groups in treatment failure (20% versus 17.1%), early rebleeding (25% versus 17.2%) or 6-week mortality (28.5% versus 22.8%). The sclerotherapy group, however, experienced significantly more complications resulting in two deaths. Somatostatin is as effective as sclerotherapy but safer in the control of acute variceal bleeding. The same conclusion was drawn by Burroughs [36•] in an extensive literature review on the subject. In four previous comparative trials of somatostatin or octreotide with injection sclerotherapy, no statistical difference in efficacy or mortality was noted.

## Gastric varices

Thakeb *et al.* [37•] studied retrospectively two groups of patients with oesophagogastric varices. The first group included 970 patients with documented variceal bleeding but without history of sclerotherapy. Sixty-five patients (6.7%) had concomitant gastric varices and 27.1% had direct gastric extension of oesophageal varices (mostly of grade 3). Gastric varices alone without oesophageal varices were found in five cases only (0.5%). The second group included 376 patients who had undergone eradication of oesophageal varices by sclerotherapy and were free of gastric varices at first presentation. Eleven of these patients (2.9%) developed secondary gastric varices. A morphological description of gastric varices (Fig. 4) was given: (1) a cauliflower-like mass seen at the fundus (43.1%); (2) a lobulated and clubbed cystic swelling seen along the lesser curve of the stomach below the cardia (23.1%); (3) tortuous and ruga-like varices (27.7%); and (4) a network of vessels along the length of the stomach (6.1%). The larger varieties were associated with a higher risk of bleeding (35.4% for the cauliflower type and 16.9% for the cystic ones). No bleeding was recorded in the secondary gastric varices arising after endoscopic obliteration of oesophageal varices. For the gastric varices that extended from their oesophageal counterparts,

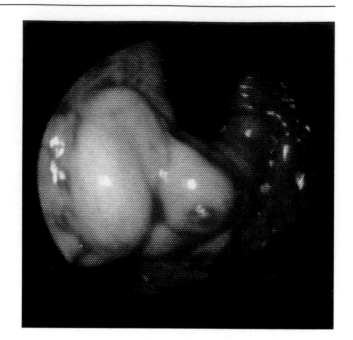

**Fig. 4.** Gastric varix with a cherry red spot.

only 5.2% had evidence of bleeding. The reported prevalence of gastric varices in the literature varies widely from 6–70% compared with around 35% from the present report. The variation arises from the lack of uniformity in the diagnostic criteria. Despite the novel description, endoscopic diagnosis of gastric varices is notoriously unreliable. Suffice it to say that the larger varieties are more likely to bleed.

The endoscopic treatment of gastric varices has been less than satisfactory. Cyanoacrylate injection has been employed with some success. Yoshida *et al.* [38] reported the use of a detachable snare (Fig. 5) in the treatment of gastric varices in 10 patients. The snare had previously been used in the endoscopic resection of elevated lesions. Eradication of gastric varices was observed endoscopically in all patients. One snare was required in seven cases and two were required in three cases. The snare allows treatment of larger varices up

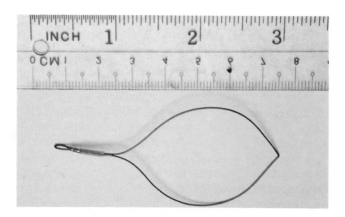

**Fig. 5.** A detachable snare for gastric varices (model MH477 from the Olympus Co.).

to 4 cm in diameter. No complication was reported except one episode of minor self-limiting haemorrhage from postligation ulceration.

## Transjugular intrahepatic portosystemic stent-stunt

Transjugular intrahepatic portosystemic stent-stunt (TIPS) is a recent and exciting addition in the therapeutic armoury of variceal haemorrhage (Fig. 6). Rössle *et al.* [39•] reported impressive results with TIPS in 100 consecutive patients with variceal bleeding due to cirrhosis. The patients were referred because of failed sclerotherapy and 22 of them belonged to Child's class C cirrhosis. Ten of the patients were treated on an emergency basis. Technical success was achieved in 93% of the patients. The major complication was haemorrhage (intraperitoneal in six, haemobilia in four and capsular haematoma in the liver in three patients). Migration of the stent into the pulmonary artery occurred in two patients. A total of 31 patients developed stent stenoses or occlusion when followed up for $12 \pm 6$ months. Only 10 of these presented with recurrent variceal haemorrhage. They were amenable to re-dilation, thrombolysis and additional stent placement. Ninety-two per cent of patients remained free of variceal bleeding at 6 months and 82% at 1 year. A quarter of the patients had encephalopathy; this was related to stent size. Inhospital 30-day mortality was 3%. One patient died from the procedure-related complication of intraperitoneal haemorrhage. None of the patients died of exanguation from varices. The cumulative survival at 1 year was 85%. This study defined the current role of TIPS in the algorithm of variceal bleeding management; those failing endoscopic treatment and, particularly, in patients of Child–Pugh C cirrhosis in whom the surgical risk is excessive. The role of TIPS is likely to expand in the era of liver transplantation and with increasing expertise in the procedure.

## Other topics

### The use of laser therapy

Laser photocoagulation has been sidelined in the management of ulcer bleeding. Its use has been relegated to the conditions of vascular ectasia and radiation mucositis. Liberski *et al.* [40] reported the use of neodymium yttrium aluminium garnet (Nd:YAG) laser in 15 patients with watermelon stomach. These patients presented with chronic blood loss and were transfusion-dependent. Both endoscopic and haematologic improvement were noted. Ten patients were no longer transfusion dependent after a mean follow-up period of 4.4 years. Five patients died of intercurrent medical illnesses but without evidence of bleeding. Potiamiano *et al.* [41•] described the successful treatment of five patients requiring transfusion with diffuse gastric antral ectasia. In contrast the treatment of three patients with so-called honeycomb stomach proved to be difficult. Here, laser treatment was successful in only one case.

### A large channel endoscope

The use of a new endoscope with a large 6-mm suction channel and a 13.7-mm outer diameter was reported in 122 out of 123 patients with upper gastrointestinal haemorrhage in whom evacuation of blood or gastric content was impossible with standard endoscopes [42]. The channel connected to a three-way stopcock which allowed alternate instillation of water and suction. Gastric emptying was achieved within 5 min in all cases. This new scope may prove useful in patients with severe bleeding obscuring endoscopic view.

## Conclusion

In peptic ulcer bleeding, endoscopic treatment emerged as the first-line treatment. Surgery plays an important supportive role. Further refinements in endoscopic techniques may add marginally to the efficacy of endoscopic haemostasis. More important is the identification of patients who require endoscopic treatment and defining the indication for emergency operation in those who rebleed after endoscopy. Preventing ulcer recurrence and therefore rebleeding by *H. pylori* eradication is likely to have a major impact on the problem of peptic ulcer haemorrhage.

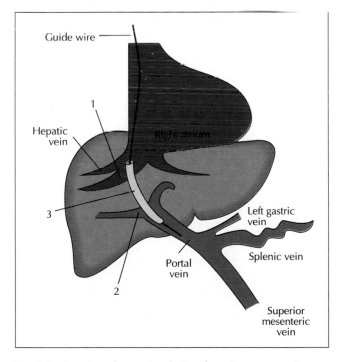

**Fig. 6.** Implantation of a transjugular intrahepatic portosystemic stent-shunt (TIPS); after transjugular catheterization of a hepatic vein (site 1) and puncture of a main branch of the portal vein (site 2), the shunt is established by the implantation of a stent (site 3) bridging the liver tissue between sites 1 and 2. Published with permission [39•].

In variceal bleeding, band ligation has been shown to be superior to sclerotherapy. Several useful pharmacological agents for prevention of bleeding or the treatment of acute episodes have been identified. Radiologists are back in the limelight with TIPS. A unifying approach combining these modalities with surgery is required to optimize the management of variceal bleeding.

## References and recommended reading

Papers of particular interest, published within the annual period of review, have been highlighted as:
- of special interest
- • of outstanding interest

1. Laine L, Peterson WL: **Bleeding peptic ulcer.** *N Engl J Med* 1994, **331**:717–727.
•• 
An excellent overview of the modern management of peptic ulcer bleeding.

2. Williams RA, Vartany A, Davis IP, Wilson SE: **Impact of endoscopic therapy on outcome of operation for bleeding peptic ulcers.** *Am J Surg* 1993, **166**:712–715.
Both the operation rate and mortality decreased with the introduction of endoscopic haemostasis compared with two historical series.

3. Benders JS, Bouwman DL, Weaver DW: **Bleeding gastroduodenal ulcers — improved outcome from a unified surgical approach.** *Am Surg* 1994, **60**:313–315.
Impressive results can be achieved with early surgery and a well-defined protocol.

4. Mueller X, Rothenbuehler JM, Amery A, Meyer B, Harder F: **Outcome of peptic ulcer hemorrhage treated according to a defined approach.** *World J Surg* 1994, **18**:406–409.
Early surgery according to well-defined clinical criteria can achieve good results.

5. Qvist P, Arnesen KE, Jacobsen CD, Rosseland AR: **Endoscopic treatment and restrictive surgical policy in the management of peptic ulcer bleeding — five years' experience in a central hospital.** *Scand J Gastroenterol* 1994, **29**:569–576.
Good results in terms of overall mortality can be achieved with endoscopic treatment. Persistence in endoscopic treatment in rebleeding patients has led to high surgical mortality.

6. Laine L, Freeman M, Cohen H: **Lack of uniformity in evaluation of**
• **endoscopic prognostic features of bleeding ulcers.** *Gastrointest Endosc* 1994, **40**:411–417.
The correct visual interpretation of SRH is related to the experience of endoscopists and could be improved after a brief session of teaching. Endoscopists disagreed more than a quarter of the time in labelling ulcer features and their agreement over colour was poor.

7. Yang CC, Shin JS, Lin XZ, Hsu PI, Chen KW, Lin CY: **The natural history (fading time) of stigmata of recent hemorrhage in peptic ulcer disease.** *Gastrointest Endosc* 1994, **40**:562–566.
A sequential endoscopic study of the evolutionary change SRH; a visible vessel took significantly longer to fade compared with an adherent clot or an old stigma.

8. Kohler B, Rieman JF: **Does Doppler ultrasound improve the prognosis of acute ulcer bleeding?** *Hepatogastroenterology* 1994, **41**:51–53.
Agreement between the visual interpretation of visible vessels and positive Doppler endoscopic signal was only 59% in 140 patients. Injection therapy was guided by Doppler signal with a 9% rebleeding rate. None of the ulcers without Doppler signal rebled.

9. Katschinski B, Logan R, Davies J, Faulkner G, Pearson J, Langman M:
• **Prognostic factors in upper gastrointestinal bleeding.** *Dig Dis Sci* 1994, **39**:706–712.
In a consecutive series of 2217 patients with upper gastrointestinal bleeding, death occurred in 189 patients (8.5%) and rebleeding in 243 patients (11%). Logistic analyses revealed that death was significantly associated with rebleeding, age greater than 60 years, and the finding of fresh blood in the stomach at endoscopy. Rebleeding was significantly associated with shock, endoscopic SRH, the identification of gastric

or duodenal ulcer and melaena. Contrary to other studies, the findings of a visible vessel was not predictive of rebleeding.

10. Hsu PI, Lin XZ, Chan SH, Lin CY, Chang TT, Shin JS, *et al.*: **Bleeding peptic**
• **ulcer — risk factors for rebleeding and sequential changes in endoscopic findings.** *Gut* 1994, **35**:746–749.
A multivariate analysis in 204 patients with ulcer bleeding indicated that a non-bleeding visible vessel, an adherent clot on the ulcer base and hypovolaemic shock were independent predictors of rebleeding. Repeat endoscopy on 19 rebleeding ulcers showed persistence in SRH.

11. Carter R, Anderson JR: **Randomised trial of adrenaline injection and laser photocoagulation in the control of haemorrhage from peptic ulcer.** *Br J Surg* 1994, **81**:869–871.
A small series confirming the efficacy of both adrenaline injection and laser photocoagulation in controlling ulcer bleeding. No difference was noted between the two modalities.

12. Choudari CP, Palmer KR: **Endoscopic injection therapy for bleeding**
• **peptic ulcer a comparison of adrenaline alone with adrenaline plus ethanolamine oleate.** *Gut* 1994, **35**:608–610.
A confirmatory report that adrenaline injection is an effective method of controlling peptic ulcer bleeding. Adding a sclerosant confers no additional benefit.

13. Lai KH, Peng SN, Guo WS, Lee FY, Chang FY, Malik U, *et al.*: **Endoscopic**
• **injection for the treatment of bleeding ulcers — local tamponade or drug effect.** *Endoscopy* 1994, **26**:338–341.
A double-blind trial of injection therapy comparing adrenaline with water. No differences in the initial control of bleeding, permanent haemostasis, overall mortality or rate of surgical intervention were noted in a small number of patients.

14. Herold G, Preclik G, Stange F: **Gastroduodenal ulcer hemorrhage: endoscopic injection therapy using a fibrin sealant.** *Hepatogastroenterology* 1994, **41**:116–119.
An uncontrolled retrospective series of 452 patients in whom bleeding peptic ulcers were treated with or without hypertonic saline plus adrenaline. It was concluded that fibrin sealing was effective and hastened ulcer healing.

15. Berg PL, Barina W, Born P: **Endoscopic injection of fibrin glue versus polidocanol in peptic ulcer hemorrhage: a pilot study.** *Endoscopy* 1994, **26**:528–530.
Fibrin glue injection is similar in efficacy in the treatment of ulcer bleeding compared with polidocanol (no statistical analysis provided). Rebleeding is less with fibrin sealant.

16. Villanueva C, Balanzo J, Torras X, Soriano G, Sainz S, Vilardell F: **Value**
• **of second-look endoscopy after injection therapy for bleeding peptic ulcer — a prospective and randomized trial.** *Gastrointest Endosc* 1994, **40**:34–39.
A trend towards better results in terms of rebleeding rate, the need for surgery, transfusion requirement, hospital stay and overall mortality was observed in the group with second-look endoscopy after enrolment of 104 patients.

17. Choudari CP, Rajgopal C, Palmer KR: **Acute gastrointestinal haemorrhage in anticoagulated patients: diagnoses and response to endoscopic treatment.** *Gut* 1994, **35**:464–466.
The most common cause of bleeding in anticoagulated patients was peptic ulcer. Endoscopic treatment is effective in this situation.

18. Rohler B, Schreiner J, Lehnert P, Walder H, Heldwein W: **Gastrointestinal intramural hematoma, a complication of endoscopic injection methods for bleeding peptic ulcers: a case series.** *Endoscopy* 1994, **26**:617–621.
Intramural haematoma occurred in five out of 227 patients following injection of adrenaline. All patients had coexisting coagulopathy and three developed intercurrent acute pancreatitis.

19. Jensen DM, Cheng S, Kovacs T, Randall G, Jensen ME, Reedy T, *et al.*: **A**
•• **controlled study of ranitidine for the prevention of recurrent hemorrhage from duodenal ulcer.** *N Engl J Med* 1994, **330**:382–386.
Maintenance ranitidine (150 mg at night) prevents recurrent bleeding from duodenal ulcers. However, 10% of patients rebled despite maintenance treatment when followed up for 3 years.

20. Graham DY, Hepps KS, Ramirez FC, Lew GM, Saeed ZA: **Treatment of**
• *Helicobacter pylori* **reduces the rate of rebleeding in peptic ulcer disease.** *Scand J Gastroenterol* 1993, **28**:939–942.
No recurrent bleeding seen in 17 patients treated with triple therapy compared with four out of 14 patients (28.6%) treated with a course of ranitidine only.

21.    Labenz J, Borsch G: **Role of** *Helicobacter pylori* **eradication in the prevention of peptic ulcer bleeding relapse.** *Digestion* 1994, **55**:19–23.
Eradication of *H. pylori* was associated with a significant reduction in ulcer recurrences and bleeding relapses.

22.    The Veterans Affairs Cooperative Variceal Sclerotherapy Group:
•    **Sclerotherapy for male alcoholic cirrhotic patients who have bled from esophageal varices: results of a randomized, multicenter clinical trial.** *Hepatology* 1994, **20**:618–625.
Sclerotherapy reduces rebleeding, transfusion requirement and the need for shunt surgery when compared with the sham group. No long-term survival was evident with sclerotherapy.

23.    Greig JD, Garden OJ, Carter DC: **Prophylactic treatment of patients with**
•    **esophageal varices — is it ever indicated?** *World J Surg* 1994, **18**:176–184.
A review of the literature on the prophylaxis of variceal bleeding. Prophylaxis with β-blockade seems to offer the best therapeutic option.

24.    Siringo S, Bolondi L, Gaiani S, Sofia S, Zironi G, Rigamanti A, *et al.*: **Timing of the first variceal hemorrhage in cirrhotic patients: prospective evaluation of Doppler flowmetry, endoscopy and clinical parameters.** *Hepatology* 1994, **20**:66–73.
Variceal size, cherry red spots, serum bilirubin and congestion index are independent predictors of variceal bleeding.

25.    Hirata M, Ishihama S, Sanjo K, Idezuki Y: **Study of new prognostic factors of esophageal variceal rupture by use of image processing with a video endoscope.** *Surgery* 1994, **116**:8–16.
Colorimetric analysis was performed on video images of oesophageal varices. The area ratio of red colour sign was significantly higher in patients with history of variceal bleeding.

26.    Moreto M, Zaballa M, Ojembarrena E, Ibancz S, Suarez MJ, Setien F, *et al.*:
•    **Combined (short term plus long term) sclerotherapy v short term only sclerotherapy: a randomized prospective trial.** *Gut* 1994, **35**:687–691.
Sclerotherapy in acute bleeding followed by planned elective treatment is superior in preventing rebleeding when compared with the on-demand sclerotherapy group. No survival advantage could be demonstrated in either group.

27.    McKee RF, Garden OJ, Anderson JR, Carter DC: **A trial of elective versus on demand sclerotherapy in poor risk patients with variceal haemorrhage.** *Endoscopy* 1994, **26**:483–485.
A prospective randomized trial in which patients with Child's C cirrhosis and proven variceal bleeding received sclerotherapy with bleeding episodes only or electively at three-week intervals; no survival difference was observed. More bleeding episodes were observed in the 'demand' sclerotherapy group.

28.    Chan ACW, Chung SCS, Sung JY, Leung JWC, Li AKC: **A double-blind**
•    **randomized controlled trial comparing sodium tetradecyl sulphate and ethanolamine oleate in the sclerotherapy of bleeding oesophageal varices.** *Endoscopy* 1993, **25**:513–517.
Both STD and ETH are effective in controlling variceal haemorrhage; the former obliterated varices in fewer sessions.

29.    Binmoeller KF, Vadeyar HJ, Soehendra N: **Treatment of esophageal**
••    **varices.** *Endoscopy* 1994, **26**:42–47.
A review of the literature on the controversy over the choice of endoscopic sclerotherapy and band ligation, pharmacological therapy, prophylactic treatment, the state-of-affairs with TIPS, the use of tissue adhesives and the secondary role of surgery.

30.    Bornman PC, Krige JE, Terblanche J: **Management of oesophageal varices.**
••    *Lancet* 1994, **343**:1079–1084.
An excellent review of the literature.

31.    Williams SGI, Westaby D: **Fortnightly review: management of variceal**
•    **haemorrhage.** *BMJ* 1994, **308**:1213–1216.
A practical guide on the management of varices.

32.    Terblanche J, Stiegmann GV, Krige JEJ, Bornman PC: **Long-term manage-**
••    **ment of variceal bleeding — the place of varix injection and ligation.** *World J Surg* 1994, **18**:185–192.
Repeated sclerotherapy is the treatment of choice in patients who have bled from oesophageal varices. A summary of four randomized trials comparing band ligation and sclerotherapy favoured band ligation. Treatment should be repeated weekly until eradication, followed by regular surveillance.

33.    Schapiro RH: **...And the bands play on.** *Hepatology* 1994, **19**:542–543.
Endoscopic variceal ligation appeared superior to sclerotherapy with fewer complications in this review of the literature.

34.    Sakai P, Maluf Filho F, Melo JM, Ishioka S: **Is endoscopic band ligation of esophageal varices contraindicated in Child Pugh C patients? [Letter].** *Endoscopy* 1994, **26**:512.
High early mortality from early rebleeding was noted in a group of Child's C patients after endoscopic band ligation.

35.    Planas R, Quer JC, Boix J, Canet J, Armengol M, Cabre E, *et al.*: **A**
•    **prospective randomized trial comparing somatostatin and sclerotherapy in the treatment of acute variceal bleeding.** *Hepatology* 1994, **20**:370–375.
Somatostatin is safer and as effective as sclerotherapy in controlling acute variceal haemorrhage.

36.    Burroughs AK: **Octreotide in variceal bleeding.** *Gut* 1994, **35**:S23–S27.
•
Octreotide is as effective as injection sclerotherapy in the treatment of variceal haemorrhage but with the advantage of fewer side effects.

37.    Thakeh F, Salem SAM, Abdallah M, El Batanouny M: **Endoscopic diagnosis**
•    **of gastric varices.** *Endoscopy* 1994, **26**:287–291.
A morphological description of gastric varices; the larger ones carry higher risks of bleeding. The risk of bleeding is negligible in secondary gastric varices arising after obliteration of oesophageal varices.

38.    Yoshida T, Hayashi N, Suzumi N, Miyazaki ST, Itoh T, Nishimura S, *et al.*: **Endoscopic ligation of gastric varices using a detachable snare.** *Endoscopy* 1994, **26**:502–505.
A new technique in the treatment of gastric varices, particularly the larger ones.

39.    Rössle M, Haag K, Ochs A, Sellinger M, Noldge G, Perarnau JM, *et al.*: **The**
•    **transjugular intrahepatic portosystemic stent-shunt procedure for variceal bleeding.** *N Engl J Med* 1994, **330**:165–171.
TIPS is a safe and effective treatment for variceal haemorrhage in patients with portal hypertension due to cirrhosis. It is a real option in patients failing endoscopic treatment and in particular patients with Child–Pugh class C cirrhosis.

40.    Liberski SM, McGarrity TJ, Hartle RJ, Varano V, Reynolds D: **The Watermelon Stomach: long-term outcome in patients treated with Nd:YAG laser therapy.** *Gastrointest Endosc* 1994, **40**:584–587.
Nd:YAG laser therapy was used in 15 patients with watermelon stomach with chronic blood loss. They were no longer transfusion-dependent following treatment.

41.    Potiamiano S, Carter CR, Anderson JR: **Endoscopic laser treatment of**
•    **diffuse gastric antral ectasia.** *Gut* 1994, **35**:461–463.
Nd:YAG laser treatment proved effective in five transfusion-requiring patients with watermelon stomach. In three more cases with diffuse gastric antral ectasia and a honeycombed stomach, results were disappointing.

42.    Hintze RE, Binmoeller KF, Adler A, Veltzke W, Thonke F, Soehendra N: **Improved endoscopic management of severe upper gastrointestinal hemorrhage using a new wide-channel endoscope.** *Endoscopy* 1994, **26**:613–616.
A new endoscope with a 6-mm wide channel allowing complete evacuation of stomach content in 122 out of 123 patients with severe bleeding. This proved impossible with standard endoscopes.

James Y.W. Lau and S.C. Sydney Chung, Department of Surgery, The Chinese University of Hong Kong, Prince of Wales Hospital, Shatin, Hong Kong.

# Endosonography

## Paul Fockens

Academic Medical Center, University of Amsterdam, Amsterdam, The Netherlands

## Introduction

More than 20 years after construction of the first instruments in which endoscopy and ultrasonography were integrated, consensus seems to be growing slowly on the name of the game. Many different names were still used in the literature of 1994, such as endoluminal ultrasonography, echoendosonography, intraductal ultrasound, transrectal ultrasonography, transanal ultrasonography and anal ultrasonography. The two names used mainly however are endoscopic ultrasonography and endosonography (ES). In view of the fact that an important number of the examinations are performed with non-optical instruments, we clearly prefer the term ES and feel that it should be used throughout the literature.

In the years to come, cost-effectiveness will be a keyword in health care. It is therefore good to see that the subject of articles on ES is slowly moving from feasibility studies and studies on the accuracy of staging of gastrointestinal malignancies, to studies in which the influence of ES on patient outcome is investigated. The publication of six original articles [1•,2••,3••,4•,5••,6•] describing the accuracy of ES-guided or ES-assisted biopsies in almost 200 patients is probably the best example of this trend. Let us not forget, on the other hand, that even for so-called 'established' examinations on 'established' indications such as computed tomography (CT) scanning in patients with oesophageal malignancies, cost-effectiveness is often not at all clear.

The ever expanding literature on ES up to 1993 was carefully reviewed by Rösch [7••], which can probably be seen as an addendum to the book he published in 1992 [8]. At the same time, the working party for the 10th World Congress of Gastroenterology in Los Angeles put down their conclusions in a special edition of the *American Journal of Gastroenterology* [9••]. In these conclusions, they made a differentiation between established indications and those that are to be regarded as investigational. Established indications are staging of gastrointestinal malignancies, examination of 'submu-cosal' abnormalities, examination of large gastric folds and detection of small pancreatic tumours. Clear indication for Doppler flow measurements was not seen by the working party and thereby classified as investigational. To ensure achievement of accuracy rates reported in literature, the working party proposes a minimum of 50 examinations for the oesophagus and stomach, and 100–150 examinations for the pancreaticobiliary tract. These figures seem to be the absolute minimum before important clinical decisions can be made on the results of ES examinations, performed by freshly trained endosonographists. ES remains one of the most difficult forms of gastrointestinal endoscopy and the fact that our knowledge is growing is not going to make it easier.

## Oesophageal carcinoma

Only a small number of articles report accuracy of staging of oesophageal carcinoma this year, which is indeed well known to almost everyone by now. Peters *et al.* [10•] proposed to use ES in selecting surgical treatment. They treated patients with a T1 or T2 carcinoma by *en bloc* oesophageal resection and patients with T3 or T4 tumour by transhiatal resection, which the authors call palliative. Out of the 42 patients in their study, three received an 'inappropriate' procedure based on the ES findings, which seems to be acceptable. Although every patient underwent extensive CT scanning as well, these results are not reported in the paper. In the discussion the authors mention the CT data as 'coming down to a guess'. A multicentre study on patients with oesophageal carcinomas, ES-stage T4, was presented by Chak *et al.* [11] during the Digestive Disease Week in New Orleans. In this retrospective study, 79 patients had been divided into two groups, group I had surgical therapy, group II different forms of palliative therapy. Survival curves for both groups were almost overlapping with a median survival for the surgical group of 5.2 months and 6.6 months for the non-surgical group. In this retrospective study, surgery did not influence survival of ES-stage T4 oesophageal carcinomas. As palliation can usually be well achieved

---

**Abbreviations**

CT—computed tomography; **EMG**—electromyography; **ERCP**—endoscopic retrograde cholangiopancreatography; **ERP**—endoscopic retrograde pancreatography; **ES**—endosonography; **MRI**—magnetic resonance imaging; **NHL**—non-Hodgkin's lymphoma.

© Current Science Ltd ISBN 1-85922-187-4 ISSN 0952-6293

without surgery, surgical exploration without adjuvant therapy is questionable for these oesophageal carcinoma patients.

Yoshikane *et al.* [12••] looked at T1 oesophageal carcinomas, using standard Olympus (Olympus Optical Co., Tokyo, Japan) echoendoscopes with 7.5 and 12 Mhz frequency. In a series of 28 patients with T1 carcinomas, they were successful in differentiating tumours limited to the mucosa from those invading the submucosa with 75% accuracy. Most tumours limited to the mucosa were invisible on ES, with a patent submucosa. When the submucosa showed an area of narrowing, however, this was regarded as a sign of invasion. The importance of the differentiation between intramucosally and submucosally infiltrating carcinoma lies in the associated percentage of lymph node metastasis: in the study of Yoshikane, 0% of the nine patents with intramucosal carcinoma, but 71% of patients with submucosal invasion. Falk *et al.* [13•] looked at nine patients with Barrett's oesophagus and high-grade dysplasia preoperatively, again with standard Olympus echoendoscopes. After resection, three of the nine patients proved to have an intramucosal carcinoma. ES was unsuccessful in detecting the intramucosal carcinoma in two out of the three patients. Of the six patients with high-grade dysplasia but without a carcinoma, ES suggested a tumour in two. The conclusion of this study was that at this point in time ES has no place in patients with Barrett's oesophagus and high-grade dysplasia. Both studies show that with the standard instruments (maximum frequency 12 Mhz) detection of intramucosal carcinoma is almost impossible and we will need higher resolution (= higher frequencies) before ES can help in screening for early oesophageal malignancies. With help of the 20-Mhz miniprobe with balloon (Olympus), some progress seems to have been made (Fig. 1). The development of a prototype echoendoscope by Olympus with switchable frequency of 7.5 and 20 Mhz, also might be an important development for these early lesions. We need to see the muscularis mucosae as a separate layer for these indications in the future. This was already shown to be possible *in vitro* by Wiersema and Wiersema [14] in 1993.

The influence of tumour reduction therapy (chemotherapy and/or radiotherapy) on the ES picture of oesophageal carcinomas was studied in two papers by Roubein *et al.* [15] and Hordijk *et al.* [16•]. A total of 19 patients were described who underwent preoperative chemotherapy. Both authors agree that quantitative tumour measurement did not correlate well with tumour reduction as assessed by other techniques such as barium oesophagogram, endoscopy, CT scanning or relief of dysphagia. Down-staging of the tumour by the chemotherapy, which occurred in five patients in the study from Hordijk *et al.* [16•], was not detected by ES

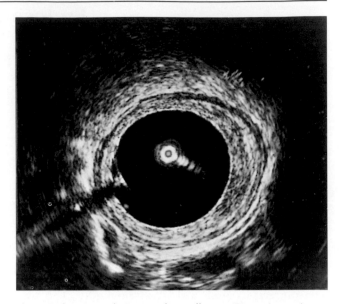

**Fig. 1.** Endosonography image of a small, stage T1 carcinoma in a Barrett's oesophagus, as visualized with a 20-Mhz balloon-fitted mini-probe (Olympus UM-3R). The second (hypoechoic) layer is markedly thickened at 4 o'clock, the third layer is somewhat thin but not interrupted.

in four patients. This was explained by the replacement of malignant cells by a dense inflammatory reaction. The other study [15] used a less effective chemotherapeutic regimen in which down-staging only occurred in two patients, both undetected by ES. Further studies on this indication only seem to be of value when using effective preoperative chemotherapy or chemoradiotherapy.

In a study from Amsterdam, Tio *et al.* [17•] described 63 patients with inoperable oesophageal carcinoma who were treated with combined intraluminal and external irradiation. ES was performed before and at regular intervals after irradiation. In oesophageal squamous cell carcinoma there was a clear correlation between the number of metastatic lymph nodes (less than five versus five or more nodes) and survival. Surprisingly, an inverse correlation between tumour thickness of squamous cell carcinomas as assessed by ES and survival was shown, when tumours with a maximum thickness of 16 mm or less were separated from those whose thickness was over 16 mm. This difference is hard to explain especially when considering the penetration depth of intraluminal radiotherapy which was focused at 6 mm. None of these differences was shown for patients with an adenocarcinoma. Not much detail is given about the follow-up ES after radiotherapy, and whether the initial response, as measured with ES, correlated with survival.

Lymph node metastases in oesophageal carcinoma were studied by Catalano *et al.* [18••]. They looked at the individual lymph node parameters: size, shape, border demarcation and central echopattern. In 100 patients who underwent surgical resection of the oesophagus with extensive lymph node dissection (14.2 per patient), the individual lymph nodes were examined. Of the four endosonographic features studied, the echopattern (homogeneous versus heterogeneous) was the single most sensitive parameter for discriminating malignant from benign. The next important feature was lymph node border (sharp versus fuzzy), followed by shape (round versus elliptical) and finally lymph node size (> 10 mm versus < 10 mm; Fig. 2). Malignant lymph nodes were found in 100% when all four features were present. It is important to note that also in most people without an oesophageal carcinoma, mediastinal lymph nodes can be visualized with ES, especially in the subcarinal area [19]. At the same time, with the use of higher frequencies the borders of these nodes become more distinct (Fig. 3). The importance of the study from Catalano *et al.* is that it shows which parameters to use in the evaluation of nodes and it also shows that size is a relatively inaccurate parameter, which should not be used solely.

## Gastric carcinoma

The good overall accuracy of ES in T- and N-staging of gastric carcinoma was again demonstrated in a study by Nattermann *et al.* [20•], who compared ES with CT scanning and transabdominal ultrasonography. Results with conventional ultrasonography were very poor with a visualization rate of the tumour of only 23%. In staging, ES was superior to CT with accuracy rates of 85% for T1–T3, but 67% for T4 tumours. In view of the fact that surgery is regarded as the best palliation even when cure is impossible, it is probably important to stress this relatively low accuracy in T4 tumours as these patients are the ones that we should try to identify before irresectability is shown at exploratory laparotomy. For this indication we probably need higher resolution imaging of the outer margin of a tumour which quite often has a thickness of 2 cm or more. The

poor overall prognosis of gastric carcinoma has led to experimental adjuvant therapy, such as preoperative chemotherapy. The early stages (T1–2), however, have a rather good prognosis with surgery alone. A study by Smith *et al.* [21•] has shown that the preoperative ES stage correlated very well with the chance of postoperative recurrence. They examined 43 patients who underwent resection of a gastric carcinoma. In the group of 13 patients with either a T1 or a T2 tumour, recurrence was shown in only two patients after a median follow-up of more than 2 years. Of the group of 30 patients with a preoperative ES stage T3 or T4, 23 presented with a recurrence during the same follow-up period and 22 of these died. Given these results, ES should be used to guide us in the selection of patients for alternative adjuvant preoperative therapies such as preoperative chemotherapy.

One of the established indications for ES is analysis of patients with enlarged gastric folds. With ES, one can identify the origin of the increased wall thickness, and define a strategy to reach a diagnosis. Increasing diameter of the second layer can be seen with severe gastritis, but also with Zollinger–Ellison's syndrome or Ménétrier's disease. And, although superficial adenocarcinoma and non-Hodgkin's lymphoma (NHL) can give the same picture, a thickened second layer on ES in these cases suggests that biopsies should be representative. More diagnostic problems arise when the third and/or fourth layer are swollen. Mendis *et al.* [22••] looked at a group of 28 patients presenting with thickened folds and performed large particle biopsies preceded by ES. In four patients, submucosal varices explained the endoscopic picture and were a reason not to perform large particle biopsies. In the group of

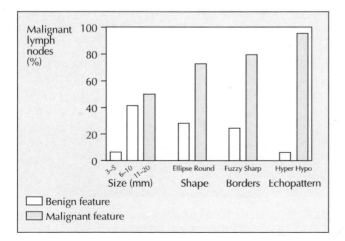

**Fig. 2.** Endosonographic features of malignant lymph nodes. Published with permission [18••].

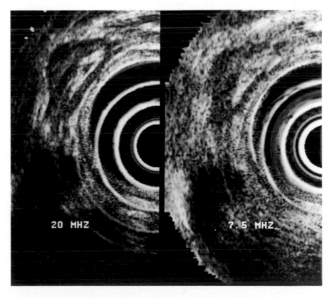

**Fig. 3.** Benign subcarinal lymph node, visualized with 7.5 Mhz (right) and 20 Mhz (left) (Olympus GF-UM20). Note the vague outer margin with 7.5 Mhz, but also the echopattern which is very suggestive of a benign lymph node.

17 patients with ES thickening of layer two and negative large particle biopsies, no malignancy developed after a mean period of almost 3 years. All three patients with negative biopsies, but with thickened layers three and four, were diagnosed with a gastric adenocarcinoma on exploratory laparotomy. The conclusion of this study was that negative biopsies with only layer two thickened can be followed, but negative biopsies with layer three and/or four thickened in the absence of ulceration is strongly suggestive of malignancy and should be followed by surgical exploration (Fig. 4). In a case report by Benamouzig *et al.* [23] a linitis-like ES picture with swelling of the third and fourth layers was described as metastasis of a bladder carcinoma. The ES picture of this form of metastatic disease was indistinguishable from primary linitis plastica. Similar ES images can be seen with metastatic breast cancer (Fig. 5).

## Gastric lymphoma

Primary gastric lymphoma was the subject of two papers this year. A multicentre French study by Palazzo *et al.* [24••] compared ES findings with histology in 24 patients who underwent a gastric resection for NHL. Penetration through the wall was correctly assessed in 91.5% of cases. Although ES was better in determining surface extension than was endoscopy, ES still underestimated surface extension in almost 40% of cases. The average length of underestimation was 10 cm (range 2–14 cm), making ES an inaccurate technique for determining surface extension in gastric NHL. The

underestimation always concerned small foci of mucosal or submucosal lymphoma and happened both in the superficial and the infiltrative type of lymphoma. In a study from Schüder *et al.* [25•], 10 patients with primary NHL of the stomach were examined with endosonography. In this group only one patient had a tumour limited to the mucosa and submucosa compared to 16 in the study by Palazzo *et al.* In this study, ES was shown to be accurate in delineating horizontal

(a)

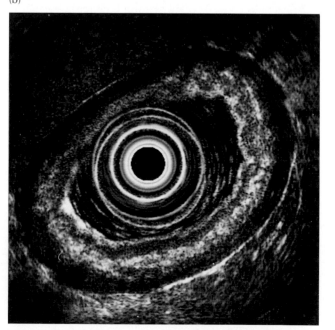

(b)

**Fig. 5.** (a) Endoscopic picture of thickened gastric folds in a patient with metastasized breast cancer. (b) Endosonographic picture of the same patient showing a markedly thickened second, third and fourth layer, typical for linitis plastica. Repeated large particle biopsies showed metastatic breast cancer.

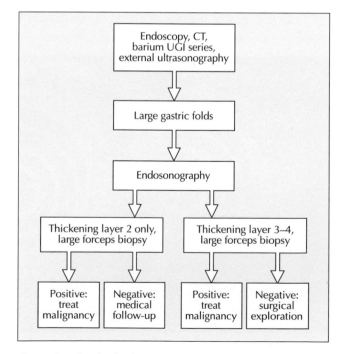

**Fig. 4.** Algorithm for the diagnostic evaluation of patients with large gastric folds. CT = computed tomography; UGI = upper gastrointestinal. Adapted from [22••].

extension, in three patients assisted by intraoperative ultrasound. Although both studies seem to be somewhat contradictory, they looked at different stages and different types of NHL. From the study of Palazzo *et al.* we must conclude that ES is currently not able to accurately guide the extent of partial resection in primary gastric NHL.

## Pancreatobiliary disease

The application of a curved array echoendoscope (Pentax Optical Co., Tokyo, Japan) in the pancreatobiliary area was shown to be accurate in the diagnosing and staging of a large number of patients (94) with a variety of abnormalities (including pancreatic cancer, ampullary cancer and common bile duct stones) by Giovannini *et al.* [26••]. The overall accuracy to provide a specific diagnosis in 25 patients with obstructive jaundice was 88%. Staging of tumours with respect to portal vein involvement was accurate in 88% of cases as well. These results are comparable to other studies utilizing echoendoscopes with rotating sector scanners.

### Choledocholithiasis

In the 1993 issue of the *Annual*, Rösch and Classen asked whether ES could replace diagnostic endoscopic retrograde cholangiopancreatography (ERCP) [27]. The results of a study concerning 62 consecutive patients with suspicion of common bile duct stones by Amouyal *et al.* [28••] gives more support for a strong yes. All patients underwent external ultrasonography, CT and ES before ERCP or intraoperative cholangiography. Sensitivity of the three procedures are listed in Figure 6, with clearly the highest sensitivity for ES (97%). Specificity was good for all three (ultrasonography and ES 100%, CT 94%). To prove its potential, ES showed a 6 mm common bile duct stone in two patients that was not apparent on fluoroscopy during ERCP but confirmed after sphincterotomy (Fig. 7).

### Pancreatic carcinoma

With the high resolution images that ES gives, it is possible to detect minute invasions in the vessel wall before abnormalities can be expected on ultrasonography combined with Doppler or on angiography. In pancreatic carcinoma, three ES criteria for vascular invasion have been described:

- peripancreatic venous collaterals in the area of a mass that obliterates the normal location of a major portal confluence vessel;
- tumour growth extending in the vessel lumen; and
- abnormal vessel contour with loss of the hyperechoic vessel–tissue interface.

| Sensitivity (%) | Ultrasound | Computed tomography | Endosonography |
|---|---|---|---|
| Total | 25 | 75 | 97 |
| Dilated CBD | 44 | 94 | 94 |
| Non-dilated CBD | 0 | 50 | 100 |
| Stone ≥ 1 cm | 42 | 79 | 95 |
| Stone < 1 cm | 0 | 69 | 100 |

**Fig. 6.** Sensitivity for choledocholithiasis of ultrasound, computed tomography and endosonography in different subgroups. CBD = common bile duct. Data from [28••].

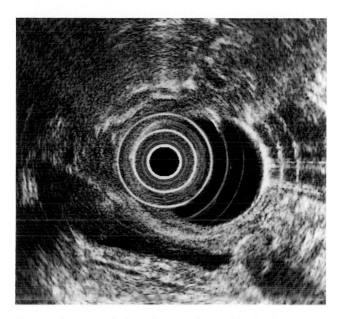

**Fig. 7.** Endosonography from the second part of the duodenum in a patient with obstructive jaundice. A dilated common bile duct is seen in the lower half of the picture. Two stones are visual as hyperechoic structures with an acoustic shadow at 5 and 8 o'clock.

It is probably the third criterion that raises the sensitivity for vascular invasion to high rates such as obtained in the paper by Snady *et al.* [29••]. In this study on 38 patients with pancreatic carcinoma, vascular invasion was present in 21 patients who all demonstrated at least one of the above criteria on ES. None of the 17 resectable patients showed any of these criteria. Arterial involvement was more difficult to visualize, but in all 7 patients in the study from Snady *et al.* every patient having arterial involvement had venous involvement as well.

Forty-nine patients with clinical suspicion of a pancreatic tumour were evaluated with ES, CT and magnetic resonance imaging (MRI; in 25 patients) in a study by Müller *et al.* [30••]. Again ES was the most sensitive (94%) and specific (100%) of the three imaging modalities in demonstrating a tumour, whether benign inflammatory or malignant. Although MRI came close with a sensitivity of 83% and the same specificity, the sensitivity of MRI dropped to 64% when only tumours of less than 3 cm were evaluated. Of the nine patients with focal pancreatitis, two were misdiagnosed as having cancer with ES. CT and MRI misdiagnosed the focal pancreatitis patients as cancer in 87 and 100%, respectively. Staging was correct in 18 out of the 22 patients with a malignancy. Two tumours were not detected, and two were understaged because invasion in the superior mesenteric vein remained undetected. At this point in time there is no competition for ES by any other imaging technique when searching for relatively small pancreatic tumours and assessing their resectability. Remember, however, the conclusion of the working party for the World Congress [9••], proposing between 100 and 150 examinations as a minimum training experience. This number of patients restricts ES of the pancreaticobiliary tract to referral centres with special expertise in this field.

### Chronic pancreatitis

Wiersema *et al.* [31] showed last year that the sensitivity of ES for diagnosing chronic pancreatitis was higher than that of endoscopic retrograde pancreatography (ERP). A study from Nattermann *et al.* [32•] gives additional information on this difficult subject. One hundred and fourteen patients, 94 pancreatitis and 20 controls, underwent ERP and ES. There are two problems with this study: one is that patients with acute oedematous pancreatitis were included as well as patients with known or suspected chronic pancreatitis, which gives a rather heterogeneous group. The second problem is that in most cases the endosonographist was not blinded to the results of ERP. Again the superb sensitivity of ES for parenchymal abnormalities was shown; in 63% of 43 patients with normal pancreatic ducts on ERP, endosonographic abnormalities were seen. These parenchymal abnormalities usually present very subtle alterations with, for instance, only a slight accentuation of the lobular pattern of the parenchyma or slight attenuation of the pancreatic duct (Fig. 8). It is unclear, however, which number of these 43 patients were recovering from an acute attack of pancreatitis. One can imagine that in these patients the appearance of the ducts will have normalized whereas the parenchyma is still inflamed. The abnormalities described above were not seen in the 20 controls.

### Colorectal carcinoma

A study by Hulsmans *et al.* [33•] described the difficulty in staging T2 rectal carcinomas. This relative difficulty and the fact that accuracy rates for T2 were up to 20% lower in the current literature than for other stages were already known [8]. Of the 55 patients in this study, 22 (40%) had a T2 tumour on pathology, but only four

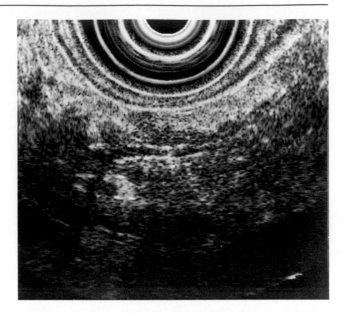

**Fig. 8.** Endosonography from the gastric body, showing the pancreas with a non-dilated pancreatic duct. The parenchyma, however, is somewhat lobulated and hypoechoic and the duct wall is slightly hyperechoic. These changes are consistent with early chronic pancreatitis.

were correctly assessed by ES. Sixteen patients were overstaged as T3 and one as T4. In the paper, explanation was sought and possibly found by the presence of peri-tumorous inflammation in six patients and also in the different ES criteria used for staging a T2 tumour. One criterion (as used with oesophageal carcinoma etc.) is the presence of an irregular outer margin of the fourth layer. A second criterion is disruption of the hyperechoic layer outside the fourth layer. This interface is, however, not always clearly visible. In order to see if staging improved by using the second criterion, hard copies of 20 patients (10 T2 and 10 T3) were blindly reviewed using both criteria, but this hardly changed the result and observer agreement was moderate. Another study on reliability and validity of ES in anorectal disorders by Solomon *et al.* [34••] also looked at ES staging of rectal cancers by having hard copies of 50 patients reviewed by four observers with different levels of expertise. Agreement with pathology rose from 44% when the observer had no experience, to (only) 64% in an observer with experience in more than 50 patients. In the same study, the authors also sent a questionnaire to referring physicians asking if ES had changed the clinical management and if ES had altered their confidence in the clinical decision. In this second part of the study, 76 patients with neoplasia or inflammatory problems or incontinence were included. Overall ES changed the therapy in 45% and changed confidence in the clinical decision in 76%.

Detection of recurrent rectal cancers was aided by ES in a study from Ramirez *et al.* [35•]. In 13 patients developing a recurrence of a lower- or middle-third

| | Total | | Oesophagus and mediastinum | | Stomach and peri-gastric lesions | | Pancreas, common bile duct and peri-pancreatic lesions | | Rectum, colon and peri-colorectal lesions | |
|---|---|---|---|---|---|---|---|---|---|---|
| | n | Acc. | n | Acc. | n | Acc. | n | Acc. | n | Acc. |
| Wiersema et al. [5••] | 50 | 37 (74%) | 20 | 15 | 23 | 15 | 1 | 1 | 6 | 6 |
| Wegener et al. [4•] | 12 | 11 (92%) | 9 | 8 | 3 | 3 | – | – | – | – |
| Vilmann et al. [6•] | 39 | 19 (49%) | 11 | 7 | 18 | 6 | 9 | 5 | 1 | 1 |
| Chang et al. [2••] | 46 | 42 (91%) | 10 | 10 | 15 | 13 | 17 | 15 | 4 | 4 |
| Wiersema et al. [3••] | 26 | 23 (88%) | 6 | 6 | 1 | 1 | 18 | 15 | 1 | 1 |
| Milsom et al. [1•] | 26 | 20 (77%) | – | – | – | – | – | – | 26 | 20 |
| **Total** | 199 | 152 (76%) | 56 | 46 (82%) | 60 | 38 (63%) | 45 | 36 (80%) | 38 | 32 (84%) |

**Fig. 9.** Diagnostic accuracy of endosonography-assisted [5••] and endosonography-guided [1•,2••,3••,4•,6•] cytological punctures published late 1993 and 1994. Divided by organ. Acc. = accuracy as shown by the number of diagnostic cytology results.

rectal cancer, all could be detected by rectal ES with a rigid 7.0 Mhz probe. Digital examination and sigmoidoscopic examination were negative in three out of these 13 patients. Salvage surgery was possible in four patents, three of whom had only been detected by ES. When follow-up of rectal cancers is performed to detect locally resectable recurrences, ES should be included in the follow-up of these patients every 6 months. The application of ES in staging and follow-up of anal squamous cell cancer was described by Roseau et al. [36•] in 20 patients. ES was performed in this study with a GF-UM3 (Olympus) echoendoscope which, because of its switchable frequency and 360° imaging, is more appropriate than the echocolonoscope (CF-UM3 or CF-UM20). The patients were initially staged by ES and followed with ES at 2–5-month intervals. Persistent hypoechoic mural thickening was noticed in 15 patients. Development of parietal nodules, increasing in size over two consecutive ES examinations, was seen in three cases with recurrent disease, who were then treated surgically. Good correlation was found between the ES images and operative findings.

## Cytology

The publication of six original articles [1•,2••,3••, 4•,5••,6•] and two case reports [37,38] on 200 patients in total, in whom ES assisted in getting a cytological or histological diagnosis, is a major step forward this year (Fig. 9). This invasive branch of ES will have a definite role in the future of ES. One of the two studies published by Wiersema et al. [5••] this year reports the results of ES followed by cytological puncture through a normal endoscope in 50 patients. Diagnostic cytology results were obtained in 37 patients (74%) after an average of four passes of a 21 Gauge needle in an endoscopically identifiable lesion (Fig. 10). The preceding ES identified an impression from spleen or splenic artery in two patients and in the other 48 patients assisted in identifying the optimal site for puncture.

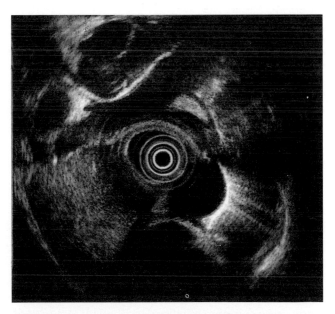

**Fig. 10.** At gastroscopy an impression in the distal oesophagus was seen in a 39-year-old man, who underwent a pneumonectomy for non-small-cell lung cancer 7 months before. Endosonography image shows a large tumour between 7 and 9 o'clock, infiltrating the oesophageal wall. Cytological puncture through a normal endoscope revealed recurrent non-small-cell lung cancer.

The other seven articles [1•,2••,3••,4•,6•,37,38] utilized direct ES guidance and therefore could also perform punctures when no endoscopic marks, such as an ulcer or bulging in the stomach or an anastomosis, were present. It is clear that for this indication a curved or linear array instruments such as the Pentax FG-32UA is preferable. The policy of Chang et al. [2••] to start the examination with a staging procedure with a 360° rotating scanner (Olympus), followed by puncture of a specific lesion with the curved array scanner (Pentax) is interesting. Vilmann et al. [6•] described the development of a needle to perform these punctures. After two unsatisfactory prototypes, their third prototype seemed to be satisfactory. The relatively low overall accuracy in this study could be attributed to the low success rate with the first two prototype needles. With prototype three, puncture was successful in seven out of eight attempts. Other studies used different catheters, sometimes with [2••] and sometimes without [3••] stylet. Wegener [4•] used a standard sclerotherapy needle with a 9 mm needle tip for puncturing lesions in the mediastinum with a maximum distance from the oesophagus of 2 cm. Chang et al. [2••] present the largest series of ES-guided fine-needle aspiration. The study was performed in two hospitals, in only one of which was a cytologist on standby during the procedure to check if representative material had been collected. With the cytologist standby, an adequate sample could be obtained in all patients during the first procedure. Without the cytologist present, 30% of samples were insufficient and the patient had to be brought back for a second procedure. The other studies also report on the importance of judging adequacy of the sample, with the echoendoscope still in the patient. The average number of needle passes was around three per patient in all studies (range 1–19!). The study by Milsom et al. [1•] looked at the possibility of puncturing para-rectal lymph nodes with the help of a rigid ES probe, also with the scanning plane in the longitudinal axis of the probe. In this study, a spring-loaded core biopsy needle was used to get a histological specimen. All lesions were punctured three to five times, and patients received antibiotics around the procedure. There was one disturbing false-positive cytology result in this series.

## Benign gastrointestinal lesions

Several case reports appeared describing the well-known use of ES in identifying the origin of submucosal abnormalities. The image of a fibrovascular polyp in the oesophagus was described [39] and that of a glomus tumour in the stomach originating from vascular smooth muscle cells [40]. A series of 19 patients with extragastric compression was described by Motoo et al. [41•]. Seven out of the 19 impressions were caused by the splenic artery, five by the spleen itself, two by a normal pancreas, one by the gallbladder and one by the colon (Fig. 11). Three tumours were identified, two

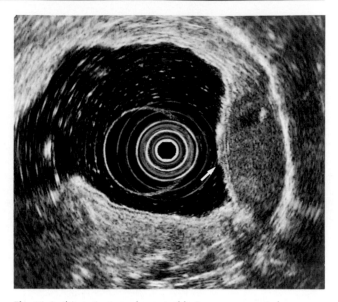

**Fig. 11.** In this patient, a submucosal lesion was suspected on routine gastroscopy. Endosonography shows an impression in the gastric body caused by the spleen (arrow).

hepatic haemangiomas and one neurogenic tumour originating from the minor omentum. Quantification of benign gastric ulcer healing by sequential ES was performed in a large group of patients by Yoshikane et al. [42] showing that the endoscopic picture strongly reflects the ulcer healing itself as seen by ES.

Three studies described benign lesions in the rectum and colon as seen with ES. Kawamoto et al. [43•] studied 20 patients with colonic submucosal tumours with ES and CT. The appearance of lipomas, carcinoid tumours, leiomyomas, lymphangiomas and haemangiomas closely resembled the images seen in the upper gastrointestinal tract. CT visualized all but one lesion. Differentiation with CT was less reliable than with ES, as to be expected. Hizawa et al. [44] described five patients with a mucosal prolapse syndrome whose rectal ES showed a thickening of the third layer sometimes with micro-cystic components. Finally Lee [45] described a case of anorectal varices in a patient with cirrhosis. In this patient, a cobble-stone appearance of the rectum on endoscopy raised suspicion of a tumour, but biopsies were negative. On ES large serpiginous rectal wall varices were seen.

ES was investigated in a group of 80 patients with portal hypertension due to alcoholic liver cirrhosis and compared to 50 controls by Boustiere et al. [46•]. They concluded that ES was inferior to endoscopy in the diagnosis of oesophageal varices but better than endoscopy for gastric varices. Of the cirrhotic patients, 70% had gastric wall thickening, endoscopically detectable as congestive gastropathy in 57.5%. Almost 80% of patients had gastric varices on ES, they were endoscopically seen in only 6% and suspected in another 6%. In the controls, no varices were seen in or around the oesophagus or stomach. Squillace *et al.* [47•] described a case in which ES showed a Dieulafoy's lesion, which had previously been reported in three patients from Japan [48]. In this case a small (3–4 mm) tortuous vessel was seen in the submucosa (Fig. 12) at the site of an endoscopically detected small mucosal defect. After treatment with epinephrine and ethanol, the calibre of the vessel had decreased on follow-up ES 30 days later.

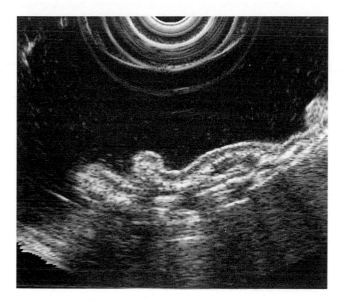

**Fig. 12.** Endosonography image of the gastric wall showing a relatively large vessel in the submucosal layer (third, hyperechoic layer), that could be followed over at least 2 cm. Image compatible with Dieulafoy's disease.

## Anal ES

### Sphincters

The anal sphincter complex is another area where ES has firmly established its role in recent years. A comparison of imaging of normal sphincters with ES and MRI [49•] resulted in a clear victory for ES, as a less costly, less elaborate and more reliable imaging technique. The main indication for ES of the sphincters is faecal incontinence. This is often related to obstetric damage, a subject accurately reviewed by Kamm [50••] in the *Lancet*. A large number of publications [51,52•, 53••,54,55,56••,57••,58] report ES findings in over 200 incontinent patients. Three studies, all from St Mark's hospital in London, are of particular importance. First, a study by Sultan *et al.* [56••] described histological confirmation of external sphincter defects with 100% accuracy, where electromyography (EMG) and manometry had 75% accuracy and clinical examination only 50%. Second, Engel *et al.* [53••] described a good correlation between ES findings and clinical symptoms after anterior anal sphincter repair in patients with obstetric trauma. Of the 35 improved patients, 32 had an endosonographically intact external sphincter. Of the 11 patients who had no improvement after surgery, only five had intact sphincters on ES. Similar results were reported by Nielsen *et al.* [59•], but in this study ES was only performed postoperatively. Finally, a retrospective study by Sultan *et al.* [57••] described third-degree obstetric sphincter tears and ES findings. Risk factors for tears were clearly identified, the most important being forceps delivery. No third-degree tears were reported in 351 vacuum extractions. Of the patients with a third-degree tear, about 50% were symptomatic after primary repair and these patients all had persistent defects on anal ES. Of the asymptomatic patients, 70% had defects on anal ES. The conclusion from these studies must be that we now have an accurate (histologically confirmed) technique to identify internal and external sphincter defects and that we can also perform follow-up examinations in this group. The effects of surgery can be imaged with ES. Long-term follow-up of the asymptomatic patients with persistent defects will tell us whether these patients need additional treatment to prevent development of 'late' incontinence.

## Inflammatory bowel disease

In 25 patients with peri-anorectal Crohn's disease, ES (transrectal and transvaginal) was compared with CT scanning by Schratter-Sehn *et al.* [60•]. CT scanning was performed with oral, rectal, vaginal and intravenous contrast and by making 4-mm slices throughout the pelvis. Even with these optimal CT preparations, ES was superior in diagnosing fistulae but of equal accuracy in diagnosing abscesses. The fact that ES is much cheaper, can easily be repeated without special preparation and uses no ionizing irradiation, make ES the investigation of choice. Similar ES results are reported by Deen *et al.* [61], who investigated 18 patients with complex fistula in ano. Surgical findings matched the ES diagnosis in all but one case (94%). The actual origin of the fistula could be visualized in only two patients (11%), probably because the frequency (7 Mhz) used in this study had insufficient resolution for detailed imaging of the wall. The only case that was missed with ES was a horseshoe track at the anal verge, which is a well known difficult area. Cheong *et al.* [62] used injection of 1–2 ml hydrogen peroxide in the external opening of the fistula to enhance the image. Both fistulas had already been visualized with ES, and were again shown after hydrogen peroxide injection. It is not yet clear if there will be an obvious advantage of this procedure over the already highly accurate technique of 'non-enhanced' ES.

## Probe technology

Five articles report the ongoing development of miniprobes that can be used through a normal endoscope. Three papers concern instruments to be used in the oesophagus, stomach, duodenum or colon [63–65]. The Olympus company is now marketing a mini-probe that can be equipped with a balloon sheath for better acoustic coupling especially important in the oesophagus [63]. The Aloka Company (Tokyo, Japan) also produces mini-probes at two frequencies (15 and 20 Mhz) which, in a study from Maruta *et al.* [65] and Frank *et al.* [64], correlated well with the images that were seen with standard echoendoscopes. Both authors describe picture quality similar to the standard echoendoscopes, but with lower penetration depth.

Two papers by Furukawa *et al.* [66,67•] discuss the use of an ultra-thin mini-probe in the pancreatic duct. The probe was originally developed for intracoronary use and utilizes a frequency of 30 Mhz. Because of this high frequency, the penetration is maximally 1 cm. The authors describe [67•] their experience in differentiating cases of chronic pancreatitis from pancreatic carcinoma and other types of pancreatic disease with this high-frequency probe, which they could successfully insert in the main pancreatic duct in 88% of cases. Whether this will indeed assist clinicians in their every day practice in the years to come remains an unanswered question.

## Conclusions

ES is assisting gastroenterologists and surgeons all around the world in their daily practice. Its role is being further defined every year and 1994 has again brought important literature on a variety of subjects. Staging of almost all gastrointestinal tumours is possible with high accuracy. Differentiation of malignancies from benign disease solely with ES is hardly ever possible, but ES can assist in selected cases, for example by guiding fine needle aspiration biopsies. The spreading of ES will continue but care has to be taken that only large numbers of examinations will lead to the high accuracy rates cited in the literature. Nothing but practice makes perfect.

## References and recommended reading

Papers of particular interest, published within the annual period of review, have been highlighted as:
- of special interest
- of outstanding interest

1. Milsom JW, Czyrko C, Hull TL, Strong SA, Fazio VW: **Preoperative biopsy of pararectal lymph nodes in rectal cancer using endoluminal ultrasonography**. *Dis Colon Rectum* 1994, **37**:364–368.
Pararectal lymph nodes of 26 patients with rectal cancer were biopsied under ES guidance using a rigid linear scanner and a spring-loaded core biopsy needle. An accuracy rate of 77% was obtained; there was one false-positive biopsy.

2. Chang KJ, Katz KD, Durbin TE, Erickson RA, Butler JA, Lin F, Wuerker RB: **Endoscopic ultrasound-guided fine-needle aspiration**. *Gastrointest Endosc* 1994, **40**:694–699.

The largest study so far, using a linear array echoendoscope (Pentax) to obtain fine needle aspiration biopsies of 46 lesions (34 extra-luminal, 12 submucosal). Overall diagnostic accuracy was 87%. The importance of a standby cytologist is illustrated from the different results of the procedure in two hospitals.

3. Wiersema MJ, Kochman ML, Cramer HM, Tao LC, Wiersema LM: **Endosonography-guided real-time fine-needle aspiration biopsy**. *Gastrointest Endosc* 1994, **40**:700–707.
In this series of 26 patients, in which ES-guided fine needle aspiration biopsy was performed using a linear array echoendoscope, an accuracy rate of 90% was achieved. In nine out of 10 patients, who had had previous unsuccessful attempts with other techniques, a diagnosis was obtained with ES.

4. Wegener M, Adamek RJ, Wedmann B, Pfaffenbach B: **Endosonographically guided fine-needle aspiration puncture of paraesophagogastric mass lesions: preliminary results**. *Endoscopy* 1994, **26**:586–591.
ES-guided fine needle aspiration biopsy of para-oesophagogastric lesions was attempted in 12 patients using a standard sclerotherapy needle. A diagnostic specimen was obtained in 11 patients.

5. Wiersema MJ, Wiersema LM, Khusro Q, Cramer HM, Tao LC: **Combined endosonography and fine-needle aspiration cytology in the evaluation of gastrointestinal lesions**. *Gastrointest Endosc* 1994, **40**:199–206.
In this study of 50 patients, fine needle aspiration biopsy was performed after ES with a rotating sector scanner (Olympus). Diagnostic results were obtained in 74% of patients. This study shows that, in the presence of an endoscopic landmark, cytology can be obtained with a normal endoscope after ES to rule out vessels and determine the optimal site for puncture.

6. Vilmann P, Hancke S, Henriksen FW, Jacobsen GK: **Endosonographically-guided fine needle aspiration biopsy of malignant lesions in the upper gastrointestinal tract**. *Endoscopy* 1993, **25**:523–527.
Description of the development of a needle to perform ES-guided fine needle aspiration biopsies with a linear array scanner (Pentax). Success rates were optimal with the third prototype although the groups were small.

7. Rösch T: **Endoscopic ultrasonography**. *Endoscopy* 1994, **26**:148–168.
Excellent overview of the literature on ES until 1993, containing 272 references. Probably best used as an addendum to the book published by the author in 1992 [8].

8. Rösch T, Classen M: *Gastroenterologic endosonography*. Stuttgart, New York: Georg Thieme Verlag; 1992.

9. Caletti G, Odegaard S, Rösch T, Sivak MV, Tio TL, Yasuda K: **Endoscopic ultrasonography (EUS): a summary of the conclusions of the working party for the tenth world congress of Gastroenterology Los Angeles, California October, 1994**. *Am J Gastroenterol* 1994, **89** (suppl).
Report of an international working party, trying to differentiate established and investigational indications for ES. Training recommendations are also suggested.

10. Peters JH, Hoeft SF, Heimbucher J, Bremner RM, De Meester TR, Bremner CG, *et al.*: **Selection of patients for curative or palliative resection of esophageal cancer based on preoperative endoscopic ultrasonography**. *Arch Surg* 1994, **129**:534–539.
ES was used to guide treatment of oesophageal carcinoma in 42 patients. Based on ES findings, three patients were treated with an 'inappropriate' procedure.

11. Chak A, Canto M, Gerdes H, Lightdale C, Hawes R, Wiersema MJ, *et al.*: **Prognosis of locally invasive esophageal cancers (esoph T4 ca) preoperatively staged by endoscopic ultrasound (EUS): a multicenter retrospective cohort study [abstract]**. *Gastrointest Endosc* 1994, **40**:P61.
Multicenter study looking at clinical outcome of oesophageal carcinomas, ES-stage T4.

12. Yoshikane H, Tsukamoto Y, Niwa Y, Goto H, Hase S, Shimodaira M, Maruta S, *et al.*: **Superficial esophageal carcinoma: evaluation by endoscopic ultrasonography**. *Am J Gastroenterol* 1994, **89**:702–707.
This study looked at 28 (!) patients with superficial oesophageal carcinoma. ES was accurate in separating mucosal from submucosal tumours in 75% of cases.

13. Falk GW, Catalano MF, Sivak MV, Rice TW, Van Dam J: **Endosonography in the evaluation of patients with Barrett's esophagus and high grade dysplasia**. *Gastrointest Endosc* 1994, **40**:207–212.
Nine patients with Barrett's oesophagus and high-grade dysplasia were examined with standard ES. ES could not detect a carcinoma in two out of the three patients with a carcinoma and was false-positive in two out of six.

14. Wiersema MJ, Wiersema LM: **High-resolution 25-megahertz ultrasonography of the gastrointestinal wall: histologic correlates.** *Gastrointest Endosc* 1993, **39**:499–504.

15. Roubein LD, DuBrow R, David C, Lynch P, Fornage B, Ajani J, *et al.*: **Endoscopic ultrasonography in the quantitative assessment of response to chemotherapy in patients with adenocarcinoma of the esophagus and esophagogastric junction.** *Endoscopy* 1993, **25**:587–591.
ES was used in this small series of eight patients to detect tumour reduction by preoperative chemotherapy in oesophageal and cardia carcinoma. No down-staging was seen with ES, but was also only present in two patients after resection.

16. Hordijk ML, Kok TC, Wilson JHP, Mulder AH: **Assessment of response of**
• **esophageal carcinoma to induction chemotherapy.** *Endoscopy* 1993, **25**:592–596.
ES was not useful for detecting the tumour response to preoperative chemotherapy in oesophageal squamous cell carcinoma in 11 patients. Pathology showed downstaging in five patients. Tumour was replaced in some patients by an inflammatory infiltrate mimicking a tumour on ES.

17. Tio TL, Blank LECM, Wijers OB, Hartog Jager FCAD, Van Dijk JDP, Tytgat
• GNJ: **Staging and prognosis using endosonography in patients with inoperable esophageal carcinoma treated with combined intraluminal and external irradiation.** *Gastrointest Endosc* 1994, **40**:304–310.
In 63 patients with irresectable oesophageal carcinoma, ES was used to monitor the effect of combined intraluminal and external irradiation. There was a correlation between survival and number of lymph nodes in squamous cell carcinoma. An inverse correlation between tumour thickness and survival was shown.

18. Catalano MF, Sivak MVJ, Rice T, Gragg LA, Van Dam J: **Endosonographic**
•• **features predictive of lymph node metastasis.** *Gastrointest Endosc* 1994, **40**:442–446.
Carefully executed study looking at four different parameters of individual lymph nodes of 100 patients with oesophageal carcinoma. Size has low discriminating capacity between malignant and benign. Best predictor of malignancy was an echo-poor texture of the lymph node.

19. Wiersema MJ, Hassig WM, Hawes RH, Wonn MJ: **Mediastinal lymph node detection with endosonography.** *Gastrointest Endosc* 1993, **39**:788–793.

20. Nattermann C, Dancygier H: **Endosonography in the diagnosis and staging**
• **of malignant gastric tumors. A prospective comparative study between endoscopic sonography, computed tomography and conventional ultrasound.** *Z Gastroenterol* 1993, **31**:719–726.
In this study of patients with gastric carcinoma, ES was compared with ultrasound and CT. As to be expected, ES was most accurate in staging. Unfortunately, a relatively low accuracy for T4 was shown.

21. Smith JW, Brennan MF, Botet JF, Gerdes H, Lightdale CJ: **Preoperative**
• **endoscopic ultrasound can predict the risk of recurrence after operation for gastric carcinoma.** *J Clin Oncol* 1993, **11**:2380–2385.
The preoperative ES stage of patients with gastric carcinoma correlated well with tumour recurrence. It could therefore be well used to select patients for adjuvant preoperative therapy.

22. Mendis RE, Gerdes H, Lightdale CJ, Botet JF: **Large gastric folds: a**
•• **diagnostic approach using endoscopic ultrasonography.** *Gastrointest Endosc* 1994, **40**:437–441.
Evaluation of large gastric folds with ES proved to be highly accurate in 29 patients. Thickening of the third and fourth layer (muscularis propria) in the absence of ulceration should lead to surgical exploration when endoscopic biopsies are negative.

23. Benamouzig R, Marteau P, Lavergne A, Palazzo L, Dahan H, Rambaud JC: **Gastroduodenal linitis plastica infiltration due to metastatic involvement from bladder cancer: Endosonographic findings correlated with histology.** *Eur J Gastroenterol Hepatol* 1994, **6**:179–182.
Case-report describing a typical linitis plastica ES image, which turned out to be metastatic disease from a bladder carcinoma.

24. Palazzo L, Roseau G, Ruskone Fourmestraux A, Rougier P, Chaussade S,
•• Rambaud J, *et al.*: **Endoscopic ultrasonography in the local staging of primary gastric lymphoma.** *Endoscopy* 1993, **25**:502–508.
ES was compared to endoscopy and histology of the resection specimen in 26 patients with primary gastric lymphoma. Infiltration depth was correctly assessed in 91.5%; surface extension, however, was underestimated in 37.5% of patients. Underestimation always concerned small mucosal or submucosal foci of lymphoma.

25. Schüder G, Hildebrandt U, Kreissler Haag D, Seitz G, Feifel G: **Role of**
• **endosonography in the surgical management of non-Hodgkin's lymphoma of the stomach.** *Endoscopy* 1993, **25**:509–512.
In 10 patients with NHL of the stomach, ES was used to assess infiltration depth and the extent of gastric resection. All resection margins were free; ES was assisted by intraoperative ultrasound in three cases.

26. Giovannini M, Seitz JF: **Endoscopic ultrasonography with a linear-type**
•• **echoendoscope in the evaluation of 94 patients with pancreatobiliary disease.** *Endoscopy* 1994, **26**:579–585.
Instead of using a rotating sector scanner as in most studies published so far, this study used a linear array echoendoscope (Pentax) in a large number of patients with pancreatobiliary disease. ES was correct in identifying the origin of cholestasis in 88% of the cases. ES also accurately staged tumours in 88% of cases. Results are comparable to those obtained with rotating sector scanners.

27. Rösch T, Classen M: **Endoscopic ultrasonography.** In *Annual of Gastrointestinal Endoscopy.* Edited by Cotton PB, Tytgat GNJ, Williams CB. 6th ed. London: Current Science Ltd; 1993:66–82.

28. Amouyal P, Amouyal G, Levy P, Tuzet S, Palazzo L, Vilgrain V, *et al.*:
•• **Diagnosis of choledocholithiasis by endoscopic ultrasonography.** *Gastroenterology* 1994, **106**:1062–1067.
Patients suspected to have common bile duct stones were examined with external ultrasound, CT, ES and ERCP or intraoperative cholangiogram. Sensitivity of ultrasound, CT and ES were 25, 75 and 97%, respectively. It is concluded that ES can replace diagnostic ERCP because of lower morbidity and mortality.

29. Snady H, Bruckner H, Siegel J, Cooperman A, Neff R, Kiefer L: **Endoscopic**
•• **ultrasonographic criteria of vascular invasion by potentially resectable pancreatic tumors.** *Gastrointest Endosc* 1994, **40**:326–333.
Using three ES criteria, a 100% accuracy for vascular involvement in pancreatic cancer is achieved in 38 patients. The criteria were: presence of venous collaterals, tumour in the vessel lumen and loss of interface between tumour and vessel. Arterial ingrowth was always accompanied by venous involvement in these patients.

30. Muller MF, Meyenberger C, Bertschinger P, Schaer R, Marincek B: **Pancre-**
•• **atic tumors: Evaluation with endoscopic US, CT, and MR imaging.** *Radiology* 1994, **190**:745–751.
Forty-nine patients with clinical suspicion of a pancreatic tumour were investigated with ES, CT and MRI. High accuracy of ES was confirmed in this study. Although overall MRI was quite accurate, the accuracy rate dropped when only results of smaller (< 3 cm) pancreatic tumours were analysed.

31. Wiersema MJ, Hawes RH, Lehman GA, Kochman ML, Sherman S, Kopecky KK: **Prospective evaluation of endoscopic ultrasonography and endoscopic retrograde cholangiopancreatography in patients with chronic abdominal pain of suspected pancreatic origin.** *Endoscopy* 1993, **25**:555–564.

32. Nattermann C, Goldschmidt AJW, Dancygier H: **Endosonography in**
• **chronic pancreatitis — A comparison between endoscopic retrograde pancreatography and endoscopic ultrasonography.** *Endoscopy* 1993, **25**:565–570.
Study comparing ERP and ES in chronic and acute pancreatitis. As in previous studies, ES was shown to more sensitive for pancreatic abnormalities than ERP. No abnormalities were seen in 20 controls.

33. Hulsmans FJH, Tio TL, Fockens P, Bosma A, Tytgat GNJ: **Assessment of**
• **tumor infiltration depth in rectal cancer with transrectal sonography: caution is necessary.** *Radiology* 1994, **190**:715–720.
In staging rectal carcinomas, very poor results were obtained in T2 carcinomas. This study focuses on this problem and investigates the different ES criteria that exist for T2 rectal carcinoma.

34. Solomon M, McLeod RS, Cohen EK, Simons ME, Wilson S: **Reliability and**
•• **validity studies of endoluminal ultrasonography for anorectal disorders.** *Dis Colon Rectum* 1994, **37**:546–551.
The first part of this study assessed the validity of ES in rectal disease by sending a questionnaire to referring physicians. This showed that ES changed clinical management in 45% and altered the doctor's confidence in 76% of cases. The second part assessed reliability of rectal cancer staging, showing a learning curve rising with experience from 44% to 64%.

35. Ramirez JM, Mortensen NJM, Takeuchi N, Humphreys MMS: **Endoluminal**
• **ultrasonography in the follow-up of patients with rectal cancer.** *Br J Surg* 1994, **81**:692–694.

Follow-up of rectal cancer patients is only of value when treatable lesions can be identified. In a group of 66 patients, four recurrences could be treated radically, three of them detectable by ES only.

36. Roseau G, Palazzo L, Colardelle P, Chaussade S, Couturier D, Paolaggi JA:
   • **Endoscopic ultrasonography in the staging and follow-up of epidermoid carcinoma of the anal canal.** *Gastrointest Endosc* 1994, **40**:447–450.
   Squamous cell carcinoma of the anus, primarily treated with irradiation, was followed up with ES in 20 patients. Six patients required surgical intervention, all correlating well with the ES images.

37. Chang KJ, Albers CG, Erickson RA, Butler JA, Wuerker RB, Lin F: **Endoscopic ultrasound-guided fine needle aspiration of pancreatic carcinoma.** *Am J Gastroenterol* 1994, **89**:263–266.
   Case-report describing successful puncture of a pancreatic neoplasm under ES guidance.

38. Wiersema MJ, Chak A, Wiersema LM: **Mediastinal histoplasmosis: evaluation with endosonography and endoscopic fine-needle aspiration biopsy.** *Gastrointest Endosc* 1994, **40**:78–81.
   Three patients with mediastinal histoplasmosis were described in whom ES assisted in making a diagnosis.

39. Lawrence SP, Larsen BR, Stacy CC, McNally PR: **Echoendosonographic and histologic correlation of a fibrovascular polyp of the esophagus.** *Gastrointest Endosc* 1994, **40**:81–84.
   A fibrovascular polyp in the oesophagus was examined with ES, showing a changing ES pattern from proximal to distal, consistent with increasing fibrous tissue components from the stalk towards the end of the polyp.

40. Imamura A, Tochihara M, Natsui K, Murashima Y, Suga T, Yaosaka T, *et al.*: **Glomus tumor of the stomach — endoscopic ultrasonographic findings.** *Am J Gastroenterol* 1994, **89**:271–272.
   Gastric submucosal tumour, which on ES was located in the third and fourth layers, was resected and turned out to be gastric glomus tumour.

41. Motoo Y, Okai T, Ohta H, Satomura Y, Watanabe H, Yamakawa O, *et al.*:
   • **Endoscopic ultrasonography in the diagnosis of extraluminal compressions mimicking gastric submucosal tumors.** *Endoscopy* 1994, **26**:239–242.
   Series of 19 patients with extra-luminal compression of the stomach. The spleen or splenic artery were responsible in 12 patients.

42. Yoshikane H, Tsukamoto Y, Niwa Y, Goto H, Hase S: **Sequential observation of gastric ulcer healing by endoscopic ultrasonography.** *Scand J Gastroenterol* 1994, **29**:665–670.
   Sequential observation by ES showed that the healing of the surface of gastric ulcers strongly reflects the healing within.

43. Kawamoto K, Ueyama T, Iwashita I, Utsunomiya T, Honda H, Onitsuka H,
   • *et al.*: **Colonic submucosal tumors: comparison of endoscopic US and target air-enema CT with barium enema study and colonoscopy.** *Radiology* 1994, **192**:697–702.
   ES was compared to CT with air-enema in suspected colonic submucosal tumours. Although almost equally accurate in detection, ES assisted more in differential diagnosis.

44. Hizawa K, Iida M, Suekane H, Mibu R, Mochizuki Y, Yao T, *et al.*: **Mucosal prolapse syndrome: diagnosis with endoscopic US.** *Radiology* 1994, **191**:527–530.
   The mucosal prolapse syndrome was visualized as hypoechoic thickening of the third ES layer in the rectum, in five patients.

45. Lee SH: **Transrectal ultrasound in the diagnosis of ano-rectal varices.** *Clin Radiol* 1994, **49**:69–70.
   Case-report of ano-rectal varices in a cirrhotic patient mimicking a rectal tumour.

46. Boustiere C, Dumas O, Jouffre C, Letard JC, Patouillard B, Etaix JP, *et al.*:
   • **Endoscopic ultrasonography-classification of gastric varices in patients with cirrhosis. Comparison with endoscopic findings.** *J Hepatol* 1993, **19**:268–272.
   ES and endoscopy were performed in 80 patients with alcoholic liver cirrhosis with portal hypertension and in 50 controls. Endoscopy is more sensitive for oesophageal varices, ES is better for gastric varices.

47. Squillace SJ, Johnson DA, Sanowski RA: **The endosonographic appearance of a Dieulafoy's lesion.** *Am J Gastroenterol* 1994, **89**:276–277.
   • At the site of a small gastric ulcer in a patient with recurrent haematemesis, a large calibre submucosal vessel was detected consistent with Dieulafoy's disease.

48. Akahoshi K, Chijiiwa Y, Misawa T, Ayukawa K, Nakamura K, Jimi M, *et al.*: **Confirmation of Dieulafoy's vascular lesion by endoscopic ultrasonography in three cases.** *Dig Endosc* 1993, **5**:383–390.

49. Schafer A, Enck P, Furst G, Kahn T, Frieling T, Lubke HJ: **Anatomy of the**
   • **anal sphincters: comparison of anal endosonography to magnetic resonance imaging.** *Dis Colon Rectum* 1994, **37**:777–781.
   Comparison of normal anal sphincter imaging with ES and MRI in eight healthy persons. The results of this small study showed that ES was clearly a better, easier and cheaper imaging method.

50. Kamm MA: **Obstetric damage and faecal incontinence.** *Lancet* 1994,
   •• **344**:730–733.
   Excellent review article on the recent literature concerning obstetric damage and faecal incontinence. The important new insights in the aetiology and therapy, gained with the help of anal ES, were summarized. Obligatory knowledge for anyone treating incontinent patients.

51. Eckardt VF, Jung B, Fischer B, Lierse W: **Anal endosonography in healthy subjects and patients with idiopathic fecal incontinence.** *Dis Colon Rectum* 1994, **37**:235–242.
   Study describing anal ES and manometry in 30 controls and 26 patients with faecal incontinence.

52. Emblem R, Dhaenens G, Stien R, Morkric L, Aasen AO, Bergan A: **The**
   • **importance of anal endosonography in the evaluation of idiopathic fecal incontinence.** *Dis Colon Rectum* 1994, **37**:42–48.
   Anal ES and anal EMG were performed in 29 patients with idiopathic incontinence and 26 controls. The results showed a negative correlation between ES and both pudendal nerve distal conduction velocity and muscle fibre density.

53. Engel AF, Kamm MA, Sultan AH, Bartram CI, Nicholls RJ: **Anterior anal**
   •• **sphincter repair in patients with obstetric trauma.** *Br J Surg* 1994, **81**:1231–1234.
   This surgical follow-up study showed that the result of anterior sphincter repair could be predicted by ES. In 91% of patients with symptomatic improvement after surgery, the external sphincter was intact. In 45% of patients without improvement there was continuity of the sphincter on ES.

54. Falk PM, Blatchford GJ, Cali RL, Christensen MA, Thorson AG: **Transanal ultrasound and manometry in the evaluation of fecal incontinence.** *Dis Colon Rectum* 1994, **37**:468–472.
   In 28 incontinent women a good correlation between internal sphincter diameter on ES and resting pressure was found, as well as an inverse relation between external sphincter defects on ES and squeeze pressure.

55. Schafer A, Enck P, Heyer T, Gantke B, Frieling T, Lubke HJ: **Endosonography of the anal sphincters — Incontinent and continent patients and healthy controls.** *Z Gastroenterol* 1994, **32**:328–331.
   Forty-two incontinent patients, 19 constipated patients and 15 healthy controls were evaluated with anal ES and manometry.

56. Sultan AH, Kamm MA, Talbot IC, Nicholls RJ, Bartram CI: **Anal en-**
   •• **dosonography for identifying external sphincter defects confirmed histologically.** *Br J Surg* 1994, **81**:463–465.
   Study showing the histological correlate to endosonographic external sphincter defects in patients with faecal incontinence, undergoing sphincter repair. The group consisted of 12 patients (11 female). Clinical evaluation was correct in 50%, EMG in 75% and ES in all patients.

57. Sultan AH, Kamm MA, Hudson CN, Bartram CI: **Third degree obstetric**
   •• **and sphincter tears: risk factors and outcome of primary repair.** *BMJ* 1994, **308**:887–891.
   Risk factors for third-degree sphincter tear were shown to be forceps delivery, primiparous delivery, birth weight over 4 kg and occiposterior position at delivery in this study. Forty-seven per cent of patients with a third-degree obstetric tear were still symptomatic after primary repair. Sonographic defects were identified in 85% of women after primary repair.

58. Yang YK, Wexner SD, Nogueras JJ, Jagelman DG: **The role of anal ultrasound in the assessment of benign anorectal diseases.** *Coloproctology* 1993, **15**:260–265.
   Heterogeneous group of 76 patients with an anorectal abscess or fistula, faecal incontinence or chronic idiopathic pain was investigated with anal ES.

59. Nielsen MB, Dammegaard L, Pedersen JF: **Endosonographic assessment**
   • **of the anal sphincter after surgical reconstruction.** *Dis Colon Rectum* 1994, **37**:434–438.

Persistent sphincter defects after anterior sphincter reconstruction were found in four out of five patients with persistent post-surgical faecal incontinence. Thus ES was useful in explaining unsatisfactory surgical results.

60. Schratter-Sehn AU, Lochs H, Vogelsang H, Schurawitzki H, Herold C,
• Schratter M. **Endoscopic ultrasonography versus computed tomography in the differential diagnosis of perianorectal complications in Crohn's disease.** *Endoscopy* 1993, **25**:582–586.
Twenty-five patents with peri-anorectal Crohn's disease were investigated with contrast-enhanced CT scanning and ES. ES was equal to CT in detecting abscesses but superior in detecting fistulae, making it the method of choice.

61. Deen KI, Williams JG, Hutchinson R, Keighley MRB, Kumar D: **Fistulas in ano: endoanal ultrasonographic assessment assists decision making for surgery.** *Gut* 1994, **35**:391–394.
This study, reporting results of ES and surgery in 18 patients with complex fistulae in ano, showed accurate delineation of the fistulae in all but one patient (94%).

62. Cheong DMO, Nogueras JJ, Wexner SD, Jagelman DG: **Anal endosonography for recurrent anal fistulas: Image enhancement with hydrogen peroxide.** *Dis Colon Rectum* 1993, **36**:1158–1160.
The possibility of hydrogen-peroxide injection in a peri-anal fistula to act as ultrasound contrast medium is illustrated by two cases.

63. Fockens P, Van Dullemen HM, Tytgat GNJ: **Endosonography of stenotic esophageal carcinomas: Preliminary experience with an ultra-thin, balloon-fitted ultrasound probe in four patients.** *Gastrointest Endosc* 1994, **40**:226–228.
Four patients with oesophageal carcinoma and high-grade stenosis were successfully examined with a balloon-fitted ES probe made by Olympus.

64. Frank N, Grieshammer B, Zimmermann W: **A new miniature ultrasonic probe for gastrointestinal scanning: feasibility and preliminary results.** *Endoscopy* 1994, **26**:603–608.
Thirty-seven patients with a variety of abnormalities, were investigated with a 2.0 mm mini-probe (Aloka) with good image quality but less penetration.

65. Maruta S, Tsukamoto Y, Niwa Y, Goto H, Hase S, Yoshikane H, *et al.*: **Evaluation of upper gastrointestinal tumors with a new endoscopic ultrasound probe.** *Gastrointest Endosc* 1994, **40**:603–608.
*In vitro* and *in vivo* study utilizing new 2.0 mm mini-probe (Aloka) with good accuracy in imaging superficial malignancy.

66. Furukawa T, Tsukamoto Y, Naitoh Y, Hirooka Y, Katoh T: **Evaluation of intraductal ultrasonography in the diagnosis of pancreatic cancer.** *Endoscopy* 1993, **25**:577–581.
Successful insertion of an intravascular 30 Mhz mini-probe (CVIS) in 17 out of 20 pancreatic cancer patients.

67. Furukawa T, Tsukamoto Y, Naitoh Y, Mitake M, Hirooka Y, Hayakawa T:
• **Differential diagnosis of pancreatic diseases with an intraductal ultrasound system.** *Gastrointest Endosc* 1994, **40**:213–219.
First attempt to use an intraductal ultrasound probe in the pancreatic duct to assist in differential diagnosis of pancreatic diseases *in vitro* and *in vivo* (40 patients). Several different echopatterns were described of different pancreatic abnormalities.

Dr Paul Fockens, Department of Gastroenterology, Academic Medical Center, University of Amsterdam, Meibergdreef 9, 1105 AZ Amsterdam, The Netherlands.

# Endoscopy and the pancreas

## Peter B. Cotton

Digestive Disease Center, Medical University of South Carolina, Charleston,
South Carolina, USA

## Introduction

Writing in the *Annual* in 1993, Lichtenstein and Carr-Locke concluded their review by stating that 'endoscopic pancreatic therapy is at an early stage of development, with largely uncontrolled reports published to date. Such techniques require a high degree of endoscopic expertise and judgement, and, even in experienced hands, carry a significant complication rate. The long-term clinical results and morbidity from these treatment modalities . . . need further clarification'. They also called for randomized controlled trials. No one can argue with these statements. Review of the relevant literature of 1994 (and a few articles published in late 1993) unfortunately reveals few major contributions to our understanding.

For endoscopists, the major issues are how best to diagnose (and exclude) early chronic pancreatitis and when endoscopic treatment may be helpful in both acute and chronic contexts. These questions cannot be answered without detailed knowledge of the diagnostic modalities, the natural history of pancreatitis, and some clearly defined objective assessment measures.

## Diagnosis, classification and prognosis in chronic pancreatitis

There is no difficulty in making a diagnosis of advanced chronic pancreatitis at a stage when imaging and functional abnormalities are grossly abnormal. Recognition at the earliest stages is much more difficult. Studies of the sensitivity and specificity of different diagnostic modalities have suffered from lack of a true gold standard, i.e. histology. Academic pancreatologists often use some form of duodenal intubation function study as a gold standard, claiming that this is more sensitive than pancreatography and other imaging modalities. The report by Bozkurt *et al.* [1•] is relevant to this debate, and reassuring for pancreatographers. This group made a comparative analysis of pancreatography (using the Cambridge classification), ultrasound scanning, computed tomography and a standardized secretin–caerulein exocrine function test. Changes on pancreatography correlated well with the functional assessments, and no patient with a normal pancreatogram had an abnormal function test. Ultrasound scans and computed tomography were less sensitive.

In this context, there is increasing interest in the use of endoscopic ultrasonography (with guided biopsy and intraductal scanning). Endosonography is reviewed in another article in the *Annual*. Several studies are claiming high sensitivity for the diagnosis of pancreatitis [2••]. The most startling imaging development is magnetic resonance cholangiopancreatography (MRCP). Using a long-echo-train fast spin-echo sequence and a surface coil, a Japanese group [3••] demonstrated remarkable cholangiograms and pancreatograms in 39 patients with chronic pancreatitis. Correlation with the standard endoscopic retrograde cholangiopancreatography (ERCP) was excellent, particularly in the case of strictures and ductal filling defects. The authors state that 'MRCP cannot replace ERCP completely'. However, if this equipment becomes widely available, it will certainly have a major impact.

There have been several recent reports concerning the prognosis of chronic pancreatitis. Ammann *et al.* [4••] published an update of their prospective long-term study of a large cohort of patients presenting with alcoholic acute pancreatitis. They showed that the disease did not progress in approximately 25% of the patients, contrary to traditional belief. These patients did not develop duct dilatation or calcification, and most obtained spontaneous lasting pain relief irrespective of alcohol intake or normal pancreatic function. A multicentre international study by Lowenfels *et al.* [5••] looked at predictors of survival amongst 2015 subjects with chronic pancreatitis. This showed that an older age and smoking and drinking were major predictors of mortality. There was no survival advantage of patients who had received surgical treatment. The Mayo Clinic group [6••] also reported long-term follow-up data. They compared patients with idiopathic chronic pancreatitis with those with alcohol-induced disease. Idiopathic pancreatitis had an equal sex distribution,

---

### Abbreviations

ERCP—endoscopic retrograde cholangiopancreatography; MRCP—magnetic resonance cholangiopancreatography.

and a much slower rate of calcification compared with alcohol-induced disease. Patients with early-onset idiopathic pancreatitis had a more severe course than those whose disease presented late.

Despite several authoritative international symposia on the subject, the classification of pancreatitis remains controversial. The main problem is in deciding whether to base a classification on pathology (which is rarely available), pathogenesis (which may be in dispute), or on the clinical stage (which may be difficult to define). Two more workshops have recently reported their conclusions. Chari and Singer from Germany [7] reviewed the previous literature, and proposed a classification of alcohol-induced chronic pancreatitis based on the clinical stage of development. Similarly, Bradley [8•] reported on a clinically based classification system for acute pancreatitis, resulting from an international consensus conference. This provides clear definitions of different stages and complications. Steinberg and Tenner [9] published a helpful comprehensive review of acute pancreatitis, covering epidemiology, causes, diagnosis, natural history and treatments.

## Endoscopic treatment of acute pancreatitis and complications

Neoptolemos *et al.* [10•] reviewed the evidence in favour of urgent endoscopic intervention for patients with acute pancreatitis, and presented a useful treatment algorithm. This included the use of pancreatography in patients with non-biliary pancreatitis who did not improve promptly to detect disruption of the main pancreatic duct. This may lead to surgical debridement, or pseudocyst drainage.

Lai and Lo [11], who also have data from randomized controlled trials, come to the same conclusion in patients with acute biliary pancreatitis. Conservative management is justified initially for patients with predicted mild disease. ERCP and sphincterotomy is warranted in patients with severe disease, and when there is any associated cholangitis.

Many authors have reported the endoscopic treatment of patients with pseudocysts by direct puncture through the stomach or duodenal wall, or with intraductal stents. Unanswered questions include the precise timing and type of intervention and the role of endoscopic as opposed to percutaneous intervention. Serious haemorrhage can occur after endoscopic cyst puncture. Binmoeller *et al.* [12] report the development of a new instrument designed to minimize this risk. Howell *et al.* [13] recommend selecting the site of puncture by first using a needle catheter to inject contrast into the cyst. On the same principle, there is increasing interest and

experience in using endoscopic ultrasound-guided needle aspiration of pseudocysts.

Whether or not to leave a stent after endoscopic pseudocyst drainage has not been clearly established. It is also not clear whether the results of endoscopic pseudocyst drainage can be predicted, for example, by knowledge of the integrity of the pancreatic duct. Surprisingly, Funnell *et al.* [14] were able to treat patients with pseudocysts after abdominal trauma, despite duct disruption in most cases.

Pancreatic fistulas develop after trauma or therapeutic intervention. Like cystic duct leaks after laparoscopic cholecystectomy, pancreatic fistulas can often be treated by improving the normal route of drainage, in other words by temporary pancreatic duct stenting as described by Saeed *et al.* [15].

A British group report the use of an expandable metal stent in this context, in a patient in whom a standard plastic prosthesis had failed due to migration [16]. Few endoscopists are prepared to use expandable metal stents in the pancreas because of uncertain long-term effects.

## 'Obstructive' pancreatitis and its treatment

Many treatments for chronic pancreatitis depend on the belief that there is increased pressure in the duct as a result of obstruction from stone, stricture or sphincter dysfunction. Most surgical and endoscopic therapies are designed to relieve the obstruction, and to improve drainage.

What is the evidence for an increased duct pressure system? Reber has been a protagonist of this hypothesis with some supportive evidence from animal experimentation. A recent study from his group [17•] supported the concept of a compartment syndrome, in which increased ductal pressure reduced pancreatic blood flow. In the cat model, duct decompression prevented the increase in main duct and interstitial pressure during secretion, and restored blood flow. The measurement of blood flow has been enhanced recently with $H_2$ gas clearance studies. Ashley *et al.* [18] developed an ERCP-based method for measuring pancreatic duct flow, using a catheter loop in the pancreatic duct. Preliminary results in a small number of patients with painful chronic pancreatitis revealed quite low basal pancreatic blood flow.

Another way to study obstruction is to measure the pancreatic duct diameter after secretin stimulation. Cavallini *et al.* [19] performed abdominal ultrasonography after maximum stimulation with secretin in several groups of patients with acute pancreatitis. Most patients with recurrent idiopathic pancreatitis, and those associated with pancreas divisum, had an abnormal test, suggesting sphincter dysfunction. The test returned to normal after sphincterotomy. Pancreatic sphincter pressure dynamics can be measured directly with endoscopic manometry. Some normal ranges have been established, and several groups have investigated patients with acute and chronic pancreatitis. Vestergaard et al. [20•] found abnormal pancreatic sphincter pressures in 11 out of 15 patients with chronic pancreatitis. In addition, Laugier [21•] found abnormalities in a substantial proportion of similar patients, using a dual solid-state micro-transducer to measure the main pancreatic duct pressure and pancreatic sphincter pressures after secretin administration. Guelrud has been a pioneer in this field, and has published a useful concise review [22].

## Pancreas divisum

The belief that pancreas divisum can cause pancreatitis is based on an obstructive hypothesis. Additional evidence comes from a recent observation [23] that a subset of patients with pancreatitis and pancreas divisum have a focal dilatation at the termination of the dorsal duct ('Santorinicele'). Excellent clinical results were obtained with endoscopic excision or balloon dilatation in a small group of patients (Fig. 1). From the same group, Coleman et al. [24•] also published their results of endoscopic stenting with or without sphincterotomy at the minor papilla in 34 symptomatic patients with pancreas divisum. Significant improvement in pain scores were found in patients with acute recurrent pancreatitis, and in those with chronic pancreatitis. These results are encouraging, but certainly need amplification in prospective, preferably randomized, studies using objective outcome measures. The only randomized trial so far reported (Lans et al., Gastrointest Endosc 1992, **38**:430–434) was helpful, but was too small to permit definitive conclusions, particularly about the correct selection of patients. As has been said repeatedly, there is a pressing need for multicentre collaboration.

## Pancreatic sphincterotomy, stenting and stone extraction

Based on good overall results of endoscopic stenting in the biliary tree, endoscopists have turned to the pancreas with enthusiasm which verges sometimes on naïveté. Stents have been used in patients with strictures and postulated sphincter dysfunction. Unfortunately, it is difficult to define obstruction precisely, and results are usually assessed subjectively. It is already clear that pancreatic stenting is not a totally benign procedure. Stent dysfunction in the biliary tree rapidly leads to cholangitis. Fortunately, infective pancreatitis is very rare after pancreatic stenting; however, stents certainly can cause substantial ductal changes. Most abnormalities are claimed to be reversible when stents are removed, but this is not always the case. A surgical case report [25] showed extensive inflammatory changes in the duct, and the area of parenchyma drained by the stent. Despite this, many authors have reportedly left pancreatic stents in place for months or even years. Little work has been done on the extent and mechanisms of pancreatic stent obstruction. Ikenberry et al. [26•] published startling results from a study of 146 pancreatic ductal stents which had been placed for a variety of reasons. Using a standardized method of assessment, they found that occlusion is much more rapid than previously reported: 50% of stents were occluded at 6 weeks and 100% at more than 9 weeks. Occlusion rates were similar for 5 F and 7 F gauge stents. Clearly, much work remains to be done on the design and materials of pancreatic stents. It is currently wise to restrict pancreatic ductal stenting to a temporary period measured in weeks.

Sphincterotomy of the main pancreatic orifice would appear to be logical if sphincter hypertension can be established (by manometry or possibly the secretin ultrasound test). Published results are difficult to assess because the criteria for patient selection are mixed; it is not clear whether clinical failures are due to poor patient selection or to restenosis. The best technique for performing a sphincterotomy is not yet established (Fig. 2). Some authors use standard sphincterotomes, others a needle knife, with or without a temporary guiding stent. Kozarek et al. [27•] published their results of pancreatic duct sphincterotomy in 56 patients. Despite the large experience, it is difficult to draw firm conclusions from this study. Most of the patients had chronic pancreatitis, but some also had obstructing ductal calculi, ductal disruption, sphincter dysfunction, and/or ductal stenosis. Complications of treatment were noted acutely in 10% of patients. Furthermore, 14% required repeat sphincterotomy for restenosis, and no fewer than 25% of all patients went on to pancreatic surgery. Technical results are easier to assess in the subset of 26 patients treated for obstructing ductal calculi. Stone extraction was ultimately successful in 23 of these patients; however, eight required extracorporeal shockwave lithotripsy, and 13 patients needed two or more endoscopic sessions. Most of the patients with stones associated with chronic relapsing pancreatitis had no further attacks within a follow-up of more than 1 year.

Van der Hul et al. [28•] reported specifically on the role of extracorporeal shockwave lithotripsy of pancreatic duct stones. They treated 17 patients in whom simple endoscopic stone removal had proved to be impossi-

(a)

(b)

(c)

(d)

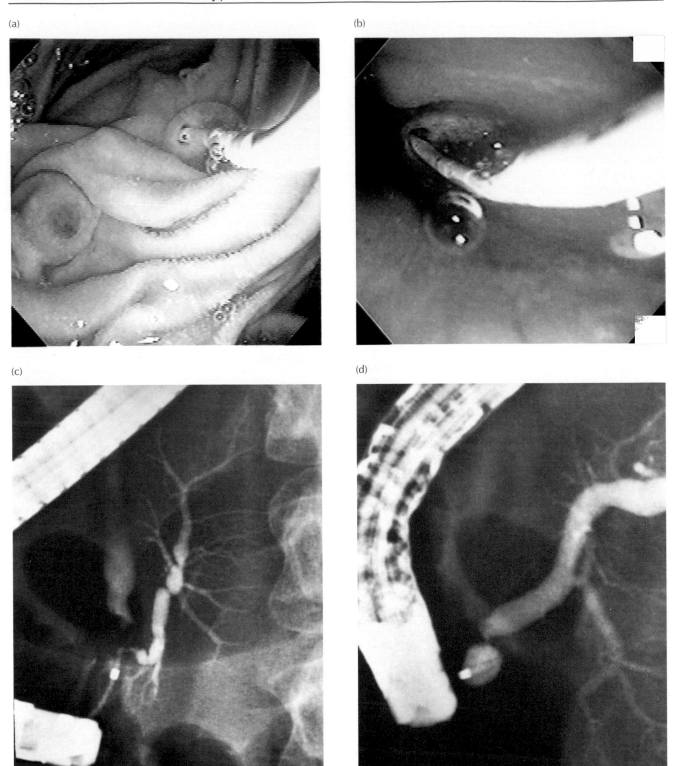

**Fig. 1.** Santorinicele. (a) Balloon inflation of the minor papilla. (b) After inflation, the orifice of the minor papilla is wide open. (c) Normal ventral pancreas (and bile duct) after cannulating the main papilla. (d) Cannulation of the minor papilla showing the dorsal duct and terminal santorinicele. (e) Balloon dilatation of the santorinicele and minor papilla. (f) Free drainage of the dorsal duct after treatment.

ble. Treatment was benign; only one patient developed an exacerbation of pancreatitis after lithotripsy, responding to conservative treatment. It was possible to clear the duct of stones completely in only seven patients, but all were free of symptoms at a mean follow-up of 30 months. These data confirm the encouraging results of prior German and Belgian studies. Stone fragmentation has also been performed by a few groups using laser and electrohydraulic lithotripsy under direct vision using pancreatoscopes. Maier *et al.* [29]

(e)

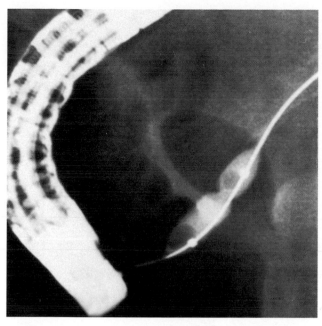

(f)

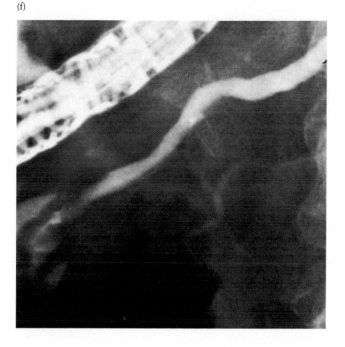

report the use of pulsed dye laser lithotripsy under fluoroscopic control, using an automatic stone tissue differentiation system. This system automatically switches off the laser on contact with tissue. Partial stone disintegration was achieved, making mechanical stone removal possible. It is clear that endoscopic and shockwave treatment of pancreatic ductal stones is a valuable technique in selected patients.

## Lessons from surgery

Lateral pancreaticojejunostomy (Peustow procedure) is commonly used for treatment of pain in patients with chronic pancreatitis and a dilated duct, on the assumption that obstruction is present. Results are usually claimed to be reasonably good. Markowitz *et al.* [30] report on an interesting case series of 15 patients with severe pain which persisted following pancreaticoje-junostomy. The causes included neuropathic changes, residual and evolving pancreatic and biliary duct obstruction, and unrecognized cancer. Good results were obtained in the majority of patients by re-operation, mostly by a Whipple-type resection of the pancreatic head. Traverso and Kozarek [31] also report on the use of the Whipple procedure in patients with chronic pancreatitis. Excellent results were obtained in 88% of 28 patients, while maintaining good endocrine function. The whole problem of choosing the best surgical procedure for patients with severe chronic pancreatitis is well discussed by Thirlby [32], commenting on the Traverso and Kozarek report [31].

## ERCP and therapy in children

Pancreatitis is not rare in children, and the same principles of diagnosis and treatment apply as in adults. The encouraging results of endoscopic therapy in six children reported by Kozarek *et al.* [33] are dwarfed by the experience of Guelrud *et al.* from Venezuela [34•]. They performed ERCP in 51 patients with recurrent pancreatitis aged 1–18 years. The cause was found in two-thirds of these cases, and endoscopic treatment was applied in 18. Fifteen (83%) had a favourable outcome and only mild complications were experienced. They conclude that endoscopic pancreatic therapy can eliminate the need for surgery in selected children, and that manipulation of the pancreatic duct is comparatively safe.

## ERCP as a cause of pancreatitis

Pancreatitis is by far the most common complication of diagnostic and therapeutic ERCP. Repeated duct manipulation and contrast injection are the most important aetiological factors. There has been much discussion concerning the relative safety of different contrast agents, with the assumption that low osmolality non-ionic contrast agents might be safer. Unfortunately, an excellent prospective randomized study by Sherman *et al.* [35••] shows that this is not the case. Sherman has also provided a comprehensive review of the causes of pancreatitis after ERCP and sphincterotomy [36], with helpful suggestions for prevention. It seems clear that the risk of pancreatitis after sphincterotomy is significantly higher in patients with sphincter of Oddi

(a)

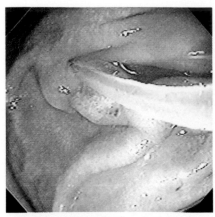

**Fig. 2.** Recurent pancreatitis after previous biliary sphincterotomy. (a) Cannulation of the stenosed biliary orifice. (b) Selective cannulation of the pancreatic orifice for manometry. (c) Wide-open biliary orifice after repeat sphincterotomy. (d) Insertion of a standard sphincterotome into the pancreatic orifice. (e) Pancreatic orifice after septotomy. (f) Insertion of a guide wire prior to stenting. (g) Temporary pancreatic stent.

(b)

(c)

(d)

(e)

(f)

(g)

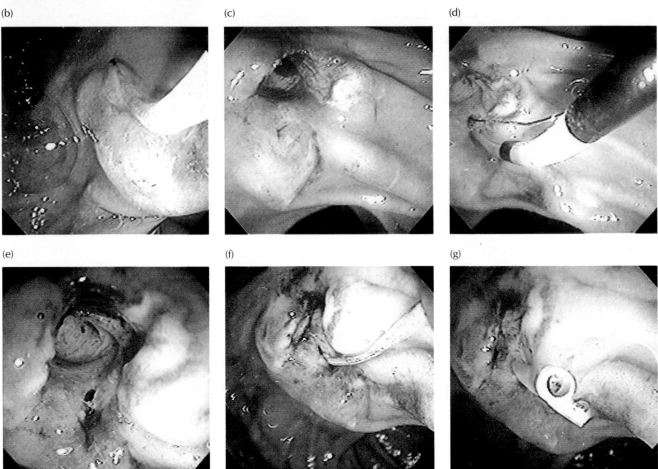

dysfunction [37•]. It has been suggested that this is related to residual pancreatic sphincter hypertension. Smithline *et al.* [38•] have tested this hypothesis. They performed a randomized study to see whether prophylactic stenting of the pancreatic duct after biliary sphincterotomy would reduce the incidence of pancreatitis in high-risk patients, i.e. those with sphincter of Oddi dysfunction, small common ducts, or after pre-cut sphincterotomy. Unfortunately it did not.

There is usually a delay of a few hours before pancreatitis develops after ERCP. For optimal patient management it would be helpful to be able to predict the onset of pancreatitis, or detect it in some way before symptoms develop. Nakae *et al.* [39] have shown that elevation of serum $\alpha_2$-macroglobulin-trypsin complex correlated better than standard enzymes with the presence of severe acute pancreatitis. Unfortunately, the elevation was not apparent before 5 h.

## Pancreatic cancer

From the endoscopist's perspective, the most interesting developments in the field of pancreatic cancer concern biliary stenting (discussed in a separate review in the *Annual*), and more precise staging and tissue diagnosis. Endosonography and targeted biopsy are gradually being accepted as useful clinical tools. Ductal brushing cytology has become easier with the development of hydrophilic guide wires and more sophisticated brush catheters. Results are good, but not perfect. Ferrari *et al.* [40] reported their experience with brush cytology of pancreaticobiliary strictures in 74 patients. Confirmation was obtained in two-thirds of the patients with pancreatic carcinoma, and there were no false-positives. Several groups have explored adjuvant methods such as flow cytometry. Ryan and Baldauf [41] showed that the addition of flow cytometry to routine cytology increased their sensitivity for the diagnosis of malignancy, but reduced the specificity. This problem of false-positive results markedly reduces the value of the technique, but other studies are justified. An additional finding of considerable interest was a greater survival in patients with pancreatic carcinoma who had a diploid cell population, as revealed by flow cytometry, compared with those with aneuploid brushings.

Endoscopic palliation of pancreatic carcinoma is usually synonymous with biliary stenting. There has been some discussion as to whether additional stenting of pancreatic duct obstruction might be helpful, for the relief of pain or improved digestion. Costamagna *et al.* [42•] have reported on an interesting group of eight patients with unresectable cancer of the pancreatic head associated with upstream dilatation of the duct and severe 'obstructive-type' pain. They were able to cross the obstruction with a stent without complications, and all patients but one were free of pain within 48 h. There was no clinical evidence of pancreatic stent clogging during follow-up. Nutritional status was not assessed.

## Conclusion

The original publications of 1994 have not been particularly helpful for endoscopists interested in pancreatic disease. The indications for endoscopic management remain unclear. However, there is an increasing groundswell of determination to develop and pursue the difficult objective and long-term studies which are needed. Careful reviews of this subject have been published this year by known experts in Seattle, Amsterdam and Milwaukee [43,44•,45]. Taken together, these provide an excellent statement of the 'state of the art', and provide a platform on which we can move gradually from art to science.

## References and recommended reading

Papers of particular interest, published within the annual period of review, have been highlighted as:
- of special interest
- of outstanding interest

1. Bozkurt T, Braun U, Leferink S, Gilly G, Lux G: **Comparison of pancreatic**
• **morphology and exocrine functional impairment in patients with chronic pancreatitis.** *Gut* 1994, **35**:1132–1136.
Remarkably good correlation between pancreatic exocrine function and pancreatography in patients with chronic pancreatitis. Diagnostic sensitivity of abdominal ultrasound and computed tomography was less. No patient with a normal pancreatogram had functional impairment.

2. Wiersema MJ, Hawes RH, Lehman GA, Kochman ML, Sherman S, Kopecky
•• KK: **Prospective evaluation of endoscopic ultrasonography and endoscopic retrograde cholangiopancreatography in patients with chronic abdominal pain of suspected pancreatic origin.** *Endoscopy* 1993, **25**:555–564.
An important attempt to define the endoscopic ultrasonographic features of chronic pancreatitis in 30 patients, in comparison with control volunteers. Endoscopic ultrasonography was more sensitive than pancreatography in patients with early chronic pancreatitis.

3. Takehara Y, Ichijo K, Tooyama N, Kodaira N, Yamamoto H, Tatami M, *et*
•• *al.*: **Breath-hold MR cholangiopancreatography with a long-echo-train fast spin-echo sequence and a surface coil in chronic pancreatitis.** *Radiology* 1994, **192**:73–78.
Thirty-nine patients with chronic pancreatitis were examined with a breath-hold fast spin-echo sequence, employing an echo-train length of 32 and a surface coil. MRCP usually visualized the pancreatic duct. Correlation with ERCP was good, particularly in the case of strictures and duct filling defects.

4. Ammann R, Muellhaupt B, Meyenberger C, Heitz P: **Alcoholic nonprogres-**
•• **sive chronic pancreatitis: prospective long-term study of a large cohort with alcoholic acute pancreatitis (1976–1992).** *Pancreas* 1994, **9**:365–373.
Remarkable long-term follow-up study of patients with alcoholic acute pancreatitis showing that almost a quarter did not progress (with no calcification, duct dilatation, or exocrine insufficiency) and lost their pain spontaneously. These results challenge the 'burning out' theory of lasting pain relief, and emphasize that the pathological mechanisms of pain in chronic pancreatitis are still ill-defined.

5. Lowenfels AB, Maisonneuve P, Cavallini G, Ammann RW, Lankisch PG,
•• Andersen JR, *et al.*: **Prognosis of chronic pancreatitis: an international multicenter study.** *Am J Gastroenterol* 1994, **89**:1467–1471.
Survival analysis among 2015 subjects with chronic pancreatitis treated in six countries. Older age and smoking and drinking were major predictors of mortality. There was no survival advantage of patients who had received surgical treatment.

6. Layer P, Yamamoto H, Kalthoff L, Clain JE, Bakken LJ, DiMagno EP: **The**
• **different courses of early- and late-onset idiopathic and alcoholic chronic pancreatitis.** *Gastroenterology* 1994, **107**:1481–1487.
Long-term follow-up from the Mayo Clinic, comparing patients with idiopathic chronic pancreatitis with those with alcohol-induced disease. Idiopathic pancreatitis had an equal sex distribution, and a much slower rate of calcification compared with alcohol-induced disease. Patients with early onset idiopathic pancreatitis had a more severe course than those whose disease presented late.

7. Chari ST, Singer MV: **The problem of classification and staging of chronic pancreatitis. Proposals based on current knowledge of its natural history.** *Scand J Gastroenterol* 1994, **29**:949–960.
Review of the problems in classifying chronic pancreatitis with a proposal for staging alcohol-induced disease.

8. Bradley EL: **A clinically based classification system for acute pancreatitis.**
• *Arch Surg* 1993, **128**:586–590.
Results of a consensus conference on classification for acute pancreatitis, based on standard clinical findings and investigations.

9. Steinberg W, Tenner S: **Acute pancreatitis.** *N Engl J Med* 1994, **330**:1198–1210.
Detailed and comprehensive review of acute pancreatitis epidemiology, causes, diagnosis, natural history and treatment. The review has 184 references.

10. Neoptolemos JP, Stonelake P, Radley S: **Endoscopic sphincterotomy for**
• **acute pancreatitis.** *Hepatogastroenterology* 1993, **40**:550–555.

Careful review of the role of urgent endoscopic intervention in patients with severe pancreatitis.

11. Lai ECS, Lo CM: **Acute pancreatitis: the role of ERCP in 1994**. *Endoscopy* 1994, **26**:488–492.
Extensive review with 54 references on the role of ERCP in diagnosis and management of patients with acute pancreatitis.

12. Binmoeller KF, Seifert H, Soehendra N: **Endoscopic pseudocyst drainage: A new instrument for simplified cystoenterostomy [letter]**. *Gastrointest Endosc* 1994, **40**:112.
A retractable injection catheter containing a diathermy wire inside a 7 F gauge sheath.

13. Howell DA, Holbrook RF, Bosco JJ, Muggia RA, Biber BP: **Endoscopic needle localization of pancreatic pseudocysts before transmural drainage**. *Gastrointest Endosc* 1993, **39**:693–698.
Endoscopic pseudocyst drainage was performed in eight patients. The correct point of puncture was determined by initial endoscopic needling of the pseudocysts for catheter injection.

14. Funnell JC, Bornman PC, Krige JEJ, Beningfield SJ, Terblanche J: **Endoscopic drainage of traumatic pancreatic pseudocyst**. *Br J Surg* 1994, **81**:879–881.
Endoscopic drainage of pseudocysts in five patients after abdominal trauma. There were no complications, and only one patient required an operation.

15. Saeed ZA, Ramirez FC, Hepps KC: **Endoscopic stent placement for internal and external pancreatic fistulas**. *Gastroenterology* 1993, **105**:1213–1217.
Five patients with pancreatic fistulas resistant to standard medical therapy were treated successfully with ductal stents.

16. Gane E, Fata'ar S, Hamilton I: **Management of a persistent pancreatic fistula secondary to a ruptured pseudocyst with endoscopic insertion of an expandable metal stent**. *Endoscopy* 1994, **26**:254–256.
Successful use of a Strecker metal stent in a patient with a pancreatic fistula resistant to prior treatment with a plastic endoprosthesis.

17. Karanjia ND, Widdison AL, Leung F, Alvarez C, Lutrin FJ, Reber HA:
• **Compartment syndrome in experimental chronic obstructive pancreatitis: effect of decompressing the main pancreatic duct**. *Br J Surg* 1994, **81**:259–264.
Studies in a cat model of chronic obstructive pancreatitis demonstrating that duct decompression prevented the increase in main duct and interstitial pressure during secretion, and restored blood flow. These studies suggest a rationale for pancreatic duct drainage treatments.

18. Ashley SW, Sherman S, Reber HA: **Endoscopic measurement of pancreatic blood flow**. *Gastrointest Clin North Am* 1994, **4**:369–382.
Discussion of the importance of pancreatic blood flow in chronic pancreatitis. Preliminary results of measuring the pancreatic blood flow using $H_2$ gas clearance, using an electrode passed into the pancreatic duct at ERCP. Preliminary results in a limited number of patients with painful chronic pancreatitis reveal quite low basal pancreatic blood flows.

19. Cavallini G, Rigo L, Bovo P, Brunori MP, Angelini GP, Vaona B, *et al.*: **Abnormal US response of main pancreatic duct after secretion stimulation in patients with acute pancreatitis of different etiology**. *J Clin Gastroenterol* 1994, **18**:298–303.
Evaluation of the secretin-stimulated ultrasound test in 21 controls and 34 patients with pancreatitis. Most patients with recurrent idiopathic pancreatitis, and those associated with pancreas divisum, had an abnormal test suggesting sphincter dysfunction.

20. Vestergaard H, Kruse A, Rokkjaer M, Frobert O, Thommesen P, Funch-Jensen P: **Endoscopic manometry of the sphincter of Oddi and the pancreatic and biliary ducts in patients with chronic pancreatitis**. *Scand J Gastroenterol* 1994, **29**:188–192.
Biliary and pancreatic sphincter pressures were measured in 15 patients with chronic pancreatitis. Eleven patients had abnormal studies, which correlated with an increase in pancreatic duct pressure.

21. Laugier R: **Dynamic endoscopic manometry in response to secretin in patients with chronic pancreatitis**. *Endoscopy* 1994, **26**:222–227.
Endoscopic manometry of the sphincter of Oddi in the main pancreatic duct was performed before and after intravenous injection of secretin in 15 control patients and 19 patients with chronic pancreatitis. Secretin significantly but transiently enhanced the duct pressure in controls, whereas chronic pancreatitis patients had an elevated basal duct pressure, and manometric evidence of sphincter of Oddi dyskinesia. The secretin-induced duct pressure was also elevated and more sustained in chronic pancreatitis patients compared with controls.

22. Guelrud M: **How good is sphincter of Oddi manometry for chronic pancreatitis?** *Endoscopy* 1994, **26**:265–267.
Authoritative review of the role of sphincter of Oddi dysfunction in causing or perpetuating chronic pancreatitis.

23. Eisen G, Schutz S, Metzler D, Baillie J, Cotton PB: **Santorinicele: new evidence for obstruction in pancreas divisum**. *Gastrointest Endosc* 1994, **40**:73–76.
Four patients with pancreatitis associated with pancreas divisum, and focal dilatation at the termination of dorsal duct. Excellent results with endoscopic treatment.

24. Coleman SD, Eisen GM, Troughton AB, Cotton PB: **Endoscopic treatment**
• **in pancreas divisum**. *Am J Gastroenterol* 1994, **89**:1152–1155.
Review of endoscopic stenting with and without sphincterotomy at the minor papilla in 34 patients with pancreas divisum and pain or pancreatitis. Significant improvement in pain scores were found in patients with acute recurrent pancreatitis, and in those with chronic pancreatitis.

25. Alvarez C, Robert M, Sherman S, Reber HA: **Histologic changes after stenting of the pancreatic duct**. *Arch Surg* 1994, **129**:765–768.
Single case report indicating severe histologic inflammatory changes in the duct and parenchyma after endoscopic stent drainage, with normal prior pancreatography. This case confirms previous reports of induced abnormalities in the pancreatic duct in man and dog.

26. Ikenberry SO, Sherman S, Hawes RH, Smith M, Lehman GA: **The occlusion**
• **rate of pancreatic stents**. *Gastrointest Endosc* 1994, **40**:611–613.
Standard assessment of the patency of 146 pancreatic ductal stents. Overall, 50% were occluded within 6 weeks, and all stents left in place for more than 9 weeks were occluded.

27. Kozarek RA, Ball TJ. Patterson DJ, Brandabur JJ, Traverso LW, Raltz S:
• **Endoscopic pancreatic duct sphincterotomy: indications, technique, and analysis of results**. *Gastrointest Endosc* 1994, **40**:592–598.
Review of endoscopic pancreatic duct sphincterotomy on 56 patients. Variable indications and combination treatments make it difficult to assess the role of sphincterotomy alone.

28. Van der Hul R, Plaisier P, Jeekel J, Terpstra O, den Toom R, Bruining H:
• **Extracorporeal shock-wave lithotripsy of pancreatic duct stones: immediate and long-term results**. *Endoscopy* 1994, **26**:573–578.
Seventeen patients with endoscopically unextractable stones in chronic pancreatitis were treated with extracorporeal shockwave lithotripsy. Complete stone removal was achieved in only seven, but all were free of symptoms subsequently. No severe complications occurred.

29. Maier M, Jakobs R, Kohler B, Riemann JF: **Fluoroscopically guided laser lithotripsy of a pancreatic duct stone**. *Endoscopy* 1994, **26**:247–249.
Successful treatment of an impacted pancreatic duct stone using a pulsed dye laser lithotriptor under fluoroscopic control. The laser had an automatic stone tissue differentiation system which automatically switches off the laser on contact with tissue.

30. Markowitz JS, Rattner DW, Warshaw AL: **Failure of symptomatic relief after pancreaticojejunal decompression for chronic pancreatitis**. *Arch Surg* 1994, **129**:374–380.
A case series of 15 patients with severe pain associated with chronic pancreatitis persisting following pancreaticojejunostomy. Causes included neuropathic changes, residual and evolving pancreatic and biliary duct obstruction, and unrecognized pancreatic cancer. Good results were obtained in the majority of patients, most of whom had a Whipple-type resection of the pancreatic head.

31. Traverso LW, Kozarek RA: **The Whipple procedure for severe complications of chronic pancreatitis**. *Arch Surg* 1993, **128**:1047–1053.
Twenty-eight patients with chronic pancreatitis treated with the Whipple procedure. Excellent results were obtained in 88%, while maintaining good pancreatic endocrine function.

32. Thirlby RC: **Choosing the best surgical procedure for patients with severe chronic pancreatitis**. *Gastroenterology* 1994, **107**:897–898.
Thoughtful review of a paper reporting the use of the Whipple procedure for severe complications of chronic pancreatitis.

33. Kozarek RA, Christie D, Barclay G: **Endoscopic therapy of pancreatitis in the pediatric population**. *Gastrointest Endosc* 1993, **39**:665–669.
Encouraging results of therapeutic ERCP in six children with pancreatitis.

34. Guelrud M, Mujica C, Jaen D, Plaz J, Arias J: **The role of ERCP in the**
• **diagnosis and treatment of idiopathic recurrent pancreatitis in children and adolescents**. *Gastrointest Endosc* 1994, **40**:428–436.
ERCP was performed in 51 children with recurrent pancreatitis. Good results were obtained after endoscopic therapy in 18 patients with ductal abnormalities. There were no severe complications.

35. Sherman S, Hawes RH, Rathgaber SW, Uzer MF, Smith MT, Khusro QE, *et*
•• *al.*: **Post-ERCP pancreatitis: randomized, prospective study comparing a low- and high-osmolality contrast agent**. *Gastrointest Endosc* 1994, **40**:422–427.
Randomized study of ERCP-induced pancreatitis in 690 patients showing no difference in the risk comparing a low-osmolality, non-ionic contrast agent with a standard high-osmolality, ionic contrast agent.

36. Sherman S: **ERCP and endoscopic sphincterotomy-induced pancreatitis**. *Am J Gastroenterol* 1994, **89**:303–305.
An editorial reviewing the causes of pancreatitis after ERCP and endoscopic sphincterotomy, with suggestions for prevention.

37. Chen YK, Foliente RL, Santoro MJ, Walter MH, Collen MJ: **Endoscopic**
• **sphincterotomy-induced pancreatitis: increased risk associated with nondilated bile ducts and sphincter of Oddi dysfunction**. *Am J Gastroenterol* 1994, **89**:327–333.
Prospective study of 210 patients undergoing sphincterotomy. The risk of pancreatitis was significantly higher (12.5%) in patients with sphincter of Oddi dysfunction. The rate of all complications combined was significantly correlated with small duct diameter.

38. Smithline A, Silverman W, Rogers D, Nisi R, Wiersema M, Jamidar P, *et al.*:
• **Effect of prophylactic main pancreatic duct stenting on the incidence of biliary endoscopic sphincterotomy-induced pancreatitis in high-risk patients**. *Gastrointest Endosc* 1993, **39**:652–657.
Randomized study showing that prophylactic stenting of the main pancreatic duct after biliary sphincterotomy did not decrease the incidence of pancreatitis in high-risk patients: those with sphincter of Oddi dysfunction, small common ducts, or pre-cut sphincterotomy.

39. Nakae Y, Hayakawa T, Kondo T, Shibata T, Kitagawa M, Sakai Y, *et al.*: **Serum $\alpha_2$-macroglobulin-trypsin complex and early recognition of severe acute pancreatitis after endoscopic retrograde pancreatography**, *J Gastroenterol Hepatol* 1994, **9**:272–276.
Serum $\alpha_2$-macroglobulin-trypsin complex measurement correlated better with severe acute pancreatitis than standard enzymes, but elevations did not occur earlier.

40. Ferrari AP, Lichtenstein DR, Slivka A, Chang C, Carr-Locke DL: **Brush cytology during ERCP for the diagnosis of biliary and pancreatic malignancies**. *Gastrointest Endosc* 1994, **40**:140–145.
Report of 74 patients with pancreatic or biliary strictures undergoing ERCP brush cytology. Confirmation was obtained in 65% of patients with pancreatic carcinoma, with no false-positives.

41. Ryan ME, Baldauf MC: **Comparison of flow cytometry for DNA content and brush cytology for detection of malignancy in pancreaticobiliary strictures**. *Gastrointest Endosc* 1994, **40**:133–139.
The addition of flow cytometry to standard cytology increased the sensitivity for the diagnosis of cancer in patients with malignant pancreatic or biliary strictures, but substantially reduced the specificity.

42. Costamagna G, Gabbrielli A, Mutignani M, Perri V, Crucitti F: **Treatment**
• **of 'obstructive' pain by endoscopic drainage in patients with pancreatic head carcinoma**. *Gastrointest Endosc* 1993, **39**:774–777.
Stenting of the pancreatic duct in eight patients with cancer and upstream duct dilatation with excellent pain relief.

43. Kozarek RA: **Chronic pancreatitis in 1994: Is there a role for endoscopic treatment?** *Endoscopy* 1994, **26**:625–628.
Review of endoscopic treatment in chronic pancreatitis by one of its protagonists, concluding that endoscopic therapy is now established in a subset of patients, and calling for comparative studies against other treatment modalities.

44. Huibregtse K, Smits ME: **Endoscopic management of diseases of the**
• **pancreas**. *Am J Gastroenterol* 1994, **89**:S66–S77.
Authoritative review of endoscopic therapy of acute and chronic pancreatitis emphasizing the need for more studies to define the subgroups of patients most likely to benefit.

45. Bedford RA, Howerton DH, Geenen JE: **The current role of ERCP in the management of benign pancreatic disease**. *Endoscopy* 1994, **26**:113–119.
Careful discussion of different forms of therapeutic endoscopy for pancreatic diseases, emphasizing the need for randomized control trials and suggesting that these techniques should currently be offered only to a very select group of patients by endoscopists well trained in therapeutic pancreatic endoscopy, in established research protocols.

Professor Peter B. Cotton, Director, Digestive Disease Center, Medical University of South Carolina, 171 Ashley Avenue, 910 CSB, Charleston, SC 29425-2220, USA.

# Endoscopy and gallstones

## Alan N. Barkun

Division of Gastroenterology, The Montreal General Hospital, McGill University, Montreal, Quebec, Canada

## Introduction

The place of endoscopy in the management of gallstone disease has always been dependent upon ongoing technological evolutions in the fields of endoscopy, surgery and radiology. Unfortunately, proper comparative assessments of new technologies have often been hindered by their premature widespread, and sometimes inappropriate, diffusion. The following review discusses the validity of the published data in 1994 and attempts to define the present role of endoscopy in gallstone disease.

## Natural history and pathophysiology

A better understanding of the pathophysiology and natural history of choledocholithiasis is fundamental in the selection of patients for treatment, and could possibly help identify preventive measures. Unfortunately, only a disappointingly small number of studies addressed these issues in 1994.

Vracko et al. [1] found that levels of trypsin in bile were highest in patients with mobile common bile duct (CBD) stones or following the removal of obstructing CBD stones. Normal levels of trypsin were seen in patients with cholelithiasis or stones obstructing the lower CBD. The authors therefore suggested that retrograde propulsive activity of the sphincter of Oddi may play a role in the occurrence of CBD stones. The stones may have damaged the sphincter, however, and causation therefore remains unproven.

Wetter et al. [2••] described differences in outer membrane characteristics between gallstone-associated and normal gut bacterial flora. Scanning electron microscopy demonstrated the presence of bacteria in pigmented and mixed stones but not cholesterol stones. The presence and absence of certain bacterial fimbriae, thought to play a role in adherence to host tissues, were characterized. Interestingly, the bacteria isolated from the stones were discordant with those identified from the blood and bile in septic patients. The investigators postulated that an initial subclinical infection is required, particularly for the formation of brown pigment and mixed stones. These bacteria possess the ability to survive in bile and in the stone matter for years. Different bacterial species are responsible for later clinical sepsis.

A study which assessed a cohort of 109 patients using intraoperative cholangiography identified 12 patients with CBD stones [3••]. At endoscopic retrograde cholangiopancreatography (ERCP), performed 4–96 days later, duct stones were found in only four patients, suggesting spontaneous passage of the majority (assuming no false-positive intraoperative cholangiographies). CBD stones in six out of eight additional patients also appeared to pass on their own. Further research is required to predict which stones will pass spontaneously without causing symptoms.

The relationship between sludge and symptomatic gallbladder or bile duct stones requires further characterization as evidenced by a case series of three patients in whom CBD sludge may have caused suppurative cholangitis, although stone migration prior to ERCP could not be ruled out [4].

### Microbiology of the biliary tract

Leung et al. [5•] cultured the bile and blood of 579 patients with ductal stones. Associated bacteraemia was noted in 121 patients (21%). Pharmacokinetic studies of the hepatic biliary excretion profiles of five antibiotics commonly used for cholangitis, coupled to in vitro susceptibility testing, were carried out. In an obstructed biliary system, only ciprofloxacillin was excreted in bile (at levels equivalent to 20% of the peak serum value) confirming the pivotal need for early biliary decompression in addition to appropriate antibiotic coverage. Clinical trials are in progress to confirm the apparent clinical superiority of ciprofloxacillin for active cholangitis or prophylaxis.

---

### Abbreviations

CBD—common bile duct; ERCP—endoscopic retrograde cholangiopancreatography; MRCP—magnetic resonance cholangiopancreatography; Nd:YAG—neodymium yttrium aluminium garnet.

Niederau *et al.* [6**] reported on a randomized prospective trial assessing the benefit of prophylactic intravenous cefotaxime administration in patients undergoing therapeutic or 'complicated' diagnostic ERCP. None of the 50 patients receiving cefotaxime developed a bacteraemia with or without sepsis compared with eight out of 50 patients (16%) who did not receive antibiotics (*P* < 0.01). The results of the study are confounded in the control group by four patients who developed cholangitis or sepsis (all within 1–3 days of the ERCP) because of unrelieved biliopancreatic obstruction or persistent CBD stones. Furthermore, there was no blinding as the control group did not receive a placebo. Nonetheless, all patients had serial blood cultures performed for 2 h following the procedure, and all were followed for at least 3 days. The data therefore appear valid and support the use of prophylactic antibiotics in this endoscopic setting as one cannot be assured of complete biliary drainage at the start of the procedure (Figs 1 and 2).

## The approach to a patient suspected of choledocholithiasis prior to laparoscopic cholecystectomy

The introduction of laparoscopic cholecystectomy has resulted in an early 28% increase in surgical procedures [7**] and has also caused, correctly or incorrectly, a reappraisal of the treatment of choledocholithiasis. In a recent audit from New Zealand, 72% of 152 general surgeons had deliberately abandoned a policy of routine intraoperative cholangiography for one of selective cholangiography in the laparoscopic era [8•]. This change in clinical practice was forced by the limited

availability of specialized expertise and sophisticated technology rather than being based on scientific evidence. Such considerations also affect the applicability of published results where the expertise and equipment available at the study centres may not reflect that present in the reader's practice. For example, a very active laparoscopic biliary institution reported a limited role for ERCP in bile duct stone management prior to cholecystectomy [9•], yet the ERCP cannulation and stone clearance rates were 76% and 54%, respectively. These results are much inferior to many other published endoscopic experiences which reached different conclusions [10**,11,12•,13,14].

Recent reviews on this topic have highlighted the difficulties in identifying an optimal approach at the present time while summarizing the performance of specific endoscopic and laparoscopic CBD stone removal techniques [15**,16,17•,18•,19].

There are many possible approaches when presented with a patient with symptomatic gallbladder stones suspected of choledocholithiasis prior to laparoscopic cholecystectomy (Fig. 3). The three main competing approaches are selective preoperative ERCP versus intraoperative cholangiography followed, if positive, by laparoscopic CBD exploration or postoperative ERCP.

There are many reports in the 1994 literature describing the results of a policy of selective preoperative ERCP [10**,11,12•,13,14]. One describes a systematic clinical strategy adopted at the time of the introduction of laparoscopic cholecystectomy [10**]. The results show that approximately 5–10% of all patients scheduled for surgery underwent preoperative ERCP for a CBD stone yield which varied between 45% and 65%. Overall, the

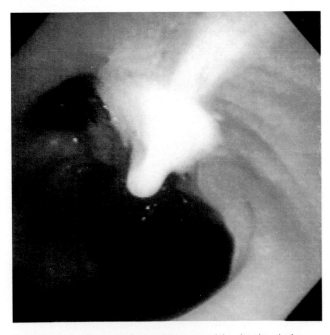

**Fig. 1.** Endoscopic view of pus coming out of the distal end of a biliary stent in a patient with cholangitis.

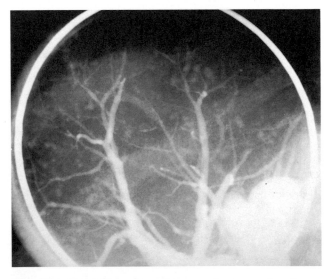

**Fig. 2.** Magnified radiographic appearance of numerous hepatic microabscesses in a patient with ascending cholangitis undergoing endoscopic retrograde cholangiopancreatography (ERCP).

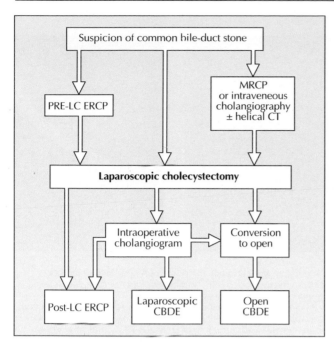

**Fig. 3.** Different reported approaches to the management of suspected choledocholithiasis in patients scheduled for laparoscopic cholecystectomy (LC), and the list is not complete! ERCP = endoscopic retrograde cholangiopancreatography; MRCP = magnetic resonance cholangiopancreatography; CT = computed tomography; CBDE = common bile duct exploration.

performance of ERCP was similar, with a 90–95% success rate of endoscopic stone extraction and a 2–10% complication rate. The overall CBD stone prevalence rate varied from 4% to 6% with one notable exception where 21% of all patients were found to have choledocholithiasis [12•]. This latter report may have reflected a selection bias with more ill patients receiving earlier medical care in the British health-care system [12•].

Some studies reported the use of intravenous cholangiography [20,21], which proved unnecessary in low-risk patients with a yield of only 1.8% [21]. Voyles *et al.* [9•] used, as others have suggested, a multi-tier stratification of patients at risk for CBD stones where low-risk patients did not undergo cholangiography, high-risk patients underwent preoperative ERCP or intraoperative cholangiography, and patients at intermediate risk could receive some intraoperative intervention. This approach theoretically decreases the number of negative ERCP examinations, and replaces them with a less morbid intraoperative cholangiography. As the difficulty resides in defining a cut-off between the high- and medium-risk groups, models of CBD stone prediction may be helpful [10••]. Voyles *et al.* [9•] also noted, with increased laparoscopic experience, a drop in the number of ERCP examinations performed (which displayed only a modest success rate in this study) and a corresponding increase in intraoperative interventions. The retained stone rate with up

to 45 months follow-up was 2.8 per thousand, a surprisingly small number compared to most other published series.

A non-randomized, prospective analysis of two patient cohorts that were referred to two units was performed [3••]. Unit A carried out selective preoperative ERCP for patients at 'very high' risk of choledocholithiasis and routine intraoperative cholangiography. Unit B only performed selective preoperative ERCP. In unit A, ERCP was performed in seven out of 114 patients (6%) and stones were found and successfully removed in five patients. Twelve patients were found to have CBD stones at intraoperative cholangiography (successfully performed in 98 out of 109 patients), and spontaneous passage occurred in eight. The remaining four patients underwent successful endoscopic extraction postoperatively. In unit B, ERCP was carried out in 76 out of 236 patients (32%) and common bile duct stones were found in 47 (62%). They were successfully removed endoscopically in all but five patients who went on to have open cholecystectomy. Eight patients treated in unit A were found to have CBD stones at intraoperative cholangiography, with spontaneous passage (before postoperative ERCP) in six. There were no ERCP-related complications, and the operative complication rates were low and comparable in both groups. Only one patient returned (in unit B) with a retained stone. Both approaches with their associated high procedural success and low complication rates therefore appear feasible. The study underlines the difficulties of setting up a randomized trial assessing this clinical problem; the numbers of patients required is large because of the low rate of outcomes (complication, retained stones), the treatment arms need to be many and the technologies studied may quickly be outdated, in addition to the problems attributable to the acceptability of randomization.

Although still limited in availability [22•], selected laparoscopists are reporting excellent success rates (> 90%) in achieving clearance of duct stones at surgery [19,23•,24,25•]. Unfortunately, adequate comparison with ERCP in some of these studies is not available because of its modest performance [9•,24]. There is no doubt that increased experience, and sophistication, of the equipment will spread the use of this technology.

One group reported its experience with intraoperative ERCP [26] but the poor quality of the fluoroscopy, unfamiliar surroundings with suboptimal availability of endoscopic equipment, limitations in patient positioning and the difficulty in scheduling, coupled to the high success rate of postoperative ERCP, limit the use of this approach in most centres.

(a)        (b)        (c)        (d)

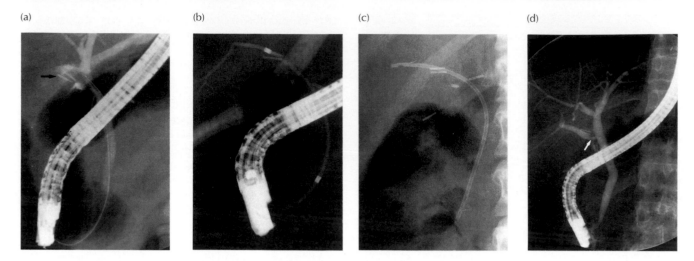

**Fig. 4.** Endoscopic treatment of a bile leak originating from transection of an anomalous right intrahepatic duct draining into the common hepatic duct following laparoscopic cholecystectomy. (a) Bile leak originating from the transected right intrahepatic duct (arrow) which failed to be repaired at a repeat laparotomy. (b) Selective cannulation of the disrupted duct with proximal opacification. (c) A 7 F, 9-cm biliary polyethylene stent was inserted across the disruption with the proximal tip in the anomalous right intrahepatic duct. (d) The stent was removed after 6 weeks with successful healing of the leak. A low-grade residual stricture with mild proximal dilatation of the right intrahepatic duct is present (arrow). This dilatation has not progressed, and the patient remains asymptomatic with normal liver enzymes 18 months after stent removal.

## The role of ERCP following cholecystectomy

Numerous reports have described the role of ERCP following laparoscopic cholecystectomy [10••,11, 12•,13,14,19,27–31,32•]. The success rate at stone removal has been close to 100% in many studies. The role of ERCP in the postlaparoscopic cholecystectomy setting is not limited to CBD stone removal. Indeed, ERCP has been confirmed as the treatment of choice for postoperative biliary leaks [28–31,32•] (Figs 4 and 5). Stent insertion, sphincterotomy or both have all been used successfully. The ease of insertion of a 10 F stent in the absence of a sphincterotomy with its associated lower risk of bleeding and perforation suggests this approach as initial treatment in the absence of comparative trials (Fig. 6). The duration of stent insertion (or nasobiliary drain) is unknown, but brief periods (as short as 3 days) have been reported to be successful [28].

A full discussion on the treatment of complex bile duct injuries is beyond the scope of this review. Reports with a short follow-up highlighted the common need for a multidisciplinary approach which yielded variable success rates [30,32•].

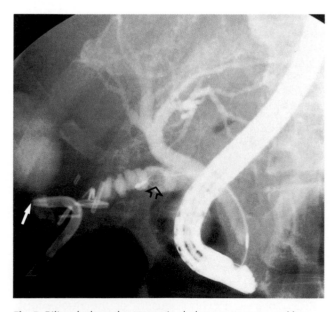

**Fig. 5.** Biliary leak postlaparoscopic cholecystectomy treated by percutaneous drainage of a large biloma (the solid arrow indicates the catheter tip near the area of dye extravasation). At endoscopic retrograde cholangiopancreatography (ERCP), a cystic duct stone acting as a ball valve and causing intermittent leakage from the proximal end of the cystic duct was removed with a basket (open arrow).

## Predictors of choledocholithiasis

As discussed above, about four out of every 10 cholangiographies will be negative using accepted criteria [15••]. A number of reports in 1994 attempted to identify better clinical predictors of a CBD stone.

A prospective analysis of 1746 patients undergoing laparoscopic cholecystectomy showed that a raised level of serum bilirubin (34–86 μmol/l) and amylase occurred in 25% and 4% of patients, respectively, with acute calculous cholecystitis in the absence of any CBD or pancreatic anomalies [33]. This finding was much more unusual in chronic calculous cholecystitis (2.9 and

0.7%, respectively). Recent CBD stone passage could not be ruled out.

Patients with gallstone pancreatitis who exhibit persistent hyperamylasaemia or hyperbilirubinaemia should be suspected of carrying a CBD stone [34].

Cystic duct size at ERCP (visualized in 118 out of 168 patients) was found to be significantly greater in patients with CBD stones with or without gallbladder stones when compared to patients with cholelithiasis alone [35].

Based on previously reported clinical criteria [15••], a study examined results from 139 patients prior to or following laparoscopic cholecystectomy in whom there existed a suspicion of choledocholithiasis [10••]. Using multivariate analysis, four independent predictors of a CBD stone at ERCP were identified using a database of clinical parameters and ERCP results. These included age > 55 years, an elevated bilirubin level > 30 μmol/l and the presence of CBD dilatation or choledocholithiasis at ultrasonography. These predictors were prospectively validated in a separate series of 49 patients. The logistic regression equation was derived only from data on patients with a suspicion of CBD stone which explains why patients with no predictors

in the model still had an 18% probability of choledocholithiasis (Figs 7 and 8).

## New imaging modalities for choledocholithiasis

Endoscopic ultrasonography was found to be an excellent imaging test for choledocholithiasis [36••]. It was superior to both ultrasonography and computed tomography with a 97% sensitivity and negative predictive value, and 100% specificity and positive predictive value when studied in 62 consecutive patients with suspected choledocholithiasis [36••]. In two patients, CBD stones seen on endoscopic ultrasonography were missed on the initial ERCP cholangiogram. Because the maximal depth display of this technique is 5–7 cm, its performance is not as good in the detection of intrahepatic and perihilar stones. Limitations of this very promising technique also include its significant operator dependency and availability of the equipment.

Intraoperative laparoscopic ultrasonography has been well described [37–41,42•]. In a prospective study of 100 consecutive patients, it displayed a sensitivity of 100% and specificity of 98% [42•]. This technique

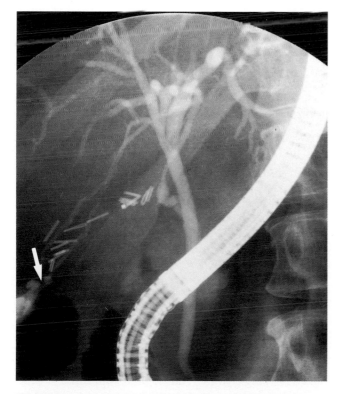

**Fig. 6.** Extravasation of dye from a duct of Luschka leak into the gallbladder bed (arrow) in a patient following laparoscopic cholecystectomy. A 10 F, 9-cm polyethylene stent was inserted without a sphincterotomy. Following successful healing, the stent was removed 2 weeks later.

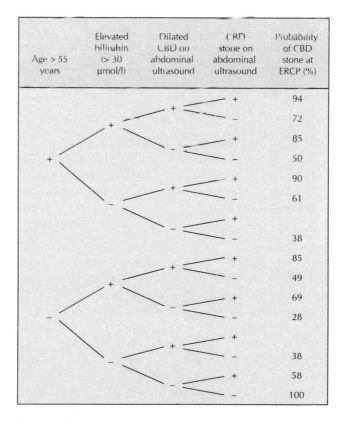

| Age > 55 years | Elevated bilirubin (> 30 μmol/l) | Dilated CBD on abdominal ultrasound | CBD stone on abdominal ultrasound | Probability of CBD stone at ERCP (%) |
|---|---|---|---|---|
| | | | + | 94 |
| | | + | – | 72 |
| | + | | + | 85 |
| | | – | – | 50 |
| + | | | + | 90 |
| | | + | – | 61 |
| | – | | | |
| | | – | | 38 |
| | | | + | 85 |
| | + | + | – | 49 |
| | | | + | 69 |
| – | | – | – | 28 |
| | | + | + | |
| | – | + | – | 38 |
| | | | + | 58 |
| | | – | – | 100 |

**Fig. 7.** Probabilities of common bile duct (CBD) stone at endoscopic retrograde cholangiopancreatography (ERCP) depending on the presence or absence of four independent predictors. These were identified using logistic regression analysis for patients in whom there exists some suspicion of choledocholithiasis prior to laparoscopic cholecystectomy.

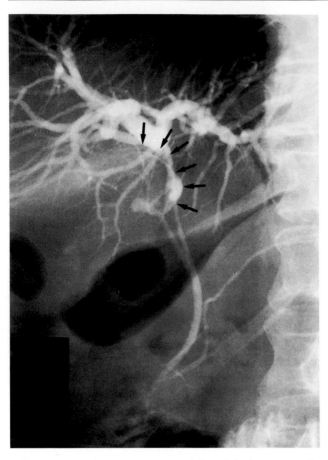

**Fig. 8.** Mirizzi syndrome in a patient with hyperbilirubinaemia and symptomatic cholelithiasis undergoing preoperative endoscopic retrograde cholangiopancreatography (ERCP). Note the large impacted cystic duct stone (arrows) compressing the common bile duct with resulting proximal intrahepatic bile duct dilatation.

performed better than intraoperative cholangiography (75% and 99%) while adding a shorter time to the operation (5.4 versus 16.4 min) [42•]. These data require confirmation as this technique is also very operator dependent.

Three-dimensional cholangiography with helical computed tomography was also studied with promising preliminary results [43,44•]. The use of intravenous cholangiographic dye and the lack of opacification in patients with elevated bilirubin may, however, limit its applicability.

Finally, a preliminary report described 10 patients with confirmed CBD stones who were studied with magnetic resonance cholangiopancreatography (MRCP) [45•]. MRCP yielded a sensitivity of 100%. A larger, blinded observer study of patients with and without CBD stones is now under way (Barkun *et al.*, personal communication). The advantages of this technique include the avoidance of contrast administration and the lack of operator dependency (Fig. 9).

## Advances in the endoscopic treatment of choledocholithiasis

Although evidence for significant long-term complications of endoscopic sphincterotomy is sparse [46], some authors have encouraged the preservation of the sphincter of Oddi, especially in younger patients. MacMathuna *et al.* [47••] presented preliminary data on endoscopic sphincteroplasty, a procedure whereby the sphincter of Oddi is dilated endoscopically with a balloon (with or without adjuvant pharmacologic relaxation) prior to stone or fragment removal with a balloon or basket (Fig. 10). Stones measuring 1.5–2 cm were removed after intracorporeal mechanical lithotripsy. Four of the 32 patients (13%) assessed in this study had CBD stones measuring more than 20 mm and were excluded [47••]. Successful balloon dilatation was carried out in 22 of the remaining 28 patients (79%). Papillotomy or stent insertion for a variety of reasons were required in the remaining six patients. Pancreatitis in one patient (4%) was the only complication. In a subsequent correspondence [48], the same group of investigators reported a 75% success rate in over 100 patients treated. This technique represents a novel and promising alternative to conventional endoscopic treatment of CBD stones. Caution should be exercised, however, before adopting any unproven technology (based on uncontrolled studies), particularly when the existing gold standard is excellent and has stood the test of time. Critical questions which need to be addressed include the applicability of this technique (perhaps limited to few and small CBD stones), the complication rates related to lithotripsy and the morbidity and cost of repeated sessions which may be required to complete CBD clearance or necessitated by recurrent stone migration. Finally, long-term follow-up is lacking; it is unclear whether this procedure preserves normal sphincter function.

Published case series have confirmed the usefulness, in expert hands, of intracorporeal laser lithotripsy in treating difficult CBD stones. In one report, 14 out of 16 patients were treated successfully under direct visual guidance [49]. Neuhaus *et al.* [50•] reported on the use of a previously described rhodamine-6G laser system in 18 patients. This laser is equipped with a special stone-tissue recognition system whereby the firing mechanism will shut off after a brief energy emission if the CBD wall has been targeted instead of the stone surface. The laser positioning was carried out in some patients under fluoroscopic control, but mostly with direct cholangioscopy. Although complications were minimal, the data are very preliminary and controlled trials comparing fluoroscopic to cholangioscopic guidance are required to confirm the added safety of the new 'smart laser' system.

(a)

(b)

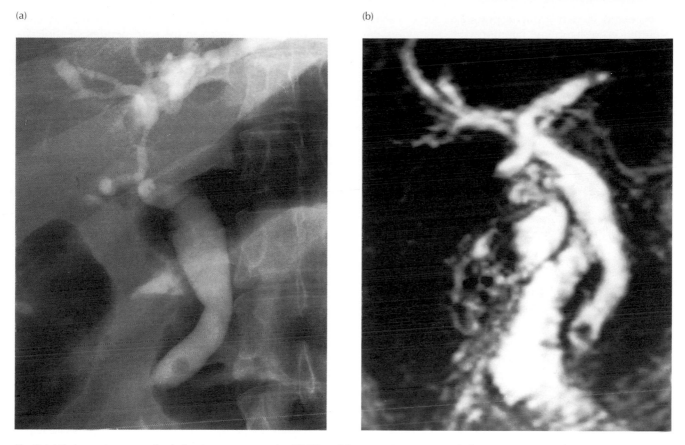

**Fig. 9.** (a) Endoscopic retrograde cholangiopancreatography (ERCP) and (b) magnetic resonance cholangiopancreatography (MRCP) demonstrating a small lower common bile duct stone in a patient scheduled for laparoscopic cholecystectomy.

Predictors of ERCP complications remain unclear. In a prospective analysis of 242 patients undergoing endoscopic sphincterotomy, post-ERCP pancreatitis was

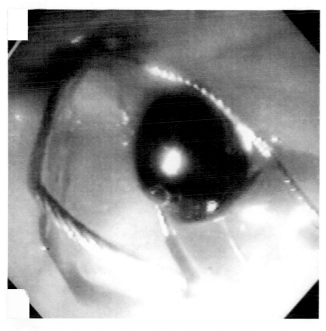

**Fig. 10.** Preliminary experience with endoscopic sphincteroplasty of small common bile duct stones was described in 1994. In this procedure, the stone is removed with a basket or balloon following endoscopic balloon dilatation of the sphincter of Oddi.

found to occur more frequently in patients whose lower CBD diameters were < 10 mm (5.6 versus 0%, $P = 0.007$) [51•]. For patients in whom a pre-cut papillotomy was performed, those with small ducts were at increased risk for both pancreatitis and perforation. In addition, bleeding following endoscopic sphincterotomy was found to be more frequent in patients in whom the papilla was juxta- or intradiverticular (16.2% versus 2.7%, $P = 0.004$, and 26.7% versus 2.7%, $P < 0.001$, respectively). In another prospective study of 210 patients undergoing endoscopic sphincterotomy, predictors of pancreatitis included a small CBD diameter when dealing with patients with CBD stones and sphincter of Oddi dyskinesia [52•]. A statistically significant inverse trend was also noted between CBD diameter and the occurrence of a postsphincterotomy complication. The conclusion of these studies has not been shared by other preliminary results [53••]. Discrepant findings may be attributable to inadequacies of follow-up, variable definitions of complications, differing endoscopic expertise and heterogeneous patient populations. In addition, in this type of clinical question, certain possible predictors (known and unknown) may be inter-related, for example, if there is an increased rate of pre-cut papillotomy in patients with small ducts. These can lead to the discovery of incorrect associations and require multivariate analysis for the generation of correct statistical inferences.

A respected French group reported its large 10-year experience in handling haemorrhage following endoscopic sphincterotomy [54•]. This complication occurred only in 0.65% of 2462 sphincterotomies. Bleeding was delayed (1–8 days, mean 2 days) in 11 patients. Of 10 patients requiring treatment, endoscopic sclerotherapy was successful in five: arteriography with or without embolization of the gastroduodenal artery was performed in the remainder. No patient required surgery.

Costamagna et al. [55•] discussed the performance of ERCP in 175 patients with Billroth II gastrectomies. The overall diagnostic success rate in 274 procedures was 88%, and therapy was carried out successfully in 93%. The endoscopic morbidity and mortality were 5.1% and 0%, respectively. These figures compare favourably with previously reported experiences.

## Other endoscopic approaches to biliary stones

Neuhaus [56•] reviewed the applications and results of intraoperative, percutaneous and peroral cholangioscopy.

A respected group reviewed its experience in the management of 54 patients with intrahepatic stones by using a combination of percutaneous transhepatic drainage, surgery and postoperative percutaneous cholangioscopy [57•].

Kalloo et al. [58•] reported on endoscopic gallbladder stenting in four high-risk patients with symptomatic cholelithiasis. Following access to the cystic duct and gallbladder with a steerable, angled tip hydrophilic wire, a 5 F nasobiliary pigtail catheter was coiled in the gallbladder and the proximal end brought out through the nose. The tube was then divided using a neodymium yttrium aluminium garnet (Nd:YAG) laser. All patients did well with, in one case, 17 months follow-up.

Agarwal et al. [59] suggested that microscopic examination of bile may help distinguish patients with cholesterol and pigment stones and may therefore improve results of direct contact solvent treatment.

Long et al. [60] studied the in vitro effects of different gallstone solvents on catheters used for direct contact dissolution and concluded that polyethylene catheters performed best under the conditions adopted in the study.

Two groups reiterated the utility of extracorporeal shock wave lithotripsy in the management of choledocholithiasis, particularly in high-risk patients [61,62].

## Case reports

Two groups reported on rare complications including a cholecysto-pleural fistula treated surgically, and a bronchobiliary fistula treated by endoscopic stone removal [63,64]. Axelrad et al. [65•] described an ERCP suite link-up to limit radiation in pregnant patients where the fluoroscopy monitor video output was relayed to a still capture device which could be accessed at will, thus avoiding the need for spot films with their attendant higher radiation exposure. Plaisier et al. [66] reported the use of extracorporeal shock wave lithotripsy to free an impacted Dormia basket. Finally, Guelrud et al. [67] reported on the performance of preoperative sphincterotomy in a 9-month-old infant with laparoscopic cholecystectomy 1 year later.

## Conclusion

1994 proved to once again be rich with endoscopic work in the management of gallstone disease. Important developments this past year included the assessment of already existing endoscopic, radiologic and surgical technologies, and their role in the management of choledocholithiasis. The overall paucity of comparative studies is disappointing yet reflects the difficulty in undertaking such trials. This will hopefully not deter endoscopic investigators from carrying out much needed technology assessments and outcome research in the coming year.

## References and recommended reading

Papers of particular interest, published within the annual period of review, have been highlighted as:

•       of special interest
••      of outstanding interest

1.      Vracko J, Zemva Z, Pegan V, Wiechel KL: **Sphincter of Oddi function studied by radioimmunoassay of biliary trypsin in patients with bile duct stones and in controls.** Surg Endosc 1994, **8**:389–392.
Bile trypsin measurements were highest in patients with non-obstructing CBD stones, or following the removal of obstructing stones. Retrograde contractions of the sphincter of Oddi may contribute to the pathogenesis of CBD stones.

2.      Wetter LA, Hamadeh RM, Griffiss JM, Oesterle A, Aagaard B Way LW:
••      **Differences in outer membrane characteristics between gallstone-associated bacteria and normal bacterial flora.** Lancet 1994, **343**:444–448.
A fascinating study of outer membrane characteristics of gallstone-associated bacteria. The data suggest that bacterial contamination of bile is a first step in the pathogenesis of brown pigment and mixed stones.

3.      Hainsworth PJ, Rhodes M, Gompertz RH, Armstrong CP, Lennard TW:
••      **Imaging of the common bile duct in patients undergoing laparoscopic cholecystectomy.** Gut 1994, **35**:991–995.
Comparative prospective study of two cohorts of patients in two separate units undergoing selective preoperative ERCP or highly selective preoperative ERCP and routine intraoperative cholangiography. Both approaches resulted in low morbidity

and low retained stone rates. Spontaneous CBD stone passage was noted in 70% of selected patients.

4.    Grier JF, Cohen SW, Grafton WD, Gholson CF: **Acute suppurative cho-**
      **langitis associated with cholesterol sludge.** *Am J Gastroenterol* 1994, **89**:
      617–619.
A case series of three patients who may have suffered from bile duct sludge-induced cholangitis.

5.    Leung JWC, Ling TKW, Chan RCY, Cheung SW, Lai CW, Sung JJY, *et al.*:
●     **Antibiotics, biliary sepsis, and bile duct stones.** *Gastrointest Endosc* 1994,
      **40**:716–721.
Ciprofloxacillin was the antibiotic most secreted (20% of peak plasma values) in a obstructed bile duct. In conjunction with susceptibility studies, these data suggest its theoretical advantage over other antibiotics in cholangitis.

6.    Niederau C, Pohlmann U, Lübke H, Thomas L: **Prophylactic antibiotic**
●●    **treatment in therapeutic or complicated diagnostic ERCP: results of a**
      **randomized controlled clinical study.** *Gastrointest Endosc* 1994, **40**:533–
      537.
A randomized controlled trial which, despite some methodological limitations, demonstrates the efficacy of prophylactic cefotaxime in decreasing bacteraemia when performing therapeutic and 'difficult' diagnostic ERCP.

7.    Steiner CA, Bass EB, Talamini MA, Pitt HA, Steinberg EP: **Surgical rates**
●●    **and operative mortality for open and laparoscopic cholecystectomy in**
      **Maryland.** *N Engl J Med* 1994, **330**:403–408.
Results of a large database which estimates surgical and mortality rates. The increase in cholecystectomy rates in the early period following introduction of laparoscopic cholecystectomy is quantified.

8.    Windsor JA, Vokes DE: **Early experience with minimally invasive sur-**
●     **gery: a New Zealand audit.** *Aust N Z J Surg* 1994, **64**:81–87.
Of 152 general surgeons, 72% deliberately abandoned a policy of routine intraoperative cholangiography for one of selective cholangiography in the laparoscopic era.

9.    Voyles CR, Sanders DL, Hogan R: **Common bile duct evaluation in the**
●     **era of laparoscopic cholecystectomy. 1050 cases later.** *Ann Surg* 1994,
      **219**:744–750.
The authors performed a three-tier stratification of patients at risk for CBD stones. High-risk patients had ERCP or intraoperative cholangiography, medium-risk patients had some operative intervention, and low-risk patients had no cholangiography. The frequency of ERCP examinations decreased over time in favour of laparoscopic techniques as, in this study, the ERCP stone clearance rate was modest.

10.   Barkun AN, Barkun JS, Fried GM, Ghitulescu G, Steinmetz O, Pham C, *et*
●●    *al.*, and the McGill Gallstone Treatment Group: **Useful predictors of bile**
      **duct stones in patients undergoing laparoscopic cholecystectomy.** *Ann*
      *Surg* 1994, **220**:32–39.
Multivariate logistic regression analysis which identifies four predictors of choledocholithiasis at ERCP in patients suspected of a CBD stone. The model was prospectively validated in a separate cohort of 49 patients.

11.   Newman L III, Newman C, Baird DR, Eubanks S, Mason E, Duncan T, *et*
      *al.*: **An institutional review of the management of choledocholithiasis in**
      **1616 patients undergoing laparoscopic cholecystectomy.** *Am Surg* 1994,
      **60**:273–277.
Seventy-nine preoperative, and 24 postoperative ERCP examinations were performed. Endoscopic sphincterotomy with stone extraction was performed in 49 patients (4.7%). Four patients failed stone extraction preoperatively, and two postoperatively (5.7%).

12.   Widdison AL, Longstaff AJ, Armstrong CP: **Combined laparoscopic and**
●     **endoscopic treatment of gallstones and bile duct stones: a prospective**
      **study.** *Br J Surg* 1994, **81**:595–597.
This prospective trial included a population with a marked increased prevalence in choledocholithiasis (21%). The authors postulated that this was because of a selection bias of more ill patients with symptomatic gallstone disease.

13.   Frazee RC, Roberts J, Symmonds R, Hendricks JC, Snyder S, Smith R, *et al.*:
      **Combined laparoscopic and endoscopic management of cholelithiasis**
      **and choledocholithiasis.** *Am J Surg* 1993, **166**:702–705.
A prospective study of 706 patients which assessed a policy of selective preoperative ERCP in 31 patients and intraoperative cholangiography in 19 prior to laparoscopic cholecystectomy.

14.   Rieger R, Sulbacher H, Woisetschläger R, Schrenk P, Wayand W: **Selective**
      **use of ERCP in patients undergoing laparoscopic cholecystectomy.**
      *World J Surg* 1994, **18**:900–905.
Description of a recent experience on the use of selective preoperative ERCP in patients undergoing laparoscopic cholecystectomy.

15.   Perissat J, Huibregtse K, Keane FBV, Russell RCG, Neoptolemos JP: **Man-**
●●    **agement of bile duct stones in the era of laparoscopic cholecystectomy.**
      *Br J Surg* 1994, **81**:799–810.
An excellent and up-to-date review of the management of choledocholithiasis. The article is written by authorities in both endoscopy and laparoscopy. These are the proceedings of a consensus conference.

16.   Leander P, Ekberg O, Almqvist P: **Radiology in laparoscopic cholecystec-**
      **tomy. A retrospective study.** *Acta Radiol* 1994, **35**:437–441.
A retrospective study of 214 patients scheduled for laparoscopic cholecystectomy over a 2-year period undergoing ultrasonography with or without preoperative cholangiography.

17.   Binmoeller KF, Soehendra N, Liguory C: **The common bile duct stone:**
●     **time to leave it to the laparoscopic surgeon?** *Endoscopy* 1994, **26**:315–319.
A review article on the management of choledocholithiasis in the era of laparoscopic cholecystectomy. The article also discusses the authors' personal experiences.

18.   Phillips EH: **Controversies in the management of common duct calculi.**
●     *Surg Clin North Am* 1994, **74**:931–948.
A review on the management of choledocholithiasis in the era of laparoscopic cholecystectomy by a very experienced laparoscopic surgeon. Particularly interesting discussion about the different laparoscopic approaches to the CBD stone.

19.   Hunter JG: **Laparoscopic cholecystectomy and the common bile duct**
      **[editorial].** *Surg Endosc* 1994, **8**:285–286.
An editorial about the management of choledocholithiasis in the era of laparoscopic cholecystectomy by an experienced laparoscopist.

20.   Salky B, Bauer J: **Intravenous cholangiography, ERCP, and selective**
      **operative cholangiography in the performance of laparoscopic cholecys-**
      **tectomy.** *Surg Endosc* 1994, **8**:289–291.
A retrospective analysis of the role of different pre- and intraoperative cholangiographic techniques including intravenous cholangiography in 143 patients.

21.   Patel JC, McInnes GC, Bagley JS, Needham G, Krukowski ZH: **The role of**
      **intravenous cholangiography in pre-operative assessment for laparo-**
      **scopic cholecystectomy.** *Br J Radiol* 1994, **66**:1125–1127.
Intravenous cholangiography was performed in 113 patients at low risk for CBD stones. Only 1.8% of patients were found to have a CBD stone.

22.   Schlumpf R, Klotz HP, Wehrli H, Herzog U: **A nation's experience in**
●     **laparoscopic cholecystectomy: prospective multicenter analysis of 3722**
      **cases.** *Surg Endosc* 1994, **8**:35–41.
In a national prospective multicenter study, 179 surgeons performed 3722 laparoscopic cholecystectomies in 50 institutions. Amongst these, only eight patients were treated by laparoscopic common bile duct exploration. It was successful in six of these patients.

23.   Carroll BJ, Fallas MH, Phillips EH: **Laparoscopic transcystic choledocho-**
●     **scopy.** *Surg Endosc* 1994, **8**:310–314.
A review of the performance of laparoscopic CBD stone clearance techniques. The authors stratify CBD stone treatment options according to age, yet overestimate the complication rate of ERCP.

24.   Ferzli GS, Massaad A, Kiel T, Worth MH Jr: **The utility of laparoscopic**
      **common bile duct exploration in the treatment of choledocholithiasis.**
      *Surg Endosc* 1994, **8**:296–298.
The results of laparoscopic common bile duct exploration performed in 24 patients is reviewed.

25.   Petelin JB: **Clinical results of common bile duct exploration.** *Endosc Surg*
●     *All Technol* 1993, **3**:125–129.
A broad review of personal experience and published literature on laparoscopic common bile duct exploration.

26.   Siddiqui MN, Hamid S, Khan H, Ahmed M: **Per-operative endoscopic**
      **retrograde cholangiopancreatography for common bile duct stones.**
      *Gastrointest Endosc* 1994, **40**:348–350.
A group's experience with intraoperative ERCP at laparoscopic cholecystectomy.

27.   Kent AL, Cox MR, Wilson TG, Padbury RT, Toouli J: **Endoscopic retro-**
      **grade cholangiopancreatography following laparoscopic cholecystec-**
      **tomy.** *Aust N Z J Surg* 1994, **64**:407–412.
Sixty-one patients underwent ERCP examinations in the postlaparoscopic cholecystectomy setting for a variety of indications with an overall 10% complication rate.

28. Pencev D, Brady PG, Pinkas H, Boulay J: **The role of ERCP in patients after laparoscopic cholecystectomy.** *Am J Gastroenterol* 1994, **89**:1523–1527.
Report of successful endoscopic stenting of cystic duct and duct of Luschka leaks amongst 56 patients undergoing postoperative ERCP for biliary problems.

29. Kent AL, Cox MR, Wilson TG, Padbury RT, Toouli J: **Endoscopic retrograde cholangiopancreatography following laparoscopic cholecystectomy.** *Aust N Z J Surg* 1994, **64**:407–412.
Only three out of five patients with postcholecystectomy bile leaks were cured with endoscopic sphincterotomy.

30. Siegel JH, Cohen SA: **Endoscopic treatment of laparoscopic bile duct injuries [review].** *Gastroenterologist* 1994, **2**:5–13.
A review of endoscopic treatment of bile duct injuries following laparoscopic cholecystectomy.

31. Peters JH, Ollila D, Nichols KE, Gibbons GD, Davanzo MA, Miller J, *et al.*: **Diagnosis and management of bile leaks following laparoscopic cholecystectomy.** *Surg Laparosc Endosc* 1994, **4**:163–170.
A series of patients treated for bile leaks following laparoscopic cholecystectomy.

32. Kozarek RA, Ball TJ, Patterson DJ, Brandabur JJ, Raltz S, Traverso LW:
• **Endoscopic treatment of biliary injury in the era of laparoscopic cholecystectomy.** *Gastrointest Endosc* 1994, **40**:10–16.
Review of the experience of a widely respected biliary group on the management of bile leaks and injuries following laparoscopic cholecystectomy.

33. Kurzwel SM, Shapiro MJ, Andrus CH, Wittgen CM, Herrman VM, Kaminski DL: **Hyperbilirubinemia without common bile duct abnormalities and hyperamylasemia without pancreatitis in patients with gallbladder disease.** *Arch Surg* 1994, **129**:829–833.
Amongst patients presenting with acute calculous cholecystitis, 25% of patients with significant hyperbilirubinaemia and 4% of those with hyperamylasaemia were found to have no CBD or pancreatic anomalies.

34. de Virgilio C, Verbin C, Chang L, Linder S, Stabile BE, Klein S: **Gallstone pancreatitis. The role of preoperative endoscopic retrograde cholangiopancreatography.** *Arch Surg* 1994, **129**:909–913.
A retrospective analysis of 71 consecutive patients with gallstone pancreatitis suggesting that cholangitis, and persistent high bilirubin or amylase are all good predictors of a CBD stone.

35. Castelain M, Grimaldi C, Harris AG, Caroli-Bosc FX, Hastier P, Dumas R, *et al.*: **Relationship between cystic duct diameter and the presence of cholelithiasis.** *Dig Dis Sci* 1994, **38**:2220–2224.
This study of 118 ERCP examinations found that the smallest and largest cystic duct diameter increased progressively in patients with sole cholelithiasis, CBD stones or both.

36. Amouyal P, Amouyal G, Levy P, Tuzet S, Palazzo L, Vilgrain V, *et al.*:
•• **Diagnosis of choledocholithiasis by endoscopic ultrasonography.** *Gastroenterology* 1994, **106**:1062–1067.
A well-designed, properly conducted prospective study in 62 patients with suspected choledocholithiasis. Endoscopic ultrasonography exhibited a sensitivity of 97% and a specificity of 100% in the detection of CBD stones.

37. McIntyre RC Jr, Stiegmann GV, Pearlman NW: **Update on laparoscopic ultrasonography.** *Endosc Surg All Technol* 1994, **2**:149–152.
A review of the potential role of laparoscopic ultrasonography in the detection of tumours, CBD stones and ductal anomalies.

38. John TG, Garden OJ: **Clinical experience with sector scan and linear array ultrasound probes in laparoscopic surgery.** *Endosc Surg All Technol* 1994, **2**:149–152.
A discussion of the differences between the sector scan and linear array technologies in laparoscopic ultrasonography.

39. Jakimowicz JJ: **Technical and clinical aspects of intraoperative ultrasound applicable to laparoscopic ultrasound.** *Endosc Surg All Technol* 1994, **2**:119–126
A review of the technique of laparoscopic ultrasonography and a discussion of its clinical application.

40. Orda R, Sayfan J, Strauss S, Barr J, Oland J: **Intra-operative ultrasonography as a routine screening procedure in biliary surgery.** *Hepatogastroenterology* 1994, **41**:61–64.
A comparative prospective study assessing the utility of ultrasonography in 117 patients.

41. Lirici MM, Caratozzolo M, Urbano V, Angelini L: **Laparoscopic ultrasonography: limits and potential of present technologies [review].** *Endosc Surg All Technol* 1994, **2**:127–133.
The technology of laparoscopic ultrasound probes is described in this paper as well as the technique of ultrasound contact scanning via the laparoscopic approach.

42. Röthlin MA, Schlumpf R, Largiader F: **Laparoscopic sonography. An**
• **alternative to routine intraoperative cholangiography?** *Arch Surg* 1994, **129**:694–700.
A well-designed, prospective, controlled study demonstrating the superior test performance of laparoscopic ultrasonography over intraoperative cholangiography using intraoperative findings and/or postoperative ERCP as the gold standard.

43. Van Beers BE, Lacrosse M, Trigaux JP, de Canniere L, De Ronde T, Pringot J: **Noninvasive imaging of the biliary tree before or after laparoscopic cholecystectomy: use of three-dimensional spiral CT cholangiography.** *AJR Am J Roentgenol* 1994, **162**:1331–1335.
Preliminary data on the performance of three-dimensional spiral computed tomography cholangiography in a series of 26 patients. Anatomical variations were correctly noted in six out of 7 patients, and CBD stones in two patients.

44. Stockberger SM, Wass JL, Sherman S, Lehman GA, Kopecky KK: **Intrave-**
• **nous cholangiography with helical CT: comparison with endoscopic retrograde cholangiography.** *Radiology* 1994, **192**:675–680.
In a cohort of 18 patients with suspected biliary disease, the sensitivity and specificity of intravenous cholangiography with helical computed tomography were 86% and 100%, respectively.

45. Guibaud L, Bret PM, Reinhold C, Atri M, Barkun AN: **Diagnosis of**
• **choledocholithiasis: value of MR cholangiography.** *AJR Am J Roentgenol* 1994, **163**:847–850.
A case series of 10 patients with choledocholithiasis studied using the novel technique of MRCP.

46. Heinerman PM, Graf AH, Boeckl O: **Does endoscopic sphincterotomy destroy the function of Oddi's sphincter?** *Arch Surg* 1994, **129**:876–880.
A prospective controlled study of 186 patients demonstrated that the sphincter of Oddi is not totally destroyed following cholecystectomy as assessed by CBD resting pressure and normalizing time.

47. MacMathuna P, White P, Clarke E, Lennon J, Crowe J: **Endoscopic sphinc-**
•• **teroplasty: a novel and safe alternative to papillotomy in the management of bile duct stones.** *Gut* 1994, **35**:127–129.
An innovative endoscopic study where a prospective cohort of 28 patients were treated with endoscopic sphincteroplasty. Successful balloon dilatation and stone removal was carried out in 22 out of 28 (79%) patients. Only one patient developed pancreatitis.

48. MacMathuna P, Lennon J, Crowe J: **[reply].** *Gut* 1994, **35**:1010.
In a response to a letter, this group updated their results on endoscopic sphincteroplasty suggesting a 75% success rate in over 100 patients treated.

49. Prat F, Fritsch J, Choury AD, Frouge C, Marteau V, Etienne JP: **Laser lithotripsy of difficult biliary stones.** *Gastrointest Endosc* 1994, **40**:290–295.
Successful treatment under cholangioscopic guidance by intracorporeal pulsed dye laser lithotripsy in 14 out of 16 patients with difficult bile duct stones.

50. Neuhaus H, Hoffman W, Gottlieb K, Classen M: **Endoscopic lithotripsy of**
• **bile duct stones using a new laser with automatic recognition system.** *Gastrointest Endosc* 1994, **39**:755–762.
Use of a new 'smart laser' on 18 patients with difficult bile duct stones which may prove to minimize the risk of bile duct damage and obviate the need for cholangioscopic control.

51. Boender J, Nix GA, de Ridder MA, van Blankestein M, Schutte HE, Dees J,
• *et al.*: **Endoscopic papillotomy for common bile duct stones: factors influencing the complication rate.** *Endoscopy* 1994, **26**:209–216.
In a prospective analysis of 242 patients undergoing laparoscopic cholecystectomy, post-ERCP pancreatitis was found to occur more frequently in patients with CBD diameters < 10 mm (5.6% versus 0%, $P = 0.007$).

52. Chen K, Foliente RL, Santoro MJ, Walter MH, Collen MJ: **Endoscopic**
• **sphincterotomy-induced pancreatitis: increased risk associated with non dilated bile ducts and sphincter of Oddi dysfunction.** *Am J Gastroenterol* 1994, **89**:327–333.
A prospective evaluation of 210 cases where small CBD diameter was significantly associated with pancreatitis in patients with CBD stones and sphincter of Oddi dysfunction.

53.    Cotton PB, Chung SC, Davis WZ, Gibson RM, Ransohoff DF, Strasberg SM:
••    **Issues in cholecystectomy and management of duct stones.** *Am J Gastroenterol* 1994, **89** (suppl):S169–S176.
Excellent multidisciplinary review by experts on both laparoscopic cholecystectomy and the roles of biliary endoscopy in gallstone disease. Part of a consensus conference/quadrennial review for the 1994 *World Congress of Gastroenterology.*

54.    Boujouade J, Pelletier G, Fritsch J, Choury A, Lefebvre JF, Roche A, *et al.*:
•    **Management of clinically relevant bleeding following endoscopic sphincterotomy.** *Endoscopy* 1994, **26**:217–221.
Presentation of one centre's large experience in dealing with postsphincterotomy haemorrhage. Bleeding was delayed in 11 out of 16 patients. No patient required surgery.

55.    Costamagna G, Mutignani M, Perri V, Gabrielli A, Locicero P, Crucitti F:
•    **Diagnostic and therapeutic ERCP in patients with Billroth II gastrectomy.** *Acta Gastroenterol Belg* 1994, **57**:155–162.
In a series of 274 ERCP examinations performed for patients with Billroth II operations, the diagnostic success rate was 88%, the therapeutic success rate 93% and the overall morbidity 5.1% with no observed mortality.

56.    Neuhaus H: **Cholangioscopy.** *Endoscopy* 1994, **26**:120–125.
•
A review of the applications and results of intraoperative, percutaneous and peroral cholangioscopy.

57.    Pitt HA, Venbrux AC, Coleman J, Prescott CA, Johnson MS, Osterman FA
•    Jr, *et al.*: **Intrahepatic stones. The transhepatic team approach.** *Ann Surg* 1994, **219**:527–535.
Presentation of one centre's large experience in a multidisciplinary approach to the management of intrahepatic stones.

58.    Kalloo AN, Thuluvath PJ, Pasricha PJ: **Treatment of high-risk patients**
•    **with symptomatic cholelithiasis by endoscopic gallbladder stenting.** *Gastrointest Endosc* 1994, **40**:608–610.
The authors discuss the insertion of cholecystoduodenal stents in four patients with symptomatic cholelithiasis at high risk for cholecystectomy.

59.    Agarwal DK, Choudhuri G, Sarawat VA, Negi TS: **Utility of biliary microcrystal analysis in predicting composition of common bile duct stones.** *Scand J Gastroenterol* 1994, **29**:352–354.
The authors suggest that microscopic analysis of bile may be useful in identifying the chemical composition of CBD stones and therefore helpful in the selection of patients for subsequent contact dissolution.

60.    Long CA, Teplick SK, Brandon JC, Harb GH, Yan K, Baker ML: **Effects of gallstone solvents on commonly used catheters.** *J Vasc Intervent Radiol* 1994, **3**:479–484.
The *in vitro* effects of different gallstone solvents on catheters used for direct contact dissolution were studied. Polyethylene catheters performed best under the conditions adopted in the study.

61.    van der Hul RL, Plaisier PW, van Blankenstein M, Terpstra OT, den Toom R, Bruining HA: **Extracorporeal shock wave lithotripsy of common bile duct stones in patients with increased operative risk.** *Eur J Surg* 1994, **160**:31–35.
A study of 90 high-risk patients having undergone extracorporeal shock wave lithotripsy for bile duct stones. Fragmentation was successful in 69% of patients with a major complication rate of 2%.

62.    Wehrmann T, Hurst A, Lembcke B, Jung M, Caspary W: **Biliary lithotripsy with a new electromagnetic shock wave source. A 2-year clinical experience.** *Dig Dis Sci* 1994, **38**:2113–2120.
One centre's results of extracorporeal biliary stone lithotripsy in patients treated for gallbladder and CBD stones.

63.    Delco F, Domenighetti G, Kauzlaric D, Donati D, Mombelli G: **Spontaneous biliothorax (thoracobilia) following cholecystopleural fistula presenting as an acute respiratory insufficiency. Successful removal of gallstones from the pleural space [review].** *Chest* 1994, **106**:961–963.
The case report of a patient with a spontaneous cholecystopleural fistula who was treated with cholecystectomy and pleural evacuation of gallstones.

64.    Moreira VF, Arocena C, Cruz F, Alvarez M, San Roman AI: **Bronchobiliary fistula secondary to biliary lithiasis. Treatment by endoscopic sphincterotomy.** *Dig Dis Sci* 1994, **39**:1994–1999.
The case report of a patient who developed a bronchobiliary fistula treated by endoscopic sphincterotomy.

65.    Axelrad AM, Fleischer DE, Strack LL, Benjamin SB, Alkawas FH: **Perform-**
•    **ance of ERCP for symptomatic choledocholithiasis during pregnancy — Techniques to increase safety and improve patient management.** *Am J Gastroenterol* 1994, **89**:109–112.
Description of an ERCP fluoroscopic set-up which cut down on the radiation exposure for a pregnant patient and her foetus.

66.    Plaisier PW, van Buuren HR, Nix GAJ, van der Hul RL, Bruining HA: **Extracorporeal shock wave lithotripsy as a trouble shooter for a Dormia basket impacted in the common bile duct.** *Gastrointest Endosc* 1994, **40**:259–260.
Use of extracorporeal shock wave lithotripsy to help disimpact a Dormia following stone impaction at ERCP.

67.    Guelrud M, Rincones VZ, Jaen D, Toledano A, Arias Y: **Endoscopic sphincterotomy and laparoscopic cholecystectomy in a jaundiced infant.** *Gastrointest Endosc* 1994, **40**:99–102.
Case report of a preoperative sphincterotomy in a 9-month-old infant with subsequent laparoscopic cholecystectomy 1 year later.

Alan Barkun, Division of Gastroenterology, The Montreal General Hospital, McGill University, Room D7-148, 1650 Cedar Avenue, Montreal, Quebec, Canada, H3G 1A4.

# Endoscopy and non-calculus biliary obstruction

## Robert H. Hawes

Digestive Disease Center, Division of Gastroenterology, Medical University of South Carolina, Charleston, South Carolina, USA

## Introduction

This article will cover recent literature on the endoscopic management of malignant and benign biliary strictures including sphincter of Oddi dysfunction. Unfortunately, little progress has been made in these areas over the last year. The greatest deficiency in this literature is the lack of properly designed studies (most are retrospective and simply outline an institution's experience) and the failure to comprehensively measure true outcomes following intervention. Most reports describe overall success rates and short-term complications but fail to assess long-term complications, quality-of-life and cost. Furthermore, this literature lacks comparative trials between endoscopic, surgical and radiologic interventions that would help define the most effective and least costly treatment algorithms. Research in malignant biliary obstruction has involved the evaluation of tissue sampling techniques and the continued evaluation of biliary prostheses. With benign biliary strictures, focus continues on biliary complications after liver transplantation and laparoscopic cholecystectomy. Finally, the evaluation of patients with possible sphincter of Oddi dysfunction, especially the use of sphincter of Oddi manometry, remains controversial.

## Malignant biliary obstruction

### Diagnosis, tissue sampling and staging

Use of laboratory studies and non-invasive imaging (ultrasound, computed tomography [CT], magnetic resonance) accurately detect the presence of extrahepatic biliary obstruction. The specific diagnosis, particularly the differentiation between benign and malignant strictures and staging, continue to be problematic. Endoscopic cholangiography continues to be the principal technique used to clarify the cause of biliary obstruction. Differentiation of benign and malignant strictures, however, must rely on tissue sampling. Multiple techniques can be used to obtain tissue and include aspiration of bile for cytologic examination, brush and fine needle aspiration cytology and pinch biopsy. Overall sensitivity for bile cytology has been disappointing (5–25%) and previous reports have shown this technique to be inferior to the other methods. A study by Mohandas et al. [1•] suggests that dilating malignant strictures to 10 F before obtaining bile for cytologic analysis improves the yield from 27% to 63%. The hypothesis is that dilation will dislodge cancer cells which can then be successfully collected. The results of this study, however, conflict with some prior reports which concluded that stricture manipulation does not improve cytologic yield [2•].

It should be remembered that examination of indwelling plastic stents at the time of stent exchange can yield positive cytologic specimens in some cases. Presumably, movement of the stent within the stricture separates cancer cells and they can then become entrapped in the sludge and biofilm within the stent. Additionally, during stent extraction, malignant cells can be entrapped by the proximal flap. Cytopathologists can desiccate the biofilm material and look for tumour cells. This technique is useful for confirming a strong clinical impression of cancer in patients with biliary strictures.

The technique most commonly employed to diagnose biliary strictures is brush cytology. This technique has overall yields (includes bile duct and pancreatic cancer) of 40–85% [3•,4•,5]. As with other sampling techniques, none consistently obtain yields greater than 70%. Direct brushing of the pancreatic duct in pancreatic cancer has been attempted in the hope of improving sensitivity. This can be an extremely difficult technical feat, but has provided improved yields [3•]. This year, Ferrari et al. [3•] reported on brush cytology results in 74 patients with pancreaticobiliary strictures. Most specimens were obtained from the biliary tree (55 patients), but 19 pancreatic duct brushings were performed. Sensitivity was 56%, specificity 100% and the overall accuracy was 70%. These results were accomplished without complications and highlight the advantages of brush cytology; principally its simplicity and safety. As with other cytologic techniques, this study reveals that positive

**Abbreviations**

CT—computed tomography; **ERCP**—endoscopic retrograde cholangiopancreatography; **FMPSPGR**—fast multiplanar spoiled gradient recalled; **PTHC**—percutaneous transhepatic cholangiography.

results confirm cancer but negative results do not reliable rule it out.

Baron *et al.* [4•] assessed the brush cytology technique in an effort to understand how diagnostic yield might be increased. This study showed that pulling the brush through the length of the sheath results in a significant loss of cells and increases the false-negative rate. In an *in vitro* system, they studied 'salvage cytology' which involves flushing the catheter sheath after the brush has been withdrawn. This was found to significantly increase cellular yield. However, a double-lumen cytology brush (Combo-Cath; Microvasive, Natick, MA, USA) has been introduced which renders salvage cytology unnecessary. The double-lumen catheter containing a cytology brush is passed over a guide wire and, after brushings are obtained, the whole catheter is removed leaving the guide wire in place.

Most centres actively studying tissue diagnosis at endoscopic retrograde cholangiopancreatography (ERCP) use multiple sampling techniques: cytology, biopsy and/or fine needle aspiration. Yields for transpapillary fine needle aspiration cytology have been reported to be as high as 60%, but others have reported yields of 30–40% (Fig. 1). Despite these reports, fine needle aspiration is the least utilized technique. In part, this relates to the fact that most centres do not have a cytopathologist willing to process the slides in the ERCP

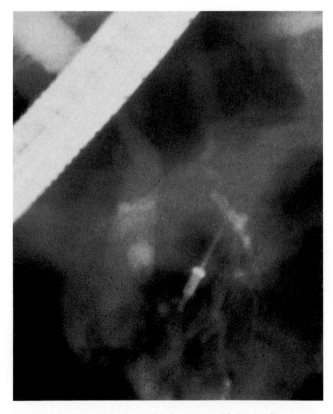

**Fig. 1.** A radiograph showing an aspiration cytology needle passed into the pancreatic duct.

suite. Without immediate feedback, an insufficient number of passes may be attempted providing inadequate cellular yield. Most reports of fine needle aspiration in conjunction with endoscopic ultrasound indicate that three or more passes are required to obtain a 90% diagnostic yield.

The most promising technique is direct transpapillary biopsy (Fig. 2). In 1994, Kubota *et al.* [6••] utilized prototype malleable forceps to perform endobiliary biopsies in 43 patients with pancreaticobiliary strictures. Adequate tissue was obtained in 95% of cases without procedure-related complications. Eighty-one per cent of patients with cancer were detected by this technique (cholangiocarcinoma, 88%; pancreatic cancer, 71%). Transpapillary biopsy usually requires sphincterotomy which is a drawback of this technique. Specials sheaths are being developed which can be passed into the bile duct without sphincterotomy and which permit repeated sampling.

Data comparing techniques are now appearing in abstract form and preliminary results favour biopsy as the single best method of sampling. Future ways to improve biopsy include:

- developing systems that will access the biliary tree without requiring a sphincterotomy;
- developing forceps that can be passed into the pancreatic duct;
- designing forceps that maximize tissue yield; and
- developing a simplified system that will allow this technique to be used by more endoscopists.

In summary, brush cytology remains the simplest method of tissue sampling and, with the new double-lumen cytology brushes, should continue to see broad utilization in the diagnosis of biliary strictures. Improvements in the brush (longer and stiffer bristles) will likely provide higher yields for this technique. Currently, the best results show only a 70% sensitivity. Fine needle aspiration systems will be simplified, but utilization of this technique will continue to be hindered by the fact that many centres do not have access to a cytopathologist who will come to the ERCP suite. Biopsy holds the greatest promise. The malleable biopsy forceps described by Kubota *et al.* [6••] should be available this year. Many experts feel, however, that for the foreseeable future, multiple sampling techniques in the same patient will be required to maximize diagnostic yield.

To date, CT, sonography and cholangiography have been the principle imaging techniques applied in patients with biliary obstruction. Cholangiography characterizes the location of the stricture and, with tissue sampling, can establish a diagnosis, but provides

(a) (b)

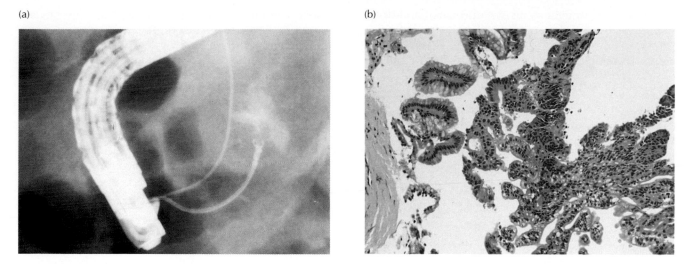

**Fig. 2.** (a) Malleable biopsy forceps passed into the pancreatic duct in a patient with a double duct sign. A guide wire has been passed into the proximal biliary tree. (b) The intraductal forceps biopsy showing pancreatic papillary cancer.

limited information about tumour extent. Sonography and CT depict dilated intrahepatic and extrahepatic bile ducts, but have difficulty in defining the extraductal extent of hilar cholangiocarcinoma and determining the cause of distal obstruction. Two recent studies suggest that application of new techniques in magnetic resonance and the use of three-dimensional CT may overcome these problems. Low *et al.* [7•] describe a new technique called contrast-enhanced fast multiplanar spoiled gradient recalled (FMPSPGR) magnetic resonance imaging and compare this with CT scan, fast spin-echo and T-1 weighted magnetic resonance and cholangiography in patients with malignant biliary obstruction. The results of this study indicate that contrast-enhanced FMPSPGR magnetic resonance imaging is a sensitive method for detecting tumours causing biliary obstruction and was particularly effective for detecting and defining tumour extent in hilar cholangiocarcinoma. There was no advantage over CT in patients with distal bile duct obstruction. This new technique uses complex technology but does have potential for providing improved imaging information. Patients with malignant obstruction involving the hilum of the biliary tree are difficult to manage surgically. There is a need for reliable imaging of tumours in this area to subselect the small group amenable to potentially curable resection.

An article by Gillams *et al.* [8•] reported their experience with three-dimensional CT cholangiography. Knowledge of segmental anatomy and intersegmental biliary connections is an essential prerequisite for effective management of patients with complex biliary strictures. It is difficult to appreciate these complex anatomic relationships on simple two-dimensional CT imaging. This study involved 14 patients with malignant biliary obstruction, all of whom underwent CT with contiguous 4-mm sections through the liver during a dynamic bolus of intravenous contrast. The biliary system was isolated from surrounding hepatic parenchyma using segmentation and contrast threshold algorithms. The authors reported excellent demonstration of the biliary anatomy, obstructed segments and intersegmental biliary connections in 13 out of the 14 patients, with the only suboptimal scan occurring in a patient with primary sclerosing cholangitis. This technique seems promising because of the ever increasing availability of spiral or helical CT scanners and because it utilizes readily available software. Clear definition of the biliary anatomy should significantly aid surgeons embarking on segmental hepatic resections and radiologists and endoscopists attempting to optimize biliary drainage in patients with hilar obstruction. Information provided by CT and magnetic resonance should improve as better scanners and software are developed. The usefulness of the images will be determined by their ability to provide information which permits more effective and less invasive therapies.

## Endoscopic stenting

Endoscopic stent placement remains the predominant palliative treatment for malignant obstructive jaundice. Expandable wire mesh stents have not replaced polyethylene stents principally because of cost. Several comparative trials have shown equal success in the relief of jaundice but higher long-term failure rates for conventional stents. It is hoped that in 1995, studies looking at quality-of-life and cost will be reported involving plastic stents and metal mesh stents as well as comparative trials between the two.

Plastic stents remain the principle tool for the biliary endoscopist in the palliation of malignant obstructive jaundice. Ten French stents are recommended and most authorities use straight stents with proximal and distal side flaps (Amsterdam-type). No study to date has shown an advantage for 11.5 F over 10 F stents. Several issues regarding plastic stents for malignant biliary obstruction should be addressed:

- Determination of the cost-effectiveness of 'prophylactic' versus 'symptomatic' stent change.
- Assessment of new materials and modification of existing materials to prolong stent patency.
- Improved measures of quality-of-life. Virtually all studies to date have measured only relief of jaundice and gross survival.

The first paper assessing symptom relief and quality of life for stenting in malignant obstructive jaundice was published by Ballinger *et al.* [9••]. Nineteen patients with malignant biliary obstruction were successfully stented and answered a three-part questionnaire used to assess symptoms and quality-of-life. The three sections of the questionnaire included the Rotterdam Symptom Checklist, the Hospital Anxiety and Depression Scale and a section to asses site and severity of pain, mood, the patient's perception of their physical health and level of activity. This questionnaire was completed before the first ERCP and then at 1, 4, 8 and 12 weeks after stent insertion. All patients had complete relief of jaundice and pruritus. There was also considerable improvement in anorexia and indigestion. Interestingly, most patients felt their mood was good/very good before stent insertion and was unchanged at the 12-week assessment. Similar results were obtained for physical health and level of activity. The evidence showed that stent insertion not only relieves jaundice and pruritus, but also improves other symptoms and quality of life with the most dramatic improvement being in appetite. This was a well-designed study which hopefully will initiate a new era in stent trials where quality-of-life is assessed in addition to immediate relief of symptoms and gross survival.

Work continues on new stent designs and materials hoping to prolong patency. Sietz *et al.* [10•] reported prolonged patency with a newly designed teflon biliary prosthesis ('Tannenbaum'; Wilson-Cook Medical, Inc., Winston-Salem, NC, USA). In a prospective, non-randomized study, 74 consecutive patients were treated with a standard 10 F teflon pigtail stent with side holes and 55 consecutive patients with a straight 10 F stent with flaps but no side holes. Immediate relief of symptoms occurred in all patients. Median survival in the two groups was not significantly different. Significantly longer patency was demonstrated for the straight stent (median patency 448 days) compared to the pigtail stent (median patency 175 days). The authors concluded that patency for the 10 F straight teflon stent compares well with published results for metallic,

self-expanding biliary stents though this was not assessed in direct comparison. The study design raises doubts about the validity of the results, particularly since patency rates for straight teflon stents are considerably longer than expected. Many studies have looked at bacterial adherence to stent material and though teflon may be 'slicker' than polyethylene, most experts have not been optimistic that this slicker surface will result in significantly less bacterial adherence and hence longer stent patency. Work continues on improved plastic stent design to reduce stent blockage.

Several advantages were anticipated when expandable metal stents were conceived. These advantages included:

- Ease of insertion, since the stents would be compressed onto small-diameter catheter systems.
- Prolonged patency due to larger luminal diameter after full expansion.
- Reduced biofilm formation because of a reduced surface area available for bacterial adherence.

To date, placement success rates have been similar between plastic and metal mesh stents. Studies have shown a longer patency for metal stents, but the cost-effectiveness of this longer patency has not been well established. A recent study looked at biofilm deposition on plastic compared with metal stents. Hoffman *et al.* [11•] used an *in vitro* bile bath system to look at biofilm formation on a polyethylene equivalent stent (C-flex; Microvasive), a new, smoother copolymer material (Percuflex; Microvasive) and a wire mesh stent (Nitinol wire mesh; Microvasive). The three stents were placed in a bile bath and perfused over a 2-week period. After a 2-week perfusion, the stents were evaluated by scanning electron microscopy. The results showed dramatically less formation of biofilm and deposition of amorphus material on the wire mesh stent and the new copolymer compared with the polyethylene stent. While this *in vitro* data is encouraging, there is no randomized prospective trial to validate the hypotheses generated from Hoffman's data.

Tumour ingrowth predominates as the limiting factor in expandable stent patency (Fig. 3) and investigators have attempted to solve this problem by putting plastic covering over part or all of the metal stent. Silvis *et al.* [12•] compared covered with uncovered wire mesh stents in the canine biliary tract. They found that mucosal hyperplasia was more marked in animals with uncovered stents and that the bare wires became deeply embedded in bile duct epithelium whereas covered stents did not. These results suggested that coatings on metal stents should prevent tumour ingrowth. No large human trials have been reported with covered stents in the biliary tree but some preliminary observations from European centres suggest that stent migration could be a problem.

An alternative solution to covered stents may be to use an expandable metal stent with narrower spaces between the struts. This is reported to be one of the potential advantages of a new coil spring expandable metal stent made from nickel-titanium alloy (Instent Inc., Israel, USA). In a very preliminary report, Goldin *et al.* [13•] reported placing this new coil spring into nine patients with pancreatic carcinoma. Clinical improvement was seen in all patients except for one who died from liver metastases 5 weeks after insertion. Two out of eight patients (25%) obstructed at 2 and 4 months after insertion (one due to tumour ingrowth and the other due to sludge formation). The other six patients had no evidence of biliary obstruction with a mean follow-up of 4.5 months. Although these preliminary results were encouraging, other investigators have reported some deployment problems. At its original conception, it was hoped that this stent would be removable and the preliminary report [13•] suggested that this might be the case. Further experience with this new stent is anticipated.

Percutaneous insertion of biliary stents for relief of low malignant obstruction has seen a steady decline in utilization. This is largely because of increased availability of expert biliary endoscopists and improvement in techniques to gain access through the papilla and across strictures (hydrophilic polymer coated guide wires, expandable stents for tight strictures, needle knife pre-cut papillotomy). These same factors have led to a decline in combined or 'rendezvous' percutaneous and endoscopic procedures. This technique has been reported extensively in the past as being advantageous in cases where endoscopic access was not possible [14•]. With the improved techniques described above, the need for percutaneous access has decreased and hence there are no new reports describing experience with the combined procedure.

Hilar tumours remain a very difficult problem. Controversy continues regarding endoscopic versus percutaneous approaches to biliary interventions in this group (Fig. 4). The availability of expandable stents, however, has strengthened the case for radiologic intervention. The principle disadvantage of percutaneous drainage has been the need to place large-bore prostheses requiring a large tract across the liver parenchyma, causing bleeding and bile leaks. Expandable metal stents can be placed through smaller catheters

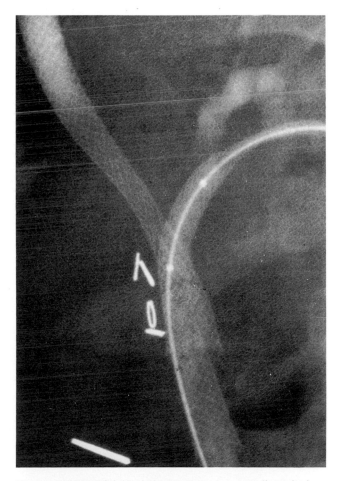

**Fig. 4.** A patient with hilar cholangiocarcinoma. A Wallstent had been placed endoscopically into the right intrahepatic system without effective drainage. Percutaneous transhepatic techniques were then used to place a second Wallstent into the left intrahepatic system.

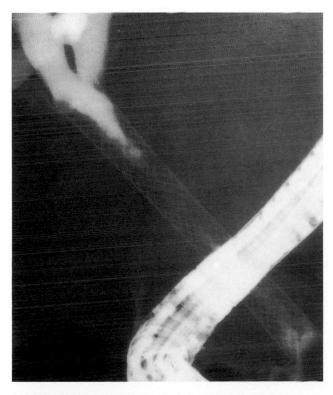

**Fig. 3.** Cholangiogram showing blockage of a Wallstent from tumour ingrowth.

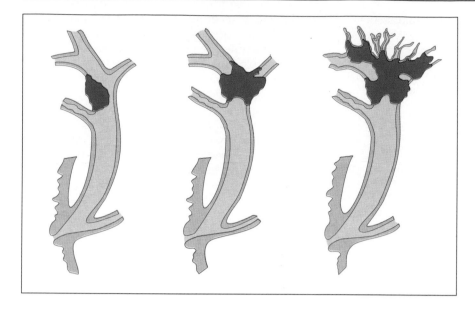

**Fig. 5.** Drawing showing the three types of hilar cholangiocarcinoma.

making percutaneous placement easier and less risky. The success of biliary drainage of hilar tumours is related to the extent to which the tumour has infiltrated proximally. Most biliary interventionists find that the Bismuth classification is helpful in determining the chances for successful biliary drainage (Fig. 5):

- Type I: tumours confined to the common hepatic duct.
- Type II: tumour infiltrates into the left and/or right intrahepatic systems.
- Type III: tumour is infiltrated into secondary branches of the left and right systems.

Success rates for biliary drainage are directly related to tumour extent (Type I > Type II > Type III). Two articles appeared in 1994 pertaining to proximal cholangiocarcinoma [15•,16•]. Both articles expressed the need for a multidisciplinary approach in these difficult patients. First, one must assess whether any benefit can be accrued to patients through intervention. If intervention is deemed potentially beneficial, then surgical, percutaneous and transpapillary methods are available. In patients with obstructive jaundice, it has been estimated that a minimum of 30% of the liver volume must be decompressed in order to relieve symptoms of jaundice and pruritus [8•]. With the advent of expandable stents for percutaneous application, comparative trials should be undertaken to assess the effectiveness of percutaneous versus endoscopic drainage in patients with malignant hilar obstruction. Such a study has been initiated in the United States in a multicentre, co-operative effort.

Surgical versus endoscopic palliation for patients with malignant obstructive jaundice remains controversial. Smith *et al.* [17••] published the final results of a prospective, randomized trial of surgical bypass versus endoscopic palliation in 204 patients with malignant low bile duct obstruction. The findings were similar to previous reports which showed high procedure-related morbidity and mortality in the surgery group while endoscopic stenting has higher long-term complications. Overall survival was the same. Cost analyses were not applied to this study. These data have not significantly altered clinical practice. Experts usually recommend endoscopic palliation in most patients except in the young, relatively healthy patients with unresectable cancer and those with duodenal impingement at high risk for gastric outlet obstruction. The new era of laparoscopic surgery may lead us to revisit this issue. Reports are now appearing describing laparoscopic gastrojejunostomy and laparoscopic cholecystoenterostomy. It is possible that the 'minimal invasiveness' of these new laparoscopic techniques will provide a cost-effective alternative to endoscopic stenting.

In patients with malignant obstructive jaundice who have resectable disease, controversy remains regarding the benefit of preoperative biliary drainage. Lai *et al.* [18••], in a prospective, randomized control trial, looked at 87 patients who were randomly assigned to elective surgery or preoperative endoscopic drainage followed by exploration. This study had a relatively high endoscopic complication rate primarily attributable to cholangitis in the subgroup of patients with hilar cholangiocarcinoma. Nevertheless, there was no significant difference in overall morbidity or mortality in the two groups and this study confirms the findings of prior trials using percutaneous stenting; preoperative biliary drainage confers no benefit.

## Postoperative biliary problems

At this time, postoperative biliary complications are seen predominantly in two clinical settings: after laparoscopic cholecystectomy and orthotopic liver transplantation. More bile duct injuries are being seen in the laparoscopic cholecystectomy era, but advocates of this procedure believe it is experience related and the incidence will decrease with time. The principle biliary complications seen after laparoscopic cholecystectomy include common bile duct strictures, bile duct or cystic duct leaks or a combination of the two [19•]. There is still considerable controversy about the treatment of bile duct injuries. Most experts agree that cystic duct stump leaks are easily managed endoscopically with success rates of approximately 90%. Interventions that equalize pressure between the duodenum and bile duct will allow the cystic duct stump to seal. This can be accomplished by endoscopic sphincterotomy or by placement of a small bore plastic stent. Sphincterotomy has the advantage of not requiring a repeat procedure while stenting preserves sphincter function in a population predominated by young females. A third alternative is nasobiliary tube placement; however, this is more cumbersome and uncomfortable to the patient and is used less often. In Kozarek's report [19•], five out of five patients with cystic duct leaks were successfully treated with small bore prostheses, and other reports have described similar success. Biliary strictures are more problematic. Kozarek et al. reported resolution of biliary strictures in 13 out of 16 patients (81%) with postoperative strictures (some with concomitant leaks as well). The follow-up, however, was relatively short and this is the basis for arguments from our surgical colleagues that endoscopic therapy has not been adequately studied. The approach taken by most endoscopists who see patients with postoperative biliary strictures is to give a trial of biliary stenting plus or minus balloon dilation. Most place one or two prostheses and exchange them every 3–4 months for a duration of 6–12 months. The stents are then removed and the patient is followed on a regular basis with liver tests. If signs of cholestasis occur, the patient is then referred for surgical treatment. A report this year from the University of Louisville describes an experience in 25 patients with bile duct injuries after laparoscopic cholecystectomy [20•]. In six cases, ERCP was used as a primary treatment and was successful in five (83%). Open surgical repair was performed in the remaining 19 patients. Operation was successful in 12 out of these 19 (10 choledocho- or hepaticojejunostomy, six primary duct repair, two repaired leaks and one completed cholecystectomy). Only one out of five patients who underwent a primary repair over a T-tube had a successful outcome. This report provides little information to help others with their decisions for treatment.

Biliary tract complications after liver transplantation and their management continue to be problematic. The incidence varies from 10% to 30% with an associated mortality rate of 10–25% [21•]. These complications can pose difficult management problems for patients who are often medically frail and invariably on high doses of immunosuppressive agents. The same endoscopic and percutaneous interventional techniques used to manage other types of benign biliary strictures have been applied to liver transplant patients. The short- and long-term results of such intervention is currently being evaluated. In a retrospective study published by Kuo et al. [21•], 157 hepatic transplants performed between January 1987 and July 1991 were reviewed. Biliary tract complications were seen in 25%. Early postoperative complications (< 30 days) were predominantly leaks while those presenting after 30 days were primarily strictures. ERCP, percutaneous transhepatic cholangiography (PTHC) and operative treatments were applied depending upon the nature of the stricture or leak. It does not appear that the percutaneous or endoscopic treatments followed a specific protocol. The 1-year patency rate for ERCP and PTHC was 44% and 46%, respectively, and for operation was 89%. These limited data collected in a retrospective manner provide little guidance on how best to manage these difficult patients.

In another publication on biliary tract strictures after liver transplantation, Theilmann et al. [22•] found that 20 out of 105 patients (19%) developed biliary strictures after liver transplantation. Eleven patients had multiple strictures involving the intra- and extrahepatic biliary tree, five patients had multiple strictures in the common bile duct not related to the bile duct anastomosis and four patients had stenosis of the common bile duct located at the site of the anastomosis. Of the eleven patients with diffuse intra- and extrahepatic biliary strictures, four were successfully treated endoscopically or percutaneously while the other seven required retransplantation. In the group with multiple extrahepatic strictures, two were treated successfully with surgery, one was treated successfully by percutaneous treatment and one out of two were successfully treated with endoscopic techniques. In the four patients with stenosis confined to the site of the bile duct anastomosis, one patient was successfully treated endoscopically, one patient was successfully treated with surgery and two had spontaneous resolution of the stricture.

Both of the articles describing post-transplantation management of biliary complications highlight the fact that no one methodology has been shown to have an advantage in all cases. Multiple techniques (endoscopic, percutaneous and surgical) can be successful, and treatment plans are largely based on local bias and expertise. This is a significant problem in liver transplant patients and deserves a vigorous multidisciplinary study to assist in finding the best algorithms of management.

## Sphincter of Oddi dysfunction

The evaluation of patients with post-cholecystectomy pain and possible sphincter of Oddi dysfunction continues to be difficult. It is clear that this young, predominantly female population are at increased risk for ERCP and sphincterotomy. Sphincter of Oddi manometry continues to be performed predominantly by expert referral centres and has not gained wide-spread use (or acceptance). Many of the technical problems in performing sphincter of Oddi manometry are related to patient sedation. Narcotics are known to cause spasm of the sphincter of Oddi and it has been assumed that meperidine cannot be used during sphincter manometry. A provocative paper was published this year in which meperidine was studied to determine its effect on sphincter of Oddi motility [23••]. This was a prospective study of 18 patients undergoing manometry for suspected sphincter of Oddi dysfunction. Manometry was first performed using only intravenous diazepam and then was repeated following the intravenous administration of 1 mg/kg meperidine. No difference in basal sphincter of Oddi pressures were found before and after meperidine in all patients. The authors did find that the frequency of phasic contractions increased after meperidine ($P = 0.001$). The authors concluded that since basal sphincter of Oddi pressures correlate best with outcome from sphincter ablation, that the use of meperidine while performing sphincter of Oddi manometry is acceptable. This article was followed by an editorial from the Indianapolis group which acknowledged the potential importance of this article, but expressed several cautions [24••]:

- Only common bile duct pressures were measured and therefore the effect on the pancreatic sphincter remains unknown.
- The sample size was small (18).
- The number of patients with abnormal basal sphincter pressures was very low (5.6%).
- There were a limited number of patients with basal sphincter pressures in the borderline range of 30–40 mmHg where a small effect of meperidine could change a normal to an abnormal study.

Some of the concerns mentioned above were studied and reported in an abstract from the same Indiana group [25••]. In 47 patients who underwent a similar protocol using meperidine, little effect was seen on the basal sphincter of Oddi pressure and there was no difference in effect between the pancreatic and biliary sphincters. Interestingly, the quality of the tracing was improved in 36% of the patients during the meperidine run. At this time, if basal sphincter of Oddi pressures are being used to diagnose sphincter of Oddi dysfunction, it would appear that meperidine can be used to improve the sedation.

Geenen and the group from Racine, Wisconsin have advocated the use of criteria to categorize patients with possible sphincter of Oddi dysfunction:

- Pancreaticobiliary type pain;
- abnormal liver or pancreatic tests during pain;
- dilated bile duct and/or pancreatic duct; and
- delayed biliary or pancreatic drainage.

Using these criteria, they have developed three categories: Type I — pain, abnormal serum tests and dilated ducts or delayed drainage; Type II — pain and one of the other three criteria; Type III — pain only.

Several studies have confirmed a relationship between the incidence of finding elevated basal sphincter of Oddi pressures and the Geenen classification (Type I > Type II > Type III). Additionally, several studies have reported a correlation between an elevation in basal sphincter of Oddi pressures and a positive outcome from sphincter ablation. Of interest is an article published this year by the Virginia Mason group that looked at long-term outcome after endoscopic sphincterotomy in Geenen Type II and III patients [26•]. In this study, no difference was found in the incidence of basal sphincter hypertension (60% versus 55%), improvement after sphincter ablation (66% versus 57%) or post-procedure pancreatitis rates (15% versus 16%) between the two groups. The incidence of abnormal sphincter of Oddi manometry in Type II patients was similar to the reported literature, but the finding was much higher in the Type III patients. Of greater importance is the effect of sphincter ablation on outcome. It is difficult to compare reports in the literature because often there are insufficient data to permit classification of patients using the Geenen criteria. Previous reports have demonstrated an improvement rate of 90% in Type II patients with abnormal sphincter of Oddi pressures. This is significantly higher than the improvement rate in the present article. There are a number of potential explanations for differences in the various investigations, not the least of which is referral bias. The study by Botoman *et al.* [26•] appears to support the importance of sphincter of Oddi manometry in Type III patients. Fifty-five per cent of patients had abnormal basal sphincter pressures and 56% of these benefited from endoscopic sphincterotomy. To date, manometry remains the only modality that can reliably detect sphincter abnormality and, more importantly, has the best correlation with outcome after sphincter ablation.

Finally, the Racine group published a report on a group of 17 patients who met criteria that categorized them in the Geenen Type I group [27•]. Sphincter of Oddi manometry was performed in all cases and was abnormal (basal sphincter pressure > 40 mmHg) in 11 patients. Sphincterotomy was performed in all patients and resulted in relief of symptoms in all (mean follow-up 28 months; range 3–46 months). The explanation for finding some patients with normal sphincter of Oddi pressures is uncertain, but the authors conclude that, because patients invariably benefit from sphincterotomy, sphincter of Oddi manometry in this group is unnecessary (and may be misleading).

## Conclusion

In 1994, we saw continued refinement in common themes that have been ongoing for several years. We are beginning to see the emergence of endoscopic trials that go beyond describing short-term success and complications to also cover cost and quality-of-life issues. This is a welcome trend which will hopefully expand in 1995.

## References and recommended reading

Papers of particular interest, published within the annual period of review, have been highlighted as:
- • of special interest
- •• of outstanding interest

1.  Mohandas KM, Swaroop VS, Gullar SU, Dave UR, Jagannath P, DeSouza
•   LJ: **Diagnosis of malignant obstructive jaundice by bile cytology: Results improved by dilating the bile duct strictures.** *Gastrointest Endosc* 1994, **40**:150–155.
Dilation of malignant biliary strictures improves cytologic yield by bile aspiration.

2   Kurzawinski T, Deery A, Dooley J, Dick R, Hobbs KEF, Davidson BR: **A**
•   **prospective study of biliary cytology in 100 patients with bile duct strictures.** *Hepatology* 1993, **18**:1399–1403.
Stricture manipulation prior to bile aspiration for cytology does not improve yield.

3.  Ferrari AP Jr, Lichtenstein DR, Slivka A, Chang C, Carr-Locke DL: **Brush**
•   **cytology during ERCP for the diagnosis of biliary and pancreatic malignancies.** *Gastrointest Endosc* 1994, **40**:140–145.
Seventy-four patients with pancreaticobiliary strictures underwent brush cytology (55 bile duct specimens, 19 pancreatic duct specimens). The overall results showed a sensitivity of 56%, specificity of 100%, positive predictive value of 100% and negative predictive value of 51% and an accuracy of 70%.

4.  Baron TH, Lee JG, Wax TD, Schmitt CM, Cotton PB, Leung JWC: **An *in***
•   ***vitro*, randomized, prospective study to maximize cellular yield during bile duct brush cytology.** *Gastrointest Endosc* 1994, **40**:146–149.
When obtaining brush cytology, pulling the brush through the length of the sheath results in a significant loss of cellular material. 'Salvage cytology' can be performed by aspirating 5 cm$^3$ fluid through the empty sheath and this significantly increases cellular yield.

5.  Ryan ME, Baldauf MC: **Comparison of flow cytometry for DNA content and brush cytology for detection of malignancy in pancreaticobiliary strictures.** *Gastrointest Endosc* 1994, **40**:133–139.

6.  Kubota Y, Takaoka M, Tani K, Ogura M, Kin H, Fujimura K, *et al.*:
••  **Endoscopic transpapillary biopsy for diagnosis of patients with pancreaticobiliary strictures.** *Am J Gastroenterol* 1993, **88**:1700–1704.
Transpapillary biopsy of the bile duct and pancreatic duct was performed with malleable forceps. Sampling was successful in 95.3% with sensitivity of 88% for cholangiocarcinoma and 71% for pancreatic carcinoma.

7.  Low RN, Sigeti JS, Francis IR, Weinman D, Bower B, Shimakawa A, *et al.*:
•   **Evaluation of malignant biliary obstruction: Efficacy of fast multi-planar spoiled gradient-recalled MR imaging vs. spin-echo MR imaging, CT and cholangiography.** *AJR Am J Roentgenol* 1994, **162**:315–323.

This paper compares contrast-enhanced FMPSPGR magnetic resonance to conventional spin-echo T-1 weighted images, fast spin-echo T-2 weighted images, CT scan and cholangiograms in patients with malignant biliary obstruction. The contrast-enhanced FMPSPGR magnetic resonance imaging appears particularly effective for detecting and defining tumour extent of hilar cholangiocarcinomas.

8.  Gillams A, Gardener J, Richards R, Tan AC, Linney A, Lees WR: **Three**
•   **dimensional computed tomography cholangiography: A new technique for biliary tract imaging.** *Br J Radiol* 1994, **67**:445–448.
Spiral CT combined with dynamic bolus intravenous contrast is used to image the biliary tree followed by three-dimensional surface reconstruction. This technique is helpful in demonstrating the intersegmental biliary anatomy which is important in planning biliary drainage in patients with hilar malignant obstruction.

9.  Ballinger AB, McHugh M, Catnach SM, Alstead EM, Clark ML: **Symptom**
••  **relief in quality of life after stenting for malignant bile duct obstruction.** *Gut* 1994, **35**:467–470.
Nineteen patients treated by endoscopic stenting for malignant obstructive jaundice were assessed for relief of symptoms and quality-of-life after stent insertion. Stent insertion was associated with relief of jaundice and pruritus and improvement in overall quality-of-life. This is the first study looking specifically at quality-of-life after stenting for malignant obstructive jaundice.

10. Seitz U, Vadeyar H, Soehendra H: **Prolonged patency with a new-designed**
•   **teflon biliary prosthesis.** *Endoscopy* 1994, **26**:478–482.
This is a prospective, non-randomized study of 74 patients treated with 10 F pigtail stents and 55 consecutive patients treated with teflon straight stents without side holes. This study revealed a significantly longer patency for the teflon stent without side holes.

11. Hoffman BJ, Cunningham JT, Marsh WH, O'Brien JJ, Watson J: **An *in vitro***
•   **comparison of biofilm formation on various biliary stent materials.** *Gastrointest Endosc* 1994, **50**:581–583.
A bile perfusion model is used to compare biofilm formation on a polyethylene-equivalent stent, a wire mesh stent (composed of Nitinol) and a stent made of percuflex which is a prototype copolymer. There was less formation of bacterial biofilm and less deposition of amorphous material on the wire mesh and copolymer stent compared with the polyethylene equivalent.

12. Silvis SE, Sievert CE, Vennes JA, Abeyta DK, Brennecke LH: **Comparison**
•   **of covered versus uncovered wire mesh stents in the canine biliary tract.** *Gastrointest Endosc* 1994, **140**:17–21.
Silicone-covered or uncovered Wallstents were placed in 22 mongrel dogs through the sphincter of Oddi for 1–3 months. Mucosal hyperplasia was more marked in animals with uncovered stents and the bare wires became deeply imbedded in the bile duct epithelium whereas the wires of the covered stents did not. The authors suggest that silicone covering may prohibit tumour ingrowth and might render covered stents removable thus enabling their use in the treatment of benign biliary strictures.

13. Goldin E, Beyar M, Safra T, Globerman O, Verstandig A, Wengrower D, *et*
•   *al.*: **A new self-expandable and removable metal stent for biliary obstruction — A preliminary report.** *Endoscopy* 1993, **25**:597–599.
The first report of a new self-expandable metallic coil spring stent made from nickel-titanium alloy; report of placement in nine patients.

14. Martin DF: **Combined percutaneous and endoscopic procedures for bile**
•   **duct obstruction.** *Gut* 1994, **35**:1011–1012.
A nice review article outlining the indications and results from combining percutaneous and endoscopic techniques for relief of bile duct obstruction.

15. Van Der Hul RL, Plaisier PW, Lameris JS, Veeze-Kuijpers B, Van Blanken-
•   stein M, Terpstra OT: **Proximal cholangiocarcinoma: A multi-disciplinary approach.** *Eur J Surg* 1994, **160**:213–218.
A retrospective study evaluating the diagnosis and treatment techniques for proximal cholangiocarcinoma. Since it is a non-randomized, retrospective study, few conclusions can be drawn from this report.

16. Helling TS: **Carcinoma of the proximal bile duct.** *J Am Coll Surg* 1994,
•   **178**:97–106.
Nice review of the diagnosis and treatment (operative and non-operative) and prognosis for patients with Hilar cholangiocarcinoma.

17. Smith AC, Dowsett JF, Russell RCG, Hatfield ARW, Cotton PB: **Random-**
••  **ized trial of endoscopic stenting versus surgical bypass in malignant low bile duct obstruction.** *Lancet* 1994, **344**:1655–1660.
Two hundred and four patients randomized to surgical bypass or endoscopic stenting. An excellent study.

18. Lai ECS, Mok FPT, Fan ST, Lo CM, Chu KM, Leio CL, *et al*.: **Preoperative**
•• **endoscopic training for malignant obstructive jaundice.** *Br J Surg* 1994,
**81**:1195–1198.
A randomized, controlled trial investigating whether preoperative endoscopic drainage benefits patients undergoing surgery for malignant obstructive jaundice. Endoscopic complications occurred in 32% (principally cholangitis in patients with hilar lesions). The overall morbidity and mortality rates were similar in the two treatment arms irrespective of the level of biliary obstruction.

19. Kozarek RA, Ball TJ, Patterson DJ, Brandebur JJ, Raltz S, Traverso LW:
• **Endoscopic treatment of biliary injury in the era of laparoscopic**
**cholecystectomy.** *Gastrointest Endosc* 1994, **40**:10–16.
Report of 33 patients with post-cholecystectomy bile duct injuries. With a minimum 1-year follow-up, 25 out of 29 patients treated endoscopically were symptom free with normal ultrasonography and serum liver function tests.

20. Vitale GC, Stephens G, Wienman TJ, Larson GM: **Use of endoscopic**
• **retrograde cholangiopancreatography in the management of biliary**
**complications after laparoscopic cholecystectomy.** *Surgery* 1993, **114**:
806–814.
A retrospective review outlining the experience using ERCP in 25 patients who suffered bile duct injuries during laparoscopic cholecystectomy. It is a retrospective summary of the authors experience, but adds little to our understanding of the best long-term approach to these unfortunate patients.

21. Kuo PC, Lewis WD, Stokes K, Pleskow D, Simpson MA, Jenkins RL: **A**
• **comparison of operation, endoscopic retrograde cholangiopancrea-**
**tography, and percutaneous transhepatic cholangiography in biliary**
**complications after hepatic transplantation.** *J Am Coll Surg* 1994,
**179**:177–181.
A retrospective study of biliary complications after liver transplantation. The overall incidence was 25%. Bile leaks occurred early and bile strictures predominated late. Treatment by ERCP and PTCH had 1-year patency rates of 45% while operative patency was 89%. Comparison of results of treatment in this study are unreliable.

22. Theilmann L, Kuppers B, Kadmon M, Roeren T, Notheisen H, Stiehl A, *et*
• *al*.: **Biliary tract strictures after orthoptic liver transplantation: Diagno-**
**sis and management.** *Endoscopy* 1994, **26**:517–522.
A retrospective review which revealed 20 biliary tract complications observed in 105 patients. Ten out of 20 biliary strictures were considered treatable and four were corrected endoscopically, three percutaneously and three by surgery. Patients with intra and extrahepatic strictures required retransplantation.

23. Elta GH, Barnett JL: **Meperidine need not be proscribed during sphincter**
•• **of Oddi manometry.** *Gastrointest Endosc* 1994, **40**:7–9.
A prospective study of 18 patients undergoing sphincter of Oddi manometry for suspected sphincter dysfunction. The manometry was performed using only intravenous diazepam followed by the administration of meperidine followed by repeat manometry. There was no difference in baseline sphincter pressures before and after meperidine in all patients, though phasic contractions were affected.

24. Sherman S, Lehman GA: **Opioids and the sphincter of Oddi.** *Gastrointest*
•• *Endosc* 1994, **49**:105–106.
This editorial reviews the effect of narcotics on the sphincter of Oddi and raises cautionary points about their use during sphincter of Oddi motility.

25. Sherman S, Rahaman S, Gottlieb K, Male R, Uzer M, Smith M, *et al*.: **Effect**
• **of meperidine on sphincter of Oddi motility [abstract].** *Gastrointest*
*Endosc* 1994, **40**:P127.
Report on some of the concerns expresses by Sherman and Lehman [24••].

26. Botoman VA, Kozarek RA, Novell LA, Patterson DJ, Ball TJ, Wechter DG,
• *et al*.: **Long-term outcome after endoscopic sphincterotomy in patients**
**with biliary colic and suspected sphincter of Oddi dysfunction.** *Gastrointest Endosc* 1994, **40**:165–170.
A study of Geenen Type II and III looking at the incidence of elevated sphincter of Oddi pressures and the results of sphincterotomy. Type II and III patients had a similar percentage with elevated basal sphincter pressures and the same results with sphincterotomy.

27. Rolny P, Geenen JE, Hogan WJ: **Post-cholecystectomy in patients with**
• **'objective signs' of partial bile outflow obstruction: Clinical charac-**
**teristics, sphincter of Oddi findings, and results of therapy.** *Gastrointest Endosc* 1993, **39**:778–781.
This report described 17 biliary group I patients (biliary-type pain, dilated common bile duct and delayed contrast drainage) who underwent sphincter of Oddi manometry and sphincter ablation (15 endoscopic sphincterotomy and two surgical sphincterplasty). Six patients (35%) had normal basal sphincter of Oddi pressures, yet all patients had relief of symptoms with a mean follow-up of 28 months. This study suggests that patients with multiple signs of partial bile outflow obstruction benefit from sphincter ablation and that sphincter of Oddi manometry is not necessary and that a normal sphincter of Oddi manometry in this group may be misleading.

Robert H. Hawes, Digestive Disease Center, Division of Gastroenterology, Medical University of South Carolina, 171 Ashley Avenue, 910 CSB, Charleston, S.C. 29425-2220 USA.

# Laparoscopy

## Lennox J. Jeffers and Carlos A. Vargas*

Division of Hepatology, Center for Liver Diseases, University of Miami School of Medicine and
Veterans Affairs Medical Center, Miami, Florida,
and *Fundaction Valle del Lili, University of del Valle, Cali, Colombia

## Introduction

The worldwide explosion in the use of the laparoscope for an expanding list of indications has been fuelled by the general surgeon's ability to adapt to, and master, minimally invasive surgery.

The majority of cholecystectomies in the Western world are now being performed laparoscopically. Colectomies, inguinal hernia repairs, drainage and marsupialization of hepatic cyst and antireflex surgery can now be performed safely in many centres (Fig. 1). The addition of the laparoscopic ultrasound will also enhance the gastroenterologist's and surgeon's ability to assess operability in patients with liver tumours. The laparoscope will play an integral role in medicine in the twenty-first century.

| | |
|---|---|
| Cholecystectomy | Small bowel resection |
| Choledochostomy | Gastrostomy |
| Appendectomy | Gastrojejunostomy |
| Herniorrhaphy | Adrenalectomy |
| Splenectomy | Nephrectomy |
| Colectomy | Hepatic cystectomy |
| Fundoplication | Duodenal diverticulectomy |
| Vagotomy | Oesophageal myotomy |
| Gastrectomy | Drainage of hepatic abscess |

Fig. 1. List of laparoscopic surgical procedures.

## Diagnostic laparoscopy

Diagnostic laparoscopy has been abandoned by the vast majority of gastroenterologists and hepatologists throughout the world. There is, however, an ongoing resurgence of this procedure among surgeons. Diagnostic laparoscopy continues to be the best method for the evaluation of patients with chronic liver disease, in the staging of patients with primary and secondary liver tumours and in the evaluation of peritoneal diseases and ascites of unknown origin. Technological breakthroughs such as the laparoscopic ultrasound and modification of existing instruments allow for better visualization of the abdominal cavity, and at the same time decreases the need for open laparotomy and its associated complications. Schrenk et al. [1••] evaluated 92 patients with diagnostic laparoscopy. Indications were 33 patients (36%) for suspected malignancy or to assess operability, 31 patients (34%) for chronic abdominal pain, 15 patients (16%) for acute abdominal pain, nine patients (10%) with abdominal trauma and four patients (4%) with miscellaneous conditions. The result of this study was impressive in that laparoscopy was able to provide a diagnosis, or assess operability of liver cancer, in 30 out of 33 patients (90%). In 24 out of 31 patients with chronic abdominal pain, laparoscopy established the diagnosis; in 14 out of 15 patients with acute abdominal pain, the diagnosis was confirmed with laparoscopy; and in all patients investigated for trauma, laparoscopy was diagnostic. The overall results of this study revealed that laparoscopy was diagnostic in 87% of the patients and a laparotomy was avoided in 85% of the patients. Diagnostic laparoscopy was converted to a therapeutic laparoscopy in 71% of the patients. This study strongly suggests that diagnostic laparoscopy leads to a decreased number of unnecessary laparotomies and, in the hands of skilled surgeons, can be easily altered to a therapeutic procedure.

Crantock et al. [2••] evaluated 200 consecutive patients with diagnostic laparoscopy using a 5-mm laparoscope in an endoscopy suite under conscious sedation. A pneumoperitoneum with nitrous oxide was obtained. The most interesting findings were unsuspected malignancy in eight out of 25 patients who had liver tumours despite a negative ultrasound, and four out of 72 patients who had a diagnosis of cirrhosis unconfirmed histologically. An additional nine patients with cirrhosis were misdiagnosed by ultrasound as having metastatic liver disease, only to be correctly diagnosed at laparoscopy to have cirrhosis of the liver. Two major complications occurred: one patient bled from the

**Abbreviations**

CT—computed tomography; HIV—human immunodeficiency virus.

© Current Science Ltd ISBN 1-85922-187-4 ISSN 0952-6293

trocar site, the other from intra-abdominal adhesions. This interesting study outlines, in detail, the technique of diagnostic laparoscopy. The finding of a malignancy in patients with a negative ultrasound is not uncommon for those who evaluate patients with laparoscopy. Rademaker *et al.* [3•] evaluated the effects of carbon dioxide and nitrous oxide pneumoperitoneum on the haemodynamic circulation. Fifteen patients were studied with nitrous oxide and carbon dioxide under general anaesthesia. During laparoscopy the heart rate, mean arterial pressure, cardiac index, cardiac output and central venous pressures were monitored. Results of this study indicated that abdominal insufflation with either carbon dioxide or nitrous oxide results in circulatory depression. Insufflation with nitrous oxide resulted in hypotension, whereas blood pressure was better preserved with carbon dioxide. This significant study demonstrated that laparoscopic insufflation with either carbon dioxide or nitrous oxide results in cardiovascular depression and, therefore, patients with a compromised cardiac system should be monitored very closely during laparoscopy. Bleeding from abdominal wall vessels during the introduction of the trocar is a recognized complication of laparoscopy and occurs more frequently than bleeding from the liver biopsy site, particularly in patients with portal hypertension. A potentially new and exciting approach was described by Whitley *et al.* [4•]. They evaluated ten volunteer patients with an 8-MHz, hand-held ultrasound probe by mapping the abdominal wall vessels. The courses of the vessels were identified and marked with an indelible ink marker and then scanned with colour flow Doppler. Forty epigastric arteries were marked successfully and confirmed by colour Doppler. An additional 75 intramural arteries were identified; however, the majority of these were too small to be confirmed by colour Doppler. This is an important study, particularly if this procedure is applied to patients with portal hypertension. A safe site can then be selected for the introduction of the trocar, thus eliminating the inaccurate transillumination procedure commonly performed by most experienced laparoscopists.

The two most common gases used to obtain an adequate pneumoperitoneum are nitrous oxide and carbon dioxide. Most gastroenterologists and hepatologists prefer the use of nitrous oxide since it has much less of an irritating effect on the peritoneum and can be performed without general anaesthesia. Surgeons prefer carbon dioxide during therapeutic and diagnostic laparoscopy. The advantage of this agent is the ability to use electrocautery during the procedure. Eisenhauer *et al.* [5•] evaluated the haemodynamic effects of argon gas in the creation of a pneumoperitoneum. They performed laparoscopy in eight anaesthetized adult pigs using argon gas to achieve an adequate pneumoperitoneum. The gas was delivered for 2 h at a constant intra-abdominal pressure after an adequate pneumo-

peritoneum was obtained. Argon gas was found to have no effects on respiratory function, but increased systemic vascular resistance and reduced the stroke volume index and cardiac index by 25% and 30% from baseline values, respectively. This small study demonstrated that argon gas can be used as an alternative insufflating agent in patients with decreased pulmonary reserve, to avoid severe hypercapnia and acidaemia. On the other hand, this gas should be avoided in patients with compromised cardiac function.

## Malignant diseases

### Staging laparoscopy

The role of diagnostic laparoscopy in the staging of hepatic malignancy is well established. Babineau *et al.* [6•] evaluated 29 patients with primary or secondary hepatic malignancies prior to laparotomy. All patients were deemed potentially resectable based upon a standard preoperative evaluation, including ultrasound and computed tomography (CT) scanning. Twelve patients had primary hepatic malignancies and 17 had metastatic disease. Laparoscopy demonstrated evidence of unresectability in 14 out of 29 patients (48%). Four patients had unsuspected cirrhosis and 10 had extrahepatic metastatic disease or satellite lesions within the liver. Only four patients had unresectable disease that was not identified by laparoscopy. All four patients had previous surgery with significant adhesions within the right upper quadrant which precluded adequate visualization of the area. This study demonstrated that diagnostic laparoscopy is associated with a 78% sensitivity rate and 100% specificity when dealing with resectability of hepatic malignancies. The authors concluded that staging laparoscopy should precede laparotomy in patients with potentially resectable hepatic malignancies since this procedure would decrease the length of stay, cost, morbidity and the outcome of a negative laparotomy.

### Peritoneal carcinomatosis

It is well established that laparoscopy is the best method to detect peritoneal metastases. Jahns *et al.* [7•] reported a case of a 72-year-old man with renal cell carcinoma treated with chemotherapy, who presented with ascites. Two paracenteses with cytological examination of the ascitic fluid failed to demonstrate malignant cells. Laparoscopy was performed which revealed extensive stranding and studding of the parietal and visceral peritoneum with nodules. Biopsies of one of the nodules revealed a poorly differentiated metastatic renal cell carcinoma. This brief case report supports the role of diagnostic laparoscopy in the definitive diagnosis of ascites of unknown origin.

Chu *et al.* [8•] reported a large series of patients who underwent diagnostic laparoscopy for the evaluation of ascites of unclear origin. A total of 129 patients were evaluated. The diagnosis of peritoneal carcinomatosis was found in 73 patients (56.6%), tuberculosis peritonitis in 31 of the cases (24%) and cirrhosis in seven of the patients (5.4%). Eighteen patients (14%) had a negative diagnostic laparoscopy. Laparoscopy with guided liver biopsy in this study established the definitive diagnosis in 86% of all cases. This study again demonstrated that diagnostic laparoscopy plays a very important role in patients with ascites of unknown origin. The majority of the patients in this study did not have cirrhosis and ascites. The aetiology of portal hypertension-induced ascites can often be established with a diagnostic paracentesis and analysis of the fluid, thus avoiding laparoscopy. In this study, unnecessary laparotomy was avoided in a large percentage of patients when laparoscopy was used to confirm the diagnosis of a malignancy.

The development of intraoperative ultrasound has had an impact on intraoperative decision making during surgical resection for primary and secondary liver tumours. The surgeon can now assess the proximity of vessels to the tumour, the extent of the tumour, and discover lesions not seen by conventional imaging studies. This technology can now be used in conjunction with laparoscopy (Fig. 2). John *et al.* [9**] evaluated 50 consecutive patients who had a potentially resectable liver tumour with laparoscopy and laparoscopic ultrasound. Laparoscopic ultrasound was performed in 43 patients. Two 10-mm laparoscopic ports were placed under general anaesthesia in the umbilical and right lumbar areas. A 7.5-MHz linear array probe with a diameter of 9 mm and a length of 40 cm was placed under direct vision to inspect the liver surface and under-surface, and the findings were monitored with an Aloca UST-5521-7.5 (Key Med Ltd, Southend-on-Sea, Essex, UK). Tumours not visible by laparoscopy were identified in 14 patients (33%) and laparoscopic ultrasonography provided additional information precluding hepatic resection in 18 patients. The decision

to resect a particular malignancy based on laparoscopic ultrasound findings resulted in a successful outcome in 13 out of 14 patients (93%). Prior to the use of laparoscopy and laparoscopic ultrasound, 38 patients underwent open laparotomy to assess their potential for hepatic resection. Only 58% of these patients underwent a successful liver resection. The results of this study strongly support the use of laparoscopic ultrasound prior to surgical resection of liver tumours (Fig. 3). The addition of colour Doppler and the introduction of flexible laparoscopic ultrasound probes will also increase the diagnostic accuracy of this new technological breakthrough.

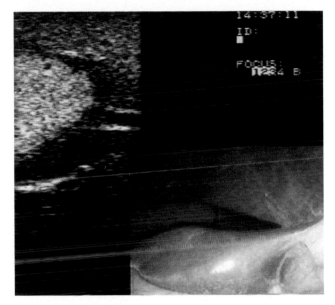

**Fig. 3.** Aloka ultrasound probe on the surface of right lobe of the liver. A small hepatocellular carcinoma not seen on the surface can be seen within the right lobe. Courtesy of T. John, University of Edinburgh Royal Infirmary.

## Laparoscopy in patients with human immunodeficiency virus

Patients infected with the human immunodeficiency virus (HIV) may present with a variety of opportunistic infections and malignancies (Fig. 4). Jeffers *et al.* [10*] presented their laparoscopic and histological findings in 54 patients who were HIV positive, 44 with AIDS. All of these patients underwent laparoscopic examination and visually guided biopsies for the assessment of clinical or biochemical evidence of liver injury. Significant abnormalities were detected in 25 out of 54 patients (46%). The most common findings were peritoneal involvement in 13 out of 54 (24%), nodular liver in seven (13%), focal lesions of the liver in three (5%) and massive adhesions in two (4%). One complication occurred in a patient with dense adhesions secondary to microbacterium tuberculosis who developed a bowel perforation during placement of the trocar. This study demonstrated that laparoscopy appears to be a

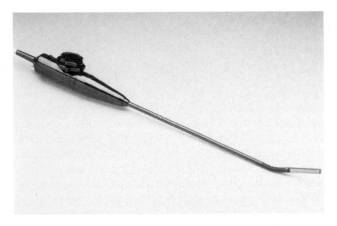

**Fig. 2.** Tetrad flexible linear array laparoscopic ultrasound probe, 10 mm in diameter.

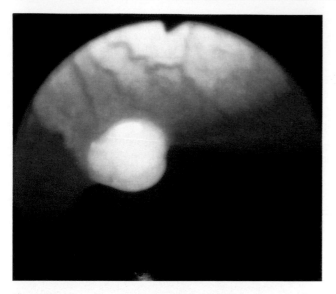

**Fig. 4.** *Mycobacterium avium*-intracellular infection. A raised soft and fleshy mass 2 mm in diameter located on the mesentery and bowel surface.

safe and accurate procedure to diagnose intra-abdominal disease in HIV-positive patients, particularly in those patients with ascites secondary to peritoneal disease or intrinsic liver disease (Fig. 5).

Acute fatty liver of pregnancy is a life-threatening process that occurs usually in the third trimester of pregnancy. A case report of a 27-year-old woman who developed foetal distress during the 38th week of pregnancy was reported [11•]. It was noticed that the patient was jaundiced with severe pitting oedema and increased liver function test. She underwent an emergency Caesarean section and delivered a normal female infant. Her postpartum course was complicated by progressive worsening of her jaundice and severe disseminated intravascular coagulopathy. The patient

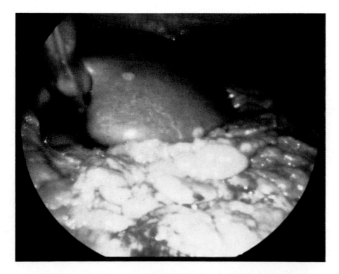

**Fig. 5.** White raised plaques are extensively distributed over the parietal and visceral aspects of the peritoneum and liver surface, in a patient with non-Hodgkin's lymphoma.

was placed on mechanical ventilation and a CT scan of the abdomen revealed a fatty liver with ascites. A bedside laparoscopy was performed which demonstrated an enlarged firm liver and ascites. A liver biopsy revealed acute fatty liver of pregnancy. There were no complications reported as a result of the laparoscopy, and the patient's liver function test improved during her hospitalization. This case, again, illustrates the effectiveness of laparoscopy in patients with ascites.

## Therapeutic laparoscopy

Since the advent of laparoscopic cholecystectomy, the number of laparoscopic procedures for the management of intra-abdominal processes has increased dramatically over the past year (Fig. 1). The amazing success of therapeutic laparoscopy is due, in part, to the shorter hospital stay required, the reduced postoperative pain, an early return to normal activities, and the significant cosmetic benefit to the patients.

### Laparoscopic cholecystectomy

Laparoscopic cholecystectomy was developed in France in 1987 and introduced into the United States in 1989. Laparoscopic cholecystectomy accounts for approximately 80–85% of cholecystectomies performed over the past year in the United States. Large series describing the experience of many surgical groups throughout the world have been reported previously in the medical literature. Cappuccino *et al.* [12•] reported their experience with 563 cases performed at a community teaching hospital and reviewed the literature of an additional 12 201 cases. In their patients, laparoscopic cholecystectomy was successfully accomplished in 536 (95.3%) of the patients and only 30 (4.7%) of the cases were converted to an open procedure. There was a total of 39 (6.9%) complications with only 14 related to technical aspects of the procedure and no deaths were reported. The mean duration of the procedure was 86.4 min and the mean hospital stay was 2.2 days. Interestingly, 41% of their cases had previous abdominal or pelvic surgery. In their review of the literature, a total of 11 638 cases were reviewed and found suitable to be included in the study. The complication rate ranged from 0 to 5% and the major problems associated with this procedure included common bile duct injuries, bowel and vascular injuries, retained stones and intraoperative bleeding. The authors concluded from their review that laparoscopic cholecystectomy is a safe procedure with acceptable morbidity and mortality rates, with the additional advantages of a shorter hospital stay, a quicker return to work, and less postoperative pain. This extensive review confirms that laparoscopic cholecystectomy is here to stay and, with the improving skills of surgeons, one would expect a decrease in the number of complications in the upcoming years. Kum and Goh [13•]

reported on 1066 cases from Singapore who underwent laparoscopic cholecystectomy. Only 57 of these patients (5.4%) had to be converted to an open laparotomy. Common bile duct injury and bile duct leaks in 17 patients (1.6%) and one death (0.09%), which occurred in an elderly man with postoperative sepsis secondary to biliary spillage during the gallbladder dissection, were the major complications. The average hospital stay from this series was 3 days. Results of this large series are comparable to others previously reported in the medical literature.

Emphysematous cholecystitis is a rare condition caused by mixed polymicrobial infections, and characterized by severe inflammation of the gallbladder associated with the production of gas within the walls and lumen. The surgical management for this condition is an open laparotomy. Barnwell *et al.* [14•] reported three cases of emphysematous cholecystitis managed by laparoscopic cholecystectomy. The preoperative diagnosis was made in all cases by ultrasound. The mean hospital stay was 6 days and two patients developed postoperative infection, but no deaths were reported. The authors concluded that, in experienced hands, laparoscopic removal of the gallbladder with emphysematous cholecystitis is feasible with no significant morbidity. The number of patients in this study was small and one should not assume that laparoscopic cholecystectomy is the treatment of choice for emphysematous cholecystitis, a potentially fatal disorder. Therefore, this study should be treated with caution until larger series are reported for this condition. Open cholecystectomy remains the treatment of choice in patients with well-established emphysematous cholecystitis. Steiner *et al.* [15••] reported an analysis of hospital discharges in all patients who underwent a cholecystectomy during the period 1985–1992 in the state of Maryland, USA. In addition, they analysed the rate of cholecystectomies with the introduction of laparoscopic cholecystectomy, characteristics of the patients, and mortality rates. The rate of cholecystectomy was essentially constant until 1989; however, with the introduction of laparoscopic cholecystectomy that same year, the overall rate of cholecystectomies increased by 28% in 1992. Seventy-six per cent of all cholecystectomies performed in Maryland were done with laparoscopic cholecystectomy. Patients undergoing laparoscopic cholecystectomy were more likely to be female, white and younger than the patients undergoing open cholecystectomy. The average hospital stay for patients who had undergone laparoscopic cholecystectomy was 65% shorter than the patients with an open procedure. The operative mortality was significantly lower for laparoscopic cholecystectomy than for open cholecystectomy. The authors suggest that the overall increase in cholecystectomies was due to the advent of laparoscopy, and more liberal indications for this procedure. This study did not analyse the non-fatal complications of laparoscopic cholecystectomy such as bile duct injuries, retained stones, biliary leaks, vascular and bile duct injuries. These findings are not unique for Maryland; they are seen throughout the Western world.

Most surgeons advocate the use of intraoperative cholangiography during laparoscopic cholecystectomy. This procedure may detect unsuspected bile duct stones and anatomical anomalies of the common bile duct which are important in order to avoid bile duct injuries during the procedure. Corbitt and Yusem [16••] reported their experience with intraoperative cholangiography. They studied 511 out of 516 patients with intraoperative cholangiography at the time of laparoscopic cholecystectomy, which was successfully completed in 99% of the cases. Unsuspected common bile duct stones were identified in a total of 29 patients (5%). The authors concluded that intraoperative cholangiography was easier to perform laparoscopically with a minimal operative time of less than 5 min. The addition of intraoperative cholangiography will identify common bile duct stones and anatomical anomalies, which will decrease complications in the management of choledocholithiasis. However, laparoscopy common bile duct exploration is entering a new era. This technique requires surgeons with excellent skills in therapeutic laparoscopy and familiarity with specialized equipment, including fluoroscopy, choledochoscope, guide wires, stone baskets and balloon-tipped catheters. The stones can be retrieved either through a transcystic duct approach or under direct vision with a stone basket placed through the choledochoscope. Franklin *et al.* [17•] reported their experience with the laparoscopic approach to common bile duct stones. They performed intraoperative cholangiography in 857 patients. Eighty-six patients (10.4%) had common bile duct stones. Laparoscopic common bile duct exploration was accomplished in 60 consecutive patients. Their technique for the removal of common bile duct stones consisted of performing a laparoscopic choledochostomy either by directly opening the common bile duct with scissors, or laparoscopic knife, or by potassium titanyl phosphate laser. The size and the number of stones determined the approach used to remove the stones either by direct vision through a choledochoscope, or a Fogarty catheter-aided removal. After exploration of the common bile duct and removal of the stones, a T-tube was placed laparoscopically and sutured in place with 40 vicryl using intracorporeal knot-tying techniques with a pre-tied loop. The T-tube was removed 10–14 days after a final cholangiogram. This procedure was accomplished satisfactorily in 96% of all patients with choledocholithiasis; however, the procedure should only be attempted by a skilled surgical operator who has considerable experience with biliary tract surgery.

### Laparoscopic herniorrhaphy

The laparoscopic approach to inguinal hernia repairs is considered a valid alternative to the traditional open procedure. The advantages of the laparoscopic approach are several, including decreased postoperative pain and the rapid rate of recovery to normal activities, but the rate of recurrence with the laparoscopic approach appears to be higher than a conventional hernia repair. Felix *et al.* [18•] presented their experience with a new technique which consists of transabdominal preperitoneal floor repair. They performed 326 laparoscopic hernia repairs in 227 patients. The technique consisted of dissecting the entire inguinal floor and using a single layer sheet of polypropylene mesh cut into an oval, large enough to cover the entire inguinal floor to buttress the direct and indirect femoral spaces. Both pieces of polypropylene were stapled to the transversalis fascia, iliopubic tract, and Cooper's ligament. The peritoneum was closed with either staples or running suture. One hundred and twenty-eight hernias were indirect, 55 were direct, 22 were pantaloon, 26 were recurrent and 22 were bilateral. Two hundred and five of these repairs were followed for a period of greater than 6 months. The incidence of complications, both major and minor, was 19%, the majority (13.9%) being seromas.

Felix *et al.* [19•] reported a series of laparoscopic repair for recurrent groin hernias. They used a laparoscopic transabdominal preperitoneal technique to repair 54 recurrent groin hernias in 50 patients. Twenty-five were direct, 19 were indirect, 10 were pantaloon and two were femoral hernias. There were no recurrences after a mean follow-up of 8 months. The only major complication was a small bowel injury in one patient. Seromas were observed in 10% of all repairs. Laparoscopic approach to recurrent groin hernias is technically feasible and the authors showed that early recurrence of the hernia was rare.

### Laparoscopic antireflux surgery

Patients with severe gastro-oesophageal reflux disease who have failed medical management are candidates for surgical repair. The laparoscopic approach appears to be a good alternative to the conventional procedure when one considers the shorter hospital stay, the rapid convalescence, the lower morbidity and the probable lower cost. Bittner *et al.* [20••] presented their results with laparoscopic Nissen fundoplication. Thirty-five patients with symptomatic gastro-oesophageal reflux and reflux-induced pulmonary diseases were evaluated for laparoscopic antireflux surgery. All patients underwent 24-h pH monitoring, upper endoscopy and manometry prior to the procedure. The indications for surgery were medical failures or the need for long-term medical treatment of reflux. The mean age of all patients was 42 years. Thirty patients underwent laparoscopic Nissen fundoplication. Four patients had to be converted to an open procedure. The average total surgical time for the laparoscopic operation was 107 min and the mean hospital stay was 3.3 days. Eighty-seven per cent of the patients described their outcome as excellent. Complications occurred in four patients, but no deaths were reported. The authors concluded that laparoscopic Nissen fundoplication is an effective antireflux operation that compares favourably with the conventional procedure.

Kraemer *et al.* [21•] reported their initial experience with laparoscopic Hill repair after extensively testing their technique in animals. The laparoscopic Hill repair technique to correct gastro-oesophageal reflux was performed in 17 patients with a mean age of 52 years. Patients were selected because of severe gastro-oesophageal reflux that was unresponsive to medical management. The preoperative evaluation consisted of upper endoscopy, oesophageal manometry and 24-h pH monitoring. There were no deaths or serious complications reported. The mean follow-up was 10.5 months and the average lower oesophageal sphincter pressure changed from 12.1 mmHg preoperatively to 22.4 mmHg postoperatively. Twenty-four-hour pH monitoring showed no evidence of gastro-oesophageal reflux. The results accomplished with this technique are as good as with the conventional procedure. The advantages of laparoscopic antireflux surgery are obvious: shortened hospital stay, early return to normal activities and less postoperative pain. In another report, Geagea [22••] reported his experience with reflux oesophagitis using the laparoscopic Nissen–Rossetti fundoplication. Fifty-nine patients underwent the laparoscopic procedure. The mean age was 49 years and the mean weight was 74.8 kg. All patients had chronic reflux oesophagitis unresponsive to medical therapy. The preoperative evaluation consisted of an upper endoscopy, 24-h pH monitoring, barium meal and oesophageal manometry. The mean operative time for the fundoplication alone was less than 1 h. One patient had to be converted to an open procedure and eight patients had concomitant posterior trunco-vagotomy with anterior seromyotomy. Four patients had cholecystectomy, and two had umbilical hernias repaired. There were no complications reported other than one patient with chest pain, which resolved in hospital, and no deaths were reported. Ten patients were lost to follow-up and all the remaining patients were asymptomatic with normal postoperative tests. The author suggested that this modified technique is the safest and easiest way of dealing with gastro-oesophageal reflux refractory in medical management.

Despite the successful removal of the colon with laparoscopy, this procedure has not gained widespread acceptance throughout the surgical community. Musser *et al.* [23••] reviewed their early experience with laparoscopic colectomy and compared their result with open colectomy. Twenty-four patients were evaluated. The indications for surgery included benign, malignant and inflammatory diseases of the colon. The mean age of the patients was 68 years. There were 17 with colon cancer, four patients had diverticular disease and there were three with benign caecal lesions. The laparoscopic procedure performed consisted of 11 right hemicolectomies, 10 sigmoidectomies and low anterior resections, two abdominal peritoneal resections and one subtotal colectomy. Six patients had to be converted to open colectomy due to adhesions. Laparoscopic-assisted colon resections were completed in 75% of the patients. There was no perioperative mortality and complications occurred in seven patients (29%). The length of the procedure averaged 169 min and the average hospital stay was 8.5 days. The total hospital cost was found to be lower in the laparoscopy group. The authors concluded that laparoscopic colectomy is a safe, effective and cost-efficient method for colon resection.

## Laparoscopic adrenalectomy

With recent advances in laparoscopic surgery, surgeons are discovering more indications for the laparoscopic approach. Laparoscopic adrenalectomy is now an additional procedure that can be performed safely through this technique. Sardi and McKinnon [24•] described their method of laparoscopic adrenalectomy in three patients presenting with primary aldosteronism. Two patients had left adrenal masses and one patient presented with a right adrenal adenoma. The left adrenal gland was approached through the root of the transverse mesocolon and the right adrenal gland through the subhepatic space. There were no complications and the patients were discharged within 24–48 h of the procedure, with normal blood pressure and no antihypertensive medication. Laparoscopic adrenalectomy is another procedure that can be performed safely with a very low morbidity and with a minimal hospital stay.

## Laparoscopic drainage of a hepatic abscess

The advent of minimally invasive surgery through the laparoscope has increased the therapeutic options in patients with hepatic abscesses. Cappuccino et al. [25•] presented a single, brief case report of laparoscopic-guided drainage of a hepatic abscess. The patient was a 45-year-old Haitian male who presented with fever, abnormal liver function test and leukocytosis. An abdominal CT scan revealed a large abscess in the posterior aspect of the right lobe of the liver. An attempt to aspirate the abscess with guided sonography failed to accomplish the complete drainage of the abscess and the patient underwent a laparoscopic-guided drainage of the hepatic abscess. Under direct vision, a 22-gauge 10-inch spinal needle was passed transabdominally into the region of the liver suspected of harbouring the

abscess. A free return of pus was noted and the needle was then changed to an 18-gauge 10-inch spinal needle and, through this needle, a flexible stainless J guide wire was introduced into the abscess cavity. A dilator was then passed over the guide wire and a Jackson Pratt drain was placed into the abscess cavity. The patient improved dramatically and a CT scan performed 48 h postprocedure revealed a decrease in the size of the abscess cavity. This brief report provides an alternative approach in patients with hepatic abscesses, particularly those abscesses located in the right posterior lobe of the liver which can be very difficult for the radiologist.

## Laparoscopic treatment of liver cysts

Parasitic and non-parasitic cysts of the liver are benign conditions that may become symptomatic and thus lead to surgical intervention. However, with the introduction of the laparoscopic approach, many surgeons have discovered this approach to be the treatment of choice in patients with symptomatic benign cysts of the liver. Khoury et al. [26•] reported a case of a 27-year-old man who presented with a 6-week history of recurrent right upper quadrant pain. An abdominal ultrasound revealed a 9.4 × 8 cm septated cystic mass in the right lobe of the liver compatible with a hydatid cyst. The indirect haemagglutination titre was 1/16 384. The patient underwent laparoscopic exploration and the cyst was visualized in the dome of the right lobe, extending inferiorly to the gallbladder fossa. The right upper quadrant was flooded with a 1% cetrimide (potent scolecoidal solution), bathing the cyst completely. A 14 F stamey superpubic bladder catheter was introduced through a 10-mm trocar into the cyst cavity while continuously irrigating the site of the puncture. The hydatid cyst was aspirated and equal amounts of cetrimide solution was injected into the cyst through the same catheter and left in place for 10 min. The cyst was opened and a 28 F chest tube was introduced into the cyst cavity and attached to high-pressure suction, evacuating all the endocysts and daughter cysts. The cyst was then marsupialized and the cavity was packed with omentum. The patient had a smooth postoperative course with no significant pain and was discharged on the third postoperative day. Although this paper reveals a novel approach to a hydatid cyst, one should keep in mind the potential danger with this procedure since spillage of the cyst content into the abdominal cavity can sometimes lead to anaphylactoid shock.

Libutti and Starker [27•] reported the case of a 75-year-old woman with symptomatic polycystic liver disease diagnosed by CT scan who underwent laparoscopic resection of the largest cyst. Laparoscopic exploration of the abdomen revealed several large cysts involving the left lobe of the liver. The largest of these cysts measured approximately 10 × 12 cm and was resected using an endogastrointestinal stapler device following aspiration of the cyst content with minimal blood loss. The operative time was approximately 90 min. These two cases demonstrated the use of minimally invasive surgery to correct a problem previously corrected with an open laparotomy.

## Laparoscopic diverticulectomy

The popularity of laparoscopic surgery and the improving skills of surgeons has led to innovative surgical procedures during laparoscopy. Callery *et al.* [28•] reported the case of a 53-year-old man on chronic anticoagulation therapy who presented with an upper gastrointestinal bleed. Endoscopic examination revealed the site of the bleeding in a duodenal diverticulum that was successfully controlled with epinephrine injections and the application of a heater probe. A definitive procedure was successfully attempted with laparoscopy. The diverticulum was localized to the lateral wall of the third portion of the duodenum and was exposed by using a Kocher manoeuvre. Intraoperative upper endoscopy was performed to assist with the anatomical location of the diverticulum. Using a 60-mm laparoscopic endogastrointestinal linear stapler, the base of the duodenal diverticulum was engaged and the diverticulum was resected. The patient recovered uneventfully and was discharged on the third postoperative day.

Heinzelmann *et al.* [29•] reported a case of a Meckel's diverticulum in a 17-year-old boy who presented with significant acute lower gastrointestinal bleeding. An upper endoscopy, colonoscopy and selective angiography were performed, but the source of the bleeding remained occult. Several days later, the patient presented with symptoms of gastrointestinal bleeding and a [99m]technetium (pertechnetate) scan demonstrated the source of the bleeding to be a Meckel's diverticulum. Laparoscopic diverticulectomy was performed using a linear stapler device. The patient recovered uneventfully and was discharged 24 h after admission in a stable condition. Both of these cases again demonstrated the role of laparoscopy in an evolving field of therapeutic laparoscopy.

## Laparoscopic repair of a perforated duodenal ulcer

Isaac *et al.* [30•] reported their early experience with laparoscopic repair of perforated duodenal ulcers. Seven patients with an average age of 34 years with perforated duodenal ulcers underwent laparoscopic procedures. Six ulcers were found on the anterior surface of the duodenal bulb and one was on the lateral surface of the second portion of the duodenum. The average size of the perforation was 3.5 mm. The technique consisted of a closure of the perforation using a patch of omentum over the hole and tied with intracorporeal knots. Metallic clips were placed above the knots to ensure tight application of the omentum to the perforation. Vigorous irrigation of the peritoneum was also carried out at the time of laparoscopy. The average operative time was 80 min. There were no postoperative complications observed and the average hospital stay was 6 days. This initial experience confirms that laparoscopic repair of perforated duodenal ulcers are feasible in most of the cases when the procedure is carried out a few hours after the diagnosis is confirmed.

## Exploratory laparoscopy

The use of exploratory laparoscopy in the evaluation and management of patients with iatrogenic colonic perforations has gained acceptance among surgeons. Chardavoyne and Wise [31•] reported the case of a 50-year-old woman who presented with diffuse abdominal distention and pain 24 h after a colonoscopy and polypectomy. On physical examination she was febrile with a markedly distended abdomen, but with no peritoneal signs. An upright chest X-ray revealed a significant pneumoperitoneum. Exploratory laparoscopy was performed and a large amount of free air escaped from the abdominal cavity when the Verres needle was introduced through the umbilicus. A thorough exploration was performed and bubbles of air were seen on the greater omentum, but no free perforation or injury were identified. The patient recovered uneventfully. Although the exact site was never found, the clinical presentation strongly indicated a perforation of the colon. Goh *et al.* [32•] reported a case of a 73-year-old man who underwent colonoscopy for iron deficiency anaemia. Colonoscopy was performed with some difficulty, particularly traversing a long tortuous sigmoid colon. Shortly after the procedure, the patient presented with abdominal pain. On physical examination, his abdomen was noted to be bloated and tender. Abdominal X-rays revealed free air under the diaphragm. An exploratory laparoscopy was performed and the peritoneal cavity was noted to be moderately soiled with colonic fluid. A perforation, 2.5 cm in diameter, was found in the upper sigmoid colon. The margins of the perforation were held by endoscopic graspers in a transverse fashion and the defect was closed using an endogastrointestinal stapler device. The colonoscope was passed into the sigmoid colon and air was insufflated to test the integrity of the closure. A vigorous lavage of the peritoneal cavity was performed under laparoscopic vision and the patient recovered with no complications. Both cases demonstrated a new role for laparoscopy in the exploration of the abdominal cavity in patients with suspected perforation following a colonoscopy. The therapeutic options available for primary closure of a colonic perforation was clearly described in the latter case.

## Laparoscopy in children

Paediatric surgeons throughout the world have used laparoscopy sparingly for many years and there are few reports detailing their experience in the medical literature. Schier and Waldschmidt [33••] have performed laparoscopy in newborns and children. They performed a total of 225 laparoscopies in children presenting with non-specific abdominal pain. The children's ages ranged from newborn to 15 years with an average age of 8 years. Although the initial procedure was initiated as a diagnostic laparoscopy, therapeutic laparoscopy was performed in the majority of patients resulting in 85 appendectomies, 52 lysis of adhesions, 27 resections of ovarian cysts, 25 interventions on the internal genitalia, three Meckel's diverticulectomies and various other interventions, including liver biopsies and cholangiograms. The authors concluded that there were several advantages in children undergoing diagnostic and therapeutic laparoscopy: the excellent visualization of the intra-abdominal organs, the decrease in postoperative pain, and an early discharge from the hospital.

## Complications

Since the advent of laparoscopic cholecystectomy, general surgeons have expanded the role of laparoscopy for many gastrointestinal disorders. As the role of laparoscopy has been expanded, the number of complications has increased over the years (Fig. 6). Many of these complications are secondary to bile duct injuries, thermal injuries, perforation of a hollow viscus and vascular injuries. One of the most common complications during laparoscopic cholecystectomy are bile duct injuries and bile leaks. Woods et al. [34••] reported a multi-institutional study of patients with biliary tract injuries occurring during laparoscopic cholecystectomy. The patients were referred to one of three tertiary referral centres for the management of laparoscopic cholecystectomy-related bile duct injuries. The authors reviewed the records of the patients and concentrated on the anatomy of the lesion, the method of injury, the timing of injury detection, the role of intraoperative cholangiography, and the treatment and outcome of these injuries. Eighty-one patients were referred to three centres during a 33-month period. Fifteen patients had cystic duct leaks, 27 had bile leaks and/or ductal strictures and 39 had ductal trans-section or excision. Only 31 of the 81 injuries (38%) were recognized at the time of procedure and converted to an open operation. The majority (62%) of the injuries were recognized after the procedure. An intraoperative cholangiogram was performed in only 63 out of 81 cases. Thirty-eight (60%) of the cases did not undergo cholangiography at the time of laparoscopy and 25 patients (40%) underwent cholangiography. In 14 patients (37%) who did not undergo intraoperative cholangiogram, their procedure was converted to an open operation, whereas 13 patients (52%) who underwent an intraoperative cholangiogram had their procedure converted to a laparotomy. Two surgical and/or endoscopic approaches were used to repair biliary tract injuries. All simple cystic duct leaks resolved with endoscopic stents and 91% of bile duct strictures resolved with endoscopic stenting and/or balloon dilatation. Patients with trans-section or excision injuries were treated with surgical procedures, primarily biliary enteric bypass. The authors clearly addressed the importance of performing intraoperative cholangiograms to detect biliary tract injuries during laparoscopic cholecystectomy and suggest that attempts be made for primary suture repair of bile duct injuries during laparoscopic cholecystectomy.

Peters et al. [35•] reported their experience with biliary tract leaks following laparoscopic cholecystectomy. They performed 854 laparoscopic cholecystectomies and reported nine (1.1%) cases with postoperative bile duct leaks. An additional six patients were referred to their institution for the management of bile duct leaks. The majority of patients presented in the first week following the procedure, with increasing abdominal pain, nausea and low-grade fever. Eleven out of 15 patients (66.7%) underwent technetium-99 imidodiacetic acid scanning to determine the presence of possible bile leaks. Predictably, the results were positive in all patients. Thirteen patients underwent endoscopic cholangiography to confirm the presence of bile leakage. The location of the bile leak was determined to be the common bile duct in two patients, the cystic duct in five patients, and small accessory ducts located close to the gallbladder bed in eight patients. Nine patients were managed endoscopically with placement of biliary stents or endoscopic sphincterotomy. Five patients were taken to the operating room for the management of their leaks. The authors emphasize that the ideal treatment of bile duct leaks following laparoscopic cholecystectomy requires further study. However, the use of non-invasive tests, coupled with endoscopic management, allows for the rapid evaluation with prompt and appropriate treatment, which will minimize further morbidity.

| Absolute | Relative |
|---|---|
| Cirrhosis and portal hypertension | Morbid obesity |
| Coagulopathy | Pregnancy |
| Severe cardiac disease (class-IV NYHA) | Ascites |
| COPD and hypercapnia | Previous abdominal surgery |
| Previous intraperitoneal chemotherapy | Diaphragmatic hernia |
| Colostomy or ileostomy | Acute pancreatitis |

**Fig. 6.** Contraindications for laparoscopic cholecystectomy: absolutes and relatives. COPD = chronic obstructive pulmonary disease; NYHA = New York Heart Association.

Two cases of biliary leakage from the accessory bile ducts, following laparoscopic cholecystectomy, were presented by Edelman [36•]. Both of these cases presented in the postoperative period with signs and symptoms suggestive of a bile duct leak. In the first case, an endoscopic cholangiogram demonstrated an aberrant duct within the liver bed and a 10 F choledochal–duodenal stent was placed with rapid resolution over several days. In a subsequent case, a hepatobiliary scan demonstrated a bile duct leak which was confirmed with endoscopic retrograde cholangiopancreatography. A 10 F stent was placed and the patient improved dramatically. Bile leaks from the accessory bile ducts following laparoscopic cholecystectomy are uncommon. However, recent reports in the literature strongly suggest that there may be an increase in this complication following laparoscopic cholecystectomy. A rare complication of laparoscopic cholecystectomy was reported by Cervantes et al. [37•]. A 51-year-old man underwent laparoscopic cholecystectomy and presented 14 days later with fever, right upper quadrant pain and chills. An abdominal ultrasound demonstrated no abnormalities in the subhepatic space, but did indicate a large defect in the right lobe of the liver. A CT scan was performed which revealed a large subcapsular collection in the lateral aspect of the right lobe of the liver. Percutaneous drainage, guided by ultrasound, was performed and 1100 cm³ of clear bile was removed. An endoscopic cholangiogram revealed no abnormalities of the intrahepatic bile ducts or communication with the biloma.

A thermal injury of the duodenum during laparoscopic cholecystectomy was reported by Berry et al. [38•]. Six days following the procedure, the patient was awakened from sleep with acute onset of severe right upper quadrant abdominal pain. On physical examination, the patient was found to have diffuse tenderness throughout the abdomen and over the right upper quadrant. An abdominal CT scan demonstrated a collection of fluid and air posterior to the duodenum. An exploratory laparotomy was performed and the duodenum was found displaced anteriorly by a posterior mass. An extensive Kocher manoeuvre was performed which revealed a 1.5-cm segment of superficial necrosis of the second portion of the duodenum posteriorly with a small 5-mm perforation in the centre of the necrotic area. This perforation was interpreted as an electrical conductive injury which occurred during the dissection of the gallbladder in the triangle of Calot close to the posterior aspect of the second portion of the duodenum. A hepatic artery aneurysm presenting with haemobilia is a rare complication of laparoscopic cholecystectomy. Bloch et al. [39•] reported a case of haemobilia occurring 1 month after laparoscopic cholecystectomy. The patient presented with upper gastrointestinal bleeding and abdominal pain radiating to her back. An upper endoscopy revealed blood in the duodenum; however, no source of bleeding was identified. An angiogram demonstrated a false aneurysm of the right hepatic artery with a surgical clip in contact with the neck of the false aneurysm. The bleeding was treated with gel-foam embolization but, because of a recurrence of bleeding, embolization with platinum coils was successfully utilized in curtailing the bleeding. The mechanism of this complication was attributed to a metallic clip that eroded into the artery wall which led to the formation of a false aneurysm. A similar case was reported by Genyk et al. [40••] in a 57-year-old woman presenting with abdominal pain, gastrointestinal bleeding, and jaundice of 2 weeks duration following laser laparoscopic cholecystectomy. A selective angiogram showed a right hepatic artery pseudoaneurysm which was subsequently embolized. Two weeks later, the patient again presented with recurrent haemobilia, resolved with two additional embolizations along with direct injection of the aneurysm with thrombogenic material. The mechanism of the formation of this pseudoaneurysm was thought to be secondary to laser beam injury to the vessels during dissection of the gallbladder.

Two cases of aortic injury from a trocar insertion during laparoscopic cholecystectomy were recently described [41•]. The first case was that of a 49-year-old man who underwent elective laparoscopic cholecystectomy for gallbladder polyps. During the insertion of the trocar, the operator had difficulty secondary to fascia resistance. Upon entry into the peritoneum, there was a small amount of blood on the omentum, but no active bleeding was observed. During the procedure, the patient became hypotensive and the pneumoperitoneum was released with no significant change in blood pressure. However, there was a suspicion of aortic injury and a laparotomy was performed. A through-and-through injury to the distal aorta was identified at the origin of the left common iliac and two small perforations were found in the small bowel. Both injuries were repaired without complications. Another similar case was also reported by the authors [41•]. The operator had significant difficulty in the placement of a 10 mm trocar. After several attempts, the trocar was inserted into the abdominal cavity and blood was noted in the omentum beneath the umbilicus and over the surface of the liver. A rapid laparotomy was performed and the haemorrhage was controlled with finger pressure. The aorta was found to have an 8-mm defect in the anterior wall and a 3-mm defect in the posterior wall, 2 cm above the bifurcation. Both injuries were repaired and the patients recovered uneventfully. These two cases of aortic injury have a common factor. The operator encountered significant resistance of the fascia during the placement of the trocar, which resulted in the application of greater force. This problem can be easily addressed by careful dissection of the fascia prior to placement of the trocar, or the use of the

Hassan procedure during laparoscopic insertion of the trocar.

## Conclusions

In 1994, numerous papers in the area of therapeutic laparoscopy and its complications were published. This has increased the awareness of many gastroenterologists and surgeons who now refer their patients for minimally invasive surgery. The addition of laparoscopic ultrasound has improved the ability of surgeons to perform hepatic resections in patients with primary and metastatic tumours of the liver.

The future is bright for young general surgeons whose laparoscopy skills will probably improve with virtual reality training as an adjunct to laparoscopic surgery. Diagnostic laparoscopy performed by gastroenterologists and surgeons continues to be an important tool in the evaluation of malignancies, ascites of unknown origin and chronic liver disease and peritoneal disease. The option to convert to a therapeutic procedure is an added benefit.

## Acknowledgement

The authors would like to thank Ana Maria Ortiz for her assistance in the preparation of this manuscript.

## References and recommended reading

Papers of particular interest, published within the annual period of review, have been highlighted as:

- of special interest
- of outstanding interest

1. Schrenk P, Woisetschläger R, Wayand WU: **Diagnostic laparoscopy: Survey of 92 patients.** *Am J Surg* 1994, **168**:348–351.
•• This excellent paper outlines the experience with diagnostic laparoscopy by a group of surgeons who apply their therapeutic experience to further evaluate patients during the course of diagnostic laparoscopy.

2. Crantock LR, Dillon FJ, Hayes PC: **Diagnostic laparoscopy in liver disease: Experience of 200 cases.** *Austr N Z J Med* 1994, **24**:258–262.
•• This paper details the experience with 200 cases of diagnostic laparoscopy performed by gastroenterologists for a wide range of indications. The authors emphasize that this procedure is safe and effective, and can be performed in an endoscopy suite under conscious sedation.

3. Rademaker BM, Odom JA, DeWitt LTH: **Hemodynamic effects of pneumoperitoneum for laparoscopic surgery: A comparison of $CO_2$ with $N_2O$ insufflation.** *Eur J Anesth* 1984, **11**:301–305.
• This important paper describes, in detail, the measurements of hemodynamic changes that occur during the course of nitrous oxide and carbon dioxide pneumoperitoneum on the cardiovascular system. The authors alert us to the fact that, in patients with a compromised cardiovascular system, caution should be applied in the use of both nitrous oxide and carbon dioxide.

4. Whitley MS, Laws SAM, Wise MH: **Use of a hand-held Doppler to avoid abdominal wall vessels in laparoscopic surgery.** *Ann R Coll Surg Engl* 1994, **76**:348–350.
• This interesting paper addressed a potential problem in patients undergoing laparoscopy. The use of this tool can help us avoid bleeding during the placement of the trocar.

5. Eisenhauer DM, Saunders CJ, Ho HS, Wolfe BM: **Hemodynamic effects of argon pneumoperitioneum.** *Surg Endosc* 1994, **8**:315–321.
• A small but important study in animals that demonstrates that argon gas can be used in special conditions as in patients with respiratory conditions who cannot tolerate pneumoperitoneum with the current gases.

6. Babineau TJ, Lewis WD, Jenkins RL, Bleday R, Steele GD Jr, Forse RA: **Role of staging laparoscopy in the treatment of hepatic malignancy.** *Am J Surg* 1994, **167**:151–155.
• An important study that demonstrates the role of laparoscopy in the staging of malignancies. This study supports the use of laparoscopy in candidates for resection of hepatic malignancies.

7. Jahns F, Reddy V, Sherman KE: **Ascites secondary to renal-cell carcinoma diagnosed at laparoscopy.** *J Clin Gastroenterol* 1994, **18**:259–260.
• An interesting, brief case report.

8. Chu CM, Lin SM, Peng SM, Wu CS, Liaw YF: **The role of laparoscopy in the evaluation of ascites of unknown origin.** *Gastrointest Endosc* 1994, **40**:285–289.
• A large series of laparoscopy in the evaluation of ascites of unknown origin. The authors found the cause of ascites in 86% of the cases and excluded other processes that may cause ascites.

9. John TG, Greig JD, Croshie JL: **Superior staging of liver tumors with laparoscopy and laparoscopic ultrasound.** *Ann Surg* 1994, **220**:711–719.
•• A new and innovative approach in the management of primary and secondary liver tumours with laparoscopic ultrasound. Although this is an expensive tool, this procedure will give invaluable information during diagnostic laparoscopy.

10. Jeffers LJ, Alzate I, Aguilar H, Reddy KR, Idrovo V, Cheinquer H, *et al.*: **Laparoscopic and histologic findings in patients with the human immunodeficiency virus.** *Gastrointest Endosc* 1994, **40**:160–164.
• An important study of the value of diagnostic laparoscopy in the evaluation of HIV-seropositive patients. This study demonstrated that laparoscopy is a safe and accurate method in the evaluation of patients with liver and peritoneal disease.

11. Crockett HC, de Virgilio C, Shimaoka E, Bongard FS, Klein SR: **Acute fatty liver of pregnancy: Laparoscopy-assisted diagnosis.** *Surg Laparosc Endosc* 1994, **4**:230–233.
• An interesting, brief case report that demonstrates the feasibility of laparoscopy as the procedure to make an accurate diagnosis in liver disease.

12. Cappuccino H, Cargill N, Nguyen T: **Laparoscopic cholecystectomy: 563 cases at a community teaching hospital and a review of 12,201 cases in the literature.** *Surg Laparosc Endosc* 1994, **4**:213–221.
• This report presents the experience with laparoscopic cholecystectomy in a teaching hospital and a good review of the experience in this procedure.

13. Kum CK, Goh PMY: **Laparoscopic cholecystectomy: The Singapore Experience.** *Surg Laparosc Endosc* 1994, **4**:22–24.
• This is one of the largest reports of laparoscopic cholecystectomy, showing excellent results with this procedure.

14. Banwell PE, Hill ADK, Menzies-Gow N, Darzi A: **Laparoscopic cholecystectomy: safe and feasible in emphysematous cholecystitis.** *Surg Laparosc Endosc* 1994, **4**:189–191.
• This is a small report of three cases of emphysematous cholecystitis managed with laparoscopic cholecystectomy. The authors demonstrated good results with this technique.

15. Steiner CA, Bass EB, Talamini MA, Pitt HA, Steinberg EP: **Surgical rates and operative mortality for open and laparoscopic cholecystectomy in Maryland.** *N Engl J Med* 1994, **330**:403–408.
•• This is an excellent analysis that compares two different approaches in the management of gallstone disease, open cholecystectomy and laparoscopic cholecystectomy for 7 years. The study demonstrated the decrease in operative mortality with laparoscopic cholecystectomy and the increase in the cholecystectomy rate.

16. Corbitt Jr JD, Yusem SO: **Laparoscopic cholecystectomy with operative cholangiogram.** *Surg Endosc* 1994, **8**:292–295.
•• This is one of the largest reports with intraoperative cholangiogram through laparoscopy. These results demonstrated the feasibility of this procedure and the benefits.

17. Franklin Jr ME, Pharand D, Rosenthal D: **Laparoscopic common bile duct exploration.** *Surg Laparosc Endosc* 1994, **4**:119–124.
• This is a remarkable report presenting the experience with this laparoscopic choledochostomy technique as an adjuvant in the management of common bile duct stones.

18.  Felix EL, Michas CA, McKnight RL: **Laparoscopic herniorrhaphy:**
•    **Trans-abdominal preperitoneal floor repair.** *Surg Endosc* 1994, **8**:100–104.
This report presents the experience with this new technique in laparoscopic herniorrhaphy. The authors described the technique in detail and present the results and complications.

19.  Felix EL, Michas CA, McKnight RL: **Laparoscopic repair of recurrent**
•    **groin hernias.** *Surg Laparosc Endosc* 1994, **4**:200–204.
This report presents a new technique in the repair of recurrent inguinal hernias with excellent results.

20.  Bittner HB, Meyers WC, Brazer SR, Pappas TN: **Laparoscopic Nissen**
••   **fundoplication: operative results and short-term follow-up.** *Am J Surg* 1994, **167**:193–200.
This report presents the experience with a new technique. The amazing results observed are encouraging and may be considered as the procedure of choice for the surgical treatment of symptomatic gastro-oesophageal reflux.

21.  Kraemer SJM, Aye R, Kozarek RA, Hill LD: **Laparoscopic Hill repair.**
•    *Gastrointest Endosc* 1994, **40**:155–159.
This is s small but remarkable report by one of the pioneers in the surgical technique for the treatment of gastro-oesophageal reflux. The authors demonstrated the advantages of this technique through laparoscopy.

22.  Geagea T: **Laparoscopic Nissen–Rossetti fundoplication.** *Surg Endosc*
••   1994, **8**:1080–1084.
This report presents the experience of the author with this technique in the treatment of gastro-oesophageal reflux. The excellent outcome confirms the feasibility of the procedure.

23.  Musser DJ, Boorse RC, Madera F, Reed III JF: **Laparoscopic colectomy:**
••   **At what cost?** *Surg Laparosc Endosc* 1994, **4**:1–5.
This report presents the experience of laparoscopic colectomy as compared with the open procedure in regards to morbidity and mortality, operative time and costs. The results showed laparoscopic colectomy is a safe, effective and cost-efficient method of colon resection.

24.  Sardi A, McKinnon WMP: **Laparoscopic adrenalectomy in patients with**
•    **primary aldosteronism.** *Surg Laparosc Endosc* 1994, **4**:86–91.
Small but important report of the experience with laparoscopic adrenalectomy for management of adrenal masses.

25.  Cappuccino H, Campanile F, Knecht J: **Laparoscopy-guided drainage of**
•    **hepatic abscess.** *Surg Laparosc Endosc* 1994, **4**:234–237.
An interesting case report that describes the simple technique for drainage of hepatic abscess by laparoscopy.

26.  Khoury G, Geagea T, Hajj A, Jabbour-Khoury S, Baraka A, Nabbout G:
•    **Laparoscopic treatment of hydatid cysts of the liver.** *Surg Endosc* 1994, **8**:1103–1104.
This is the first case report of laparoscopic treatment of hydatid cyst of the liver. The technique of evacuation and marsupialization is well described.

27.  Libutti SK, Starker PM: **Laparoscopic resection of a nonparasitic liver**
•    **cyst.** *Surg Endosc* 1994, **8**:1105–1107.
A remarkable case of the use of laparoscopy for complete resection of a benign non-parasitic liver cyst using an endoscopic gastrointestinal stapling device.

28.  Callery MP, Aliperti G, Soper NJ: **Laparoscopic duodenal diverticulec-**
•    **tomy following hemorrhage.** *Surg Laparosc Endosc* 1994, **4**:134–138.
An impressive use of laparoscopy in the treatment of a rare cause of severe upper gastrointestinal bleeding.

29.  Heinzelmann M, Schob O,Schlumpf R, Decurtins M, Himmelmann A,
•    Largiader F: **Preoperative diagnosis of Meckel's diverticulum by pertech-netate scan and laparoscopic resection.** *Surg Laparosc Endosc* 1994, **4**:378–381.
An interesting case report that describes the technique for Meckel's diveticulectomy.

30.  Isaac J, Tekant Y, Kong KC, Ngoi SS, Goh P: **Laparoscopic repair of**
•    **perforated duodenal ulcer.** *Gastrointest Endosc* 1994, **40**:68–69.
This is a small but remarkable report that demonstrates the feasibility of laparoscopic repair of perforated duodenal ulcers.

31.  Chardavoyne R, Wise L: **Exploratory laparoscopy for perforation follow-**
•    **ing colonoscopy.** *Surg Laparosc Endosc* 1994, **4**:241–243.
This is a single case to demonstrate that laparoscopy can be important in the diagnosis of suspected iatrogenic perforation.

32.  Goh PMY, Kum CK, Chia YW, Ti TK: **Laparoscopic repair of perforation**
•    **of the colon during laparoscopy.** *Gastrointest Endosc* 1994, **40**:496–497.
This is a remarkable case in the use of therapeutic laparoscopy in the management of iatrogenic colon perforation.

33.  Schier F, Waldschmidt J: **Laparoscopic in children with ill-defined ab-**
••   **dominal pain.** *Surg Endosc* 1994, **8**:97–99.
An important report on the experience of laparoscopy performed in newborns and children. The authors consider this procedure to be very useful in the evaluation of children with ill-defined abdominal pain combining both diagnostic and therapeutic laparoscopy.

34.  Woods MS, Traverso LW, Kozarek RA, Tsao J, Rossi RL, Gough D, *et al.*:
••   **Characteristics of biliary tract complications during laparoscopic cholecystectomy: A multi-institutional study.** *Am J Surg* 1994, **167**:27–34.
This report presents an excellent analysis of different types of biliary duct injuries during laparoscopic cholecystectomy. A different approach in each type of injury is given.

35.  Peters JH, Ollila D, Nichols KE, Gibbons GD, Dvanzo MA, Miller J, *et al.*:
•    **Diagnosis and management of bile leaks following laparoscopic cholecys-tectomy.** *Surg Laparosc Endosc* 1994, **4**:163–170.
This is a small but important report of biliary leaks following laparoscopic cholecystectomy. The authors present this technique in the approach to specific complications.

36.  Edelman DS: **Bile leak from the liver bed following laparoscopic cholecys-**
•    **tectomy.** *Surg Endosc* 1994, **8**:205–207.
A brief report of an uncommon complication of laparoscopic cholecystectomy.

37.  Cervantes J, Rojas GA, Ponte R: **Intrahepatic subcapsular biloma. A rare**
•    **complication of laparoscopic cholecystectomy.** *Surg Endosc* 1994, **8**:208–210.
A detailed approach to correct this complication is described in this article.

38.  Berry SM, Ose KJ, Bell RH, Fink AS: **Thermal injury of the posterior**
•    **duodenum during laparoscopic cholecystectomy.** *Surg Endosc* 1994, **8**:197–200.
This is a report of an unusual complication during laparoscopic cholecystectomy.

39.  Bloch P, Modiano P, Foster D, Bouhot F, Gompel H: **Recurrent hemobilia**
•    **after laparoscopic cholecystectomy.** *Surg Laparosc Endosc* 1994, **4**:375–377.
A rare and infrequent complication is reported.

40.  Genyk YS, Keller FS, Halpern NB: **Hepatic artery pseudoaneurysm and**
••   **hemobilia following laser laparoscopic cholecystectomy.** *Surg Endosc* 1994, **8**:201–204.
This is an unusual complication of the use of laser in laparoscopic surgery.

41.  Apelgren KN, Scheeres DE: **Aortic injury. A catastrophic complication of**
•    **laparoscopic cholecystectomy.** *Surg Endosc* 1994, **8**:689–691.
A report of two rare complications of laparoscopic cholecystectomy which occurred during trocar insertion. The authors offer suggestions for avoiding and treating this major complication.

Dr Lennox J. Jeffers, Professor of Medicine, Division of Hepatology, University of Miami School of Medicine, JMT - 1500 N.W. 12 Avenue, Suite 1101, Miami, Florida 33136, USA.

# Paediatric endoscopy

## Keith J. Benkov

Division of Pediatric Gastroenterology and Nutrition, Mount Sinai Medical Center,
New York, USA

## Introduction

While the number of articles on paediatric gastroenterology has increased over the past few years, this seems to have reached a plateau in 1994. There were, however, several notable trends in 1994. Many of the articles were case histories which, although interesting, have only limited general applicability to the practice of endoscopy in children. Several other articles did have broader implications for the subspecialty, but these were devoid of any detail regarding endoscopic procedure. There also seems to be a tendency for the majority of the articles to be published in the *Journal of Pediatric Gastroenterology and Nutrition*. Many of us in paediatric gastroenterology have benefited from a journal solely devoted to the speciality. We should not, however, lose sight of which topics deserve more general visibility.

## General endoscopy

Beginning with the more general aspects of technique, the experience of paediatric endoscopists [1] in Israel was described for 289 oesophagogastroduodonoscopies performed over a 4-year period on children between the ages of 8 months and 21 years. Almost two-thirds were performed for the evaluation of abdominal pain, of which almost half demonstrated no findings and 14% demonstrated *Helicobacter pylori*. Sixty-five per cent of the total group of patients received no intravenous sedation, contrary to the practice of many paediatric gastroenterologists.

Israel *et al.* [2••] reported on a prospective study of 40 consecutive colonoscopies performed over a 7-month period. All the aspects of indication, sedation and technique were described. In addition, the length of time of the procedure and the extent of examination were noted. The caecum was reached in 92.5% of cases in an average time of 19–37 min depending on who performed the procedure and the terminal ileum was reached in 87.5% of cases 1–23 min after the caecum was reached. Some improvement in time was seen by the trainee over the 7-month period, leading the authors to conclude that trainees can gain the necessary experience when carefully supervised. The limited number of colonoscopies performed as compared with the authors' previous reports on upper endoscopies is quite interesting. There also might be a certain bias in the length of time of the procedures when the endoscopist is aware that he or she is being timed.

## Endoscopy in neonates and young infants

There were many articles this year dealing with the interesting pathology uncovered in neonates and infants. A report from Paris [3•] presented a 4-year experience of 293 upper endoscopies performed on neonates less than 1 month of age. Disappointingly, few technical details were given and no mention was made of the sedation used, if any. No indications for the procedure were discussed, which was also rather disappointing in view of some suspicion as to why so many neonates would need this investigation. The authors stated that the procedure was well tolerated, though in over 20% the duodenum was not reached. There were no complications other than two cases of bradycardia, presumably from tracheal decompression. The findings that were reported were odd in that there were no findings in just over 25%, with just over 50% having both gastritis and oesophagitis, and oesophagitis only in about 20%. Findings were manifested by erythema, ecchymosis or petechia. Only 20 patients, however, had biopsies taken and one could question the correlation between actual pathology and the possibility of 'scope trauma'. In a smaller, but equally provocative series [4] because of unclear indications, endoscopy was performed on 17 consecutive infants at 3–7 days of age of which 14 were preterm. Only two of these infants had gastrointestinal symptoms. The authors reported 94% of infants with pathology, leading one to question the significance of their findings when so many of these were asymptomatic infants.

On the other hand, given clear indications for these procedures, a significant pathology is often encoun-

---

**Abbreviations**

ERCP—endoscopic retrograde cholangiopancreatography; CMV—cytomegalovirus; PEG—percutaneous endoscopic gastrostomy.

tered. Three otherwise healthy newborn infants, two of which passed melanotic stools and one who had haematemesis, all had significant decreases in their haematocrits [5]. Upper endoscopy revealed duodenal ulcers in the first two and haemorrhagic gastritis in the latter. Most reports of gastrointestinal bleeding in newborns have concerned sick neonates while other series have not had the availability of endoscopic examination. There is obvious endoscopic pathology that can be determined in newborns when the indications are well defined. The overuse of the procedure, however, probably leads to over reading of the histologic specimens.

A slightly older infant of 8 months with recurrent vomiting was diagnosed with breast milk allergy based on peripheral eosinophilia and eosinophilic infiltrate on endoscopic mucosal biopsies of the stomach and duodenum [6]. Persistent emesis prompted an upper gastrointestinal series that revealed partial obstruction leading to an exploratory laparotomy that showed duodenal stenosis, Ladd's bands, and a non-obstructing annular pancreas. A duodenostomy relieved the symptoms as well as the eosinophilia, proving an interesting highlight of the limitations of endoscopy and biopsy.

An interesting, incidental illustration to the use of endoscopic retrograde cholangiopancreatography (ERCP) in neonates was a series of 20 infants, less than 2 months of age. These infants were evaluated for cholestasis, and had antral biopsies performed for *H. pylori,* and histology. Only one infant, 58 days of age, demonstrated *H. pylori,* compared with 95% of the respective mothers having documented *H. pylori* on upper endoscopy [7]. Five infants were solely breast-fed, and three were both nursed and formula-fed, including the infected child. The authors attribute the high rate of infection in the mothers to the fact that they were all from lower socioeconomic groups.

Both sonography and upper endoscopy were performed in 63 infants between 1 and 10 weeks of age, later confirmed at surgery to have pyloric stenosis [8•]. Sonogram predicted 81% of the cases of pyloric stenosis while endoscopy predicted 97% based on the findings of a cauliflower-like narrowing of the pyloric channel that could not pass a 7.8 mm scope. Sedation was not used in any of these infants. While this is an exciting application, there are several reservations. The inability to pass the pylorus may be very much dependent on the skill of the endoscopist. These infants were all eventually determined to have pyloric stenosis, but no mention was made of those infants where pyloric stenosis was suspected but not confirmed surgically, namely the incidence of false-positives. The endoscopic diagnosis of this entity may even lead to further attempts of balloon dilation.

## Percutaneous endoscopic gastrostomies

Further attention was given to the technique of percutaneous endoscopic gastrostomies (PEGs). A small series of eight children who underwent the simplified 'push' technique was published [9]. This technique, which has long been used in adults, involves making a puncture in the abdomen with a needle catheter while the endoscope is already in the stomach, followed by passing a guide wire through the catheter. Using this guide wire, a series of dilators are then passed, opening the aperture, followed by a Foley-type catheter that is then inflated. All this happens under direct endoscopic vision. The advantages of this technique are that it alleviates the potential for bacteria being dragged through the mouth as well as possible damage to the oesophagus. This technique has been performed in children for almost as long as it has in adults. No series have yet been reported in the literature, however. Many endoscopists feel that this endoscopic approach is easier and may be preferable for the less experienced endoscopist. Whether there are fewer complications would be better addressed by a large series and might be better determined in adult patients.

The efficacy and safety of traditional PEG was discussed in a series of 70 children performed over 4 years [10]. Seventy per cent of the series had improved nutritional status and another 4% maintained nutritional status, with those children with congenital heart disease and cystic fibrosis receiving the most benefit. There seemed to be significant complications, with 19% having events labelled as major that required surgical intervention including gastric outlet obstruction, gastric colic fistula, peritonitis, necrotizing fasciitis, serious wound infection, aspiration pneumonia and unmanageable reflux requiring fundoplication. Minor complications occurred in 22%, including transient infections, leakage, tube dislodgement and other similar minor problems. Most complications occurred in those children with multi-system failure. The incidence of major complications seems to be in agreement with prior reports but the incidence of minor complications appears quite high, presumably reflecting a more ill population of patients. The benefits of a gastrostomy can be tremendous, but the limitations and complications must be fully understood by all the carers, both medical and parental. Werlin *et al.* [11] demonstrated that feeding could be restarted 6 h after PEG placement in 24 out of 28 consecutive children.

## Oesophageal pathology

Unusual pathology of the oesophagus via the endoscope has been reported but the number of cases was rather limited. A series of 11 children, aged 1.5–13 years with abdominal pain undergoing both oesophageal manometry and endoscopy with biopsy, received considerable attention in the lay-press, as it demonstrated that the eight who had been breast-fed from mothers with silicone implants had scleroderma-like pathology [12]. Biopsies showed non-specific findings, while manometry showed nearly absent peristalsis in the distal oesophagus and lower sphincter pressure. Sclerodermal oesophageal disease in young children is almost unheard of and the authors raised very significant concerns regarding yet another aspect of these implants.

Intralesional steroids were used in conjunction with dilation of a caustic stricture in a 2-year-old boy who had been refractory to a series of 16 dilations in 3 months [13]. A total of nine additional dilations, with injection of 3–10 mg triamcinolone acetonide per session, were performed over 5 months with the child subsequently being able to tolerate solids. A study of one patient does not change medical practice and this case, while impressive, was a little unusual in that the initial dilations were done so frequently and seemed to dilate to a 42 F fairly easily, only to stricture down again.

Ornithine decarboxylase, the rate limiting enzyme of polyamine biosynthesis and a marker for cell proliferation, was measured from oesophageal biopsy specimens in 45 children [14]. A significant correlation was seen between levels of the enzyme and severity of oesophagitis.

## Tumours and polyps

Juvenile polyps of the colon are a fairly common entity in the practice of paediatric gastroenterology, but several atypical polyp cases appeared. Two children with neurofibromatosis were found to have hyperplastic ocsophagogastric polyps on upper endoscopy after presenting with vomiting and food refusal [15]. Polypectomy revealed fibroepithelial histology and there was resolution of the symptoms. A juvenile hyperplastic polyp found on endoscopic examination in the duodenal bulb of a child who presented with anaemia and occult bleeding had to be removed by surgery because of the size [16].

A small series of three patients highlighted the rarity of gastric lesions in children but included an excellent review of the limited literature [17•]. The first case was a boy with reflux requiring a fundoplication, who coincidentally was found to have a submucosal mass on surgery that was a pancreatic rest. The next case was a young child with vomiting who had a hyperplastic polyp inducing reflux but also had a malrotation. The last child presented with significant anaemia and had multiple polypoid gastric masses which turned out to be plasma cell granuloma which, after limited surgical removal, eventually required a gastrectomy because of recurrence. Equally of concern is the child with a similar presentation who was found to have a gastric carcinoma [18].

## H. pylori in children

The articles on *H. pylori* seems to have reached a plateau. Already mentioned above was the finding of one neonate out of 20 being investigated for cholestasis with *H. pylori* [7]. The rarity in younger infants is consistent with the report of an increased frequency of *H. pylori* in older children. In 78 children diagnosed with primary antral gastritis, *H. pylori* was the aetiology in 22% [19]. However, when broken down by age, the occurrence of *H. pylori* among children with documented antritis was 4% in children between the ages of 0–4 years, 24% in children between 5–14 years and 67% between the ages of 15–20 years.

Gastric cell densities were analysed in a group of children with *H. pylori* positive gastritis, *H. pylori*-negative gastritis and healthy controls [20]. *H. pylori*-positive children had significantly higher infiltrates of all three cell types analysed: lymphocytes, neutrophils and plasma cells. They also had higher than normal *H. pylori*-negative gastritis. None of the healthy controls, and only one out of 31 children with *H. pylori*-negative gastritis, had immunoglobulin G antibodies to *H. pylori*, compared with 11 out of 12 children with *H. pylori*-positive gastritis. Furthermore, follow-up endoscopy demonstrated a decreased cell density in those children where *H. pylori* was eradicated. *H. pylori* was also found to be associated with hypergastrinaemia and elevated pepsinogen I in three out of six children [21], implying that this entity may have more than one aetiology.

The next frontier was also touched upon when the spiral bacterium *Gastrospirillium hominis* was found in two children with chronic gastritis [22]. The gastritis appeared to be milder and occurred less frequently than *H. pylori*, but may initiate a search for additional pathogens that can cause a similar gastritis.

## Role of upper endoscopy in overall gastrointestinal evaluation

Upper endoscopy has assumed a key role in evaluating many children with either primary gastrointestinal disorders or systemic complaints. Clinical practice has even progressed to the point where many general paediatricians are requesting endoscopy on their patients and, at times, even have to be dissuaded as they are frequently unaware of the limitations compared to potential benefits.

Endoscopy very often has to be performed but is frequently unrevealing. Endoscopy was of no benefit in a series of seven children with massive gastrointestinal bleeding from what was found to be ectopic gastric mucosa; nor were the initial $^{99m}$technetium pertechnetate scans revealing [23]. Small-bowel enteroscopy can be helpful, although difficult, in young children, but many of these patients still have to be surgically explored if the bleeding is significant. Endoscopy must also be performed prior to making the diagnosis of chronic idiopathic intestinal pseudo-obstruction to rule out any mucosal lesion, as was performed in 19 children where antroduodenojejunal manometry documented this motility disorder [24].

Associated histologic conditions also come to light with upper endoscopy. An interesting case of a 2-year-old boy with hypoproteinaemia secondary to Ménétrièr's disease or hypertrophic gastritis secondary to cytomegalovirus (CMV) was documented on endoscopy [25]. Small-bowel biopsy performed by endoscopic examination via either the stoma or the mouth proved crucial in the management of children with small intestinal transplantation in determining rejection compared with infection [26].

In contrast to adults, lymphocytic gastritis was associated with coeliac disease, not *H. pylori* [27•]. Of 245 consecutive children with dyspeptic symptoms undergoing upper endoscopy, 60 were found to have chronic gastritis and 25 to have coeliac disease. *H. pylori* was found in 36 children with chronic gastritis and 15 of the children with coeliac disease. A total of nine children were found to have lymphocytic gastritis, all of whom had coeliac disease, none of which had any evidence of *H. pylori* infection. While the numbers were quite convincing, it would have seemed probable that some of the patients with both gastritis and coeliac disease would have had lymphocytic gastritis.

A prospective study looked at the upper gastrointestinal mucosal lesions in 88 consecutive children diagnosed with Crohn's disease (41 patients) and ulcerative colitis (47 patients) [28•]. This study showed a high incidence of upper gastrointestinal findings (80%) as have many other studies on upper gastrointestinal findings in Crohn's disease but, in addition, 75% of those children with ulcerative colitis also had lesions. Diagnoses made included the typical oesophagitis, gastritis and duodenitis, with *H. pylori* found in 20.5% of the total group in which it was looked for. Contrast studies only revealed pathology in 10% of the cases. Granuloma were found in 24.3% of the cases of Crohn's disease,

not always associated with areas of gross inflammation. The authors make an important point that non-specific inflammation of the upper gastrointestinal tract does not necessarily signify Crohn's disease, but the documentation of granuloma may be quite useful in distinguishing hard to determine cases. Presumably the histological interpretation of these lesions is not being over read, as this is the same group who reported on cell density.

## Laparoscopy in children

Laparoscopic procedures in children do not seem to be making rapid advances, which may be advantageous as the learning curve in paediatrics always seems rather steep. The course of 26 children undergoing laparoscopic cholecystectomy were reviewed for indications, complications, length of stay and cost [29]. The authors stated several modifications they have used in recent years, including the use of routine cholangiography and several technical aspects. The actual operating costs were less for open cholecystectomies performed, as some of the instruments used in the laparoscopic procedure are disposable. The length of stay and overall costs were more favourable for the laparoscopic procedures. The authors point out that there is less of a differential in the length of stay and recuperation time in children, who tend to recover from the open procedure more readily then adults. The technique for laparoscopic splenectomy was described in seven patients, where tissue morcellation was used along with five separate trocar sites [30]. The length of this procedure was considerably longer than the open procedure and one laparoscopic procedure had to be converted to an open procedure because of inadequate homeostasis. All patients had haemolytic disease and only moderately enlarged spleens, which otherwise could have caused some problems. The Swenson pullthrough procedure, which originally was developed on a dog model, was performed successfully by laparoscope on 13 mongrel dogs [31].

## Colonoscopy in children

There were few articles discussing colonoscopy or colonic pathology this year and most of these were case reports. The report by Israel *et al.* [2••] that was discussed earlier stands out when it comes to general technique, but a series on young infants with allergic colitis was somewhat novel [32••]. Presented here were 35 consecutive infants seen over a period of 3 years with blood mixed in the stools appearing at the mean age of 4 weeks. Excluded were those infants with fissures, constipation, or necrotizing enterocolitis. Laboratory investigations and limited colonoscopy with biopsy were performed on 34 patients. Twenty-five had evidence of macroscopic colitis while 31 had histologic evidence, with the principle finding of greater than 20 eosinophils per high-power field, which was significant when compared with a smaller group of controls with rectal biopsies performed for Hirschsprung's disease. Ten infants had nodular lymphoid hyperplasia, not all with eosinophils present, but they seemed to be included as evidence of inflammatory change. There was a significant difference in the mean haemoglobin, albumin and eosinophil count of the allergic colitis group. However, when taken individually, laboratory values were only 48%, 81% and 10% sensitive, respectively. Of the 31 infants with apparent allergic colitis, 10 were solely breast-fed, two were breast-fed and supplemented, nine were on a cow's milk formula, nine were on a soy formula and one was on a casein hydrolysate. Twenty-one infants with both low haemoglobin and albumin had a feeding change, with cessation of bleeding immediately in 19 and gradually in two. In the 10 other infants with colitis but normal albumin and haemoglobin, seven of which were breast-fed, elimination of milk in the mother's diet prompted resolution of bleeding and the three others also gradually resolved.

While the above authors' contributions are greatly appreciated in this poorly defined topic of allergic colitis, their recommendations should be carefully considered. They concluded by saying that the majority of isolated rectal bleeding in this age group is 'allergic' colitis when they did not state how many other infants with rectal bleeding were encountered in this period. They based their definitive diagnosis on eosinophilia on biopsy and using controls of children with biopsies for Hirschsprung's disease might not have been adequate or have been truly double blinded. They placed too much significance on nodular lymphoid hyperplasia, which is frequently a common finding in healthy infants. The rapid resolution in many infants might even suggest other trivial aetiologies for the rectal bleeding, namely unappreciated fissures. The major concern regarding the article is that they are probably reporting on a spectrum of disease, with the minor side of it not even warranting investigation or treatment.

Two brief case histories used colonoscopy as a backdrop. An immunosuppressed infant who had undergone bone marrow transplant for severe combined immune deficiency developed diarrhoea and a maculopapular rash [33]. A small-bowel biopsy was negative for graft versus host, and the patient subsequently developed gross blood with multiple discrete ulcers seen on colonoscopy; no organisms were, however, isolated. Disseminated aspergillus was isolated at *post mortem* with granulomas in all the major organs. The unusual finding of an intramural haematoma of the transverse colon was demonstrated on colonoscopy in a preschool child who was abused and confirmed on computed tomography scan [34].

## Hepatobiliary and pancreatic disorders

Hepatobiliary and pancreatic disease continues to get a considerable share of attention in the literature, despite its relative infrequent occurrence in children. This was especially emphasized in several articles where various disorders were discussed, with endoscopy only being mentioned as a backdrop. A 35-year experience with portal–systemic shunts for extrahepatic portal hypertension in children and young adults was presented where prior treatments had failed [35]. Only 68 out of 162 patients received sclerotherapy, probably reflecting the lack of availability in the early years, and was deemed unsuccessful in all, with shunting being necessary. The 5- and 10-year survival rates were 99% and 96%, respectively, with half of the deaths resulting from unrelated sources. This was significantly better than the experience with shunts for portal hypertension from primary hepatocellular disease. The result of these shunts is quite impressive; however, the frequent necessity for shunting is not consistent with the experiences of other centres where sclerotherapy is successful in most cases of extrahepatic portal hypertension.

In just over 20 years, 56 children with sclerosing cholangitis were seen at a major centre in France [36]. Only four had endoscopic retrograde cholangiography performed, however, while 40 had percutaneous transhepatic cholangiography and 12 had operative cholangiography. As with many technically difficult procedures, the choice is usually based on the preference and the skills of the available centre, especially for an uncommon entity. This can be said to be true for other biliary tract disorders, as reported by Grosfeld *et al.* [37] on a 22-year experience. During this time, 300 children were evaluated, including 102 with biliary atresia, 29 with choledochal cyst and 169 with cholelithiasis. ERCP was performed in a handful of children with gallstones, while it may have been more useful in the children with atresia and choledochal cysts.

The only real endoscopic series on ERCP this year came out of Caracas [38••], where 51 children and adolescents aged 1–18 years were evaluated for recurrent pancreatitis for diagnosis or intervention. ERCP was successful in all but one patient and an aetiology for the chronic pancreatitis was found in 74%. Biliary anomalies were found in almost 25%, including nine patients with choledochal cysts. Pancreatic anomalies were found in another 25%, of which six patients had pancreas divisum. Chronic pancreatitis or pseudocysts were found in 20%. Endoscopic treatment was performed in 18 patients and was successful in 83% including sphincterectomy for stones, sphincter of Oddi dysfunction and pseudocysts. This 9-year experience demonstrated that similar findings are uncovered in children with chronic pancreatitis as are seen in adults, excluding those caused by obstructing cholelithiasis and alcohol abuse. An ERCP proved unsuccessful in a 3-year-old patient with chronic pancreatitis causing jaundice and a surgical sphincteroplasty was required [39].

A side-viewing ERCP endoscope was also used in a 4-year-old boy with relapsing pancreatitis [40]; a duodenal duplication near the ampulla of Vater was drained successfully via the endoscope by using a papillotome. Guelrud *et al.* [41], who have been at the forefront of the ERCP experience in children, also report on a successful sphincterotomy in a 6-month-old patient with a stone obstructing the common duct in addition to the finding of a double gallbladder that was not detected on a sonogram.

## References and recommended reading

Papers of particular interest, published within the annual period of review, have been highlighted as:

- • of special interest
- •• of outstanding interest

1. Zahavi I, Arnon R, Ovadia B, Rosenbach Y, Hirsch A, Dinari G: **Upper gastrointestinal endoscopy in the pediatric patient.** *Israel J Med Sci* 1994, **30**:664–667.
Straightforward account of the experience with 289 children undergoing upper endoscopy. The most noteworthy result was that 65% received no sedation.

2. •• Israel DM, McLain BI, Hassal E: **Successful pancolonoscopy and ileoscopy in children.** *J Pediatr Gastroenterol Nutr* 1994, **19**:283–289.
Very good account of the experience with 40 consecutive colonoscopies in children with detail given regarding indication, technique and length of time. The authors addressed the important topic of training fellows in paediatric endoscopy.

3. • de Boissieu D, Dupont C, Barbet JP, Bargaoui K, Badoual J: **Distinct features of upper gastrointestinal endoscopy in the newborn.** *J Pediatr Gastroenterol Nutr* 1994, **18**:334–338.
This article is noteworthy for the sheer numbers alone. Two hundred and ninety-three upper endoscopies were performed in a 4-year period on neonates of less than 1 month of age. However, indications were not clear, and the impression was given that the interpretation of findings was also unclear.

4. Maki M, Ruuska T, Kuusela AL, Karikoski-Leo R, Ikonen RS: **High prevalence of asymptomatic esophageal and gastric lesions in preterm infants in intensive care.** *Crit Care Med* 1993, **21**:1863–1867.
Fifteen out of 17 neonates had endoscopic findings despite only two having gastrointestinal symptoms.

5. Goyal A, Treem WR, Hyams JS: **Severe upper gastrointestinal bleeding in healthy full-term neonates.** *Am J Gastroenterol* 1994, **89**:613–616.
Three otherwise healthy newborn infants presented with gastrointestinal bleeding and significant decreases in their haematocrits, two of which were found to have duodenal ulcer and one was found to have haemorrhagic gastritis.

6. Olson AD, Fukui-Miner K: **Eosinophilic mucosal infiltrate in infants with congenital gastrointestinal obstruction.** *Am J Gastroenterol* 1994, **89**:934–936.
An infant with persistent vomiting, thought to have an allergy to breast milk, based on peripheral eosinophilia and eosinophilic infiltrate on endoscopic biopsies, was found to have duodenal stenosis, Ladd's bands and a non-obstructing annular pancreas.

7. Guelrud M, Mujica C, Jaen D, Machuc J, Essenfeld H: **Prevalence of *Helicobacter pylori* in neonates and young infants undergoing ERCP for diagnosis of neonatal cholestasis.** *J Pediatr Gastroenterol Nutr* 1994, **18**:461–464.
One infant in a series of 20 who were less than 2 months of age, being evaluated for cholestasis, was found to have *H. pylori* compared with 95% of their mothers.

8. • De Backer A, Bove T, Vandenplas Y, Peeters S, Deconinck P: **Contribution of endoscopy to early diagnosis of hypertrophic pyloric stenosis.** *J Pediatr Gastroenterol Nutr* 1994, **18**:78–81.
Both sonography and upper endoscopy were performed in 63 infants, 1–10 weeks of age, later confirmed at surgery to have pyloric stenosis. The sonogram predicted 81% of the cases of pyloric stenosis while endoscopy predicted 97% based on the findings of a cauliflower-like narrowing of the pyloric channel that could not pass a 7.8 mm scope.

9. Crombleholme TM, Jacir NN: **Simplified 'push' technique for percutaneous endoscopic gastrostomy in children.** *J Pediatr Surg* 1993, **28**:1393–1395.
A discussion of a small series of eight children who underwent the simplified 'push' technique.

10. Marin OE, Glassman MS, Schoen BT, Caplan DB: **Safety and efficacy of percutaneous endoscopic gastrostomy in children.** *Am J Gastroenterol* 1994, **89**:357–361.
Seventy per cent of 70 children who had PEGs placed showed improved nutritional status, with significant complications that required surgical intervention in 19% and minor complications in 22%.

11. Werlin S, Glicklich M, Cohen R: **Early feeding after percutaneous endoscopic gastrostomy is safe in children.** *Gastrointest Endosc* 1994, **40**:692–693.
Feedings could be restarted 6 h after PEG placement in 24 out of 28 consecutive children.

12. Levine JJ, Ilowite NT: **Scleroderma-like esophageal disease in children breast-fed by mothers with silicone breast implants.** *JAMA* 1994, **271**:213–216.
Eight children who had been breast-fed by mothers with silicone implants had scleroderma-like oesophageal pathology on biopsy, and manometry showing nearly absent peristalsis in the distal oesophagus and lower sphincter pressure.

13. Berenson GA, Wyllie R, Caulfied M, Steffen R: **Intralesional steroids in the treatment of refractory esophageal strictures.** *J Pediatr Gastroenterol Nutr* 1994, **18**:250–252.
Intralesional steroids were used in conjunction with dilation of a caustic stricture in a 2-year-old boy who had been refractory to a series of 16 dilations in 3 months.

14. Elitsur Y, Triest WE, Lin C-H: **Ornithine Decarboxylase (ODC) levels in children with reflux esophagitis.** *Dig Dis Sci* 1994, **39**:729–732.
A significant correlation was seen between ornithine decarboxylase, the rate limiting enzyme of polyamine biosynthesis and a marker for cell proliferation, and the severity of oesophagitis.

15. De Giacomo C, Gullotta R, Perrotti P, Bawa P, Cornaggia M, Fiocca R: **Hyperplastic esophagogastric polyps in two children with neurofibromatosis type I.** *J Pediatr Gastroenterol Nutr* 1994, **18**:107–110.
Two children with neurofibromatosis were found to have hyperplastic oesophagogastric polyps on upper endoscopy after presenting with vomiting.

16. Verhage J, Mulder CJ, Meyer JW, Reuvers CB: **Hyperplastic duodenal polyp in a boy.** *J Pediatr Gastroenterol Nutr* 1994, **19**:326–328.
A juvenile hyperplastic polyp was found on endoscopic examination in the duodenal bulb of a child who presented with anaemia and occult bleeding; removal was by surgery because of the size.

17. • Murphy S, Shaw K, Blanchard H: **Report of three gastric tumors in children.** *J Pediatr Surg* 1994, **29**:1202–1204.
A small series of three patients highlighting the rarity of gastric lesions in children with an excellent review of the limited literature. The pathology included a pancreatic rest, a hyperplastic polyp and polypoid gastric masses which turned out to be plasma cell granuloma.

18. McGill TW, Downey EC, Westbrook J, Wade D, de la Garza J: **Gastric carcinoma in children.** *J Pediatr Surg* 1993, **28**:1620–1621.
A child with poor feeding and vomiting was found to have gastric carcinoma.

19. Snyder JD, Hardy SC, Thorne GM, Hirsch BZ, Antonioli DA: **Primary antral gastritis in young American children: Low prevalence of _Helicobacter pylori_ infections.** _Dig Dis Sci_ 1994, **39**:1859–1863.
In 78 children diagnosed with primary antral gastritis, _H. pylori_ was the aetiology in 22%. As in adults, however, there was an increased frequency of infection with increasing age.

20. Ashorn M, Ruuska T, Karikoski R, Valipakka J, Maki M: **Gastric mucosal cell densities in _Helicobacter pylori_-positive and -negative dyspeptic children and healthy controls.** _J Pediatr Gastroenterol Nutr_ 1994, **18**:146–151.
Gastric cell densities were analysed in a group of children with _H. pylori_-positive gastritis, _H. pylori_-negative gastritis and healthy controls. _H. pylori_-positive children had significantly higher infiltrates of lymphocytes, neutrophils and plasma cells.

21. Rindi G, Annibale B, Bonamico M, Corleto V, Delle-Fave G, Solcia E: _Helicobacter pylori_ **infection in children with antral gastrin cell hyperfunction.** _J Pediatr Gastroenterol Nutr_ 1994, **18**:152–158.
_H. pylori_ was found in three out of six children with hypergastrinaemia and elevated pepsinogen I.

22. Oliva MM, Lazenby AJ, Perman JA: **Gastritis associated with _Gastrospirillium hominis_ in children. Comparison with _Helicobacter pylori_ and review of the literature.** _Mod Pathol_ 1993, **6**:513–515.
The spiral bacterium _Gastrospirillium hominis_ was found in two children with chronic gastritis.

23. Kong M-S, Huang S-C, Tzen K-Y, Lin J-N. **Repeated technetium-99 pertechnetate scanning for children with obscure gastrointestinal bleeding.** _J Pediatr Gastroenterol Nutr_ 1994, **18**:284–287.
Endoscopy, as well as the initial [99m]technetium pertechnetate scans, were unrevealing in seven children with massive gastrointestinal bleeding from ectopic gastric mucosa.

24. Cucchiara S, Annese V, Minella R, Franco MT, Iervolino C, Emiliano M, _et al._: **Antroduodenojejunal manometry in the diagnosis of chronic idiopathic intestinal pseudoobstruction in children.** _J Pediatr Gastroenterol Nutr_ 1994, **18**:294–305.
Endoscopy was performed in 19 children with chronic idiopathic intestinal pseudo-obstruction, ruling out mucosal lesions.

25. Khoshoo V, Alonzo E, Correa H, Levine S, Udall JN: **Pathological case of the month: Ménétrier's disease with cytomegalovirus gastritis.** _Arch Pediatr Adolesc Med_ 1994, **148**:611–612.
A 2-year-old boy with hypoproteinaemia secondary to Ménétrier's disease secondary to CMV documented at endoscopy.

26. De Giacomo C, Gianatti A, Negrini R, Perotti P, Bawa P, Maggiore G, _et al._: **Lymphocytic gastritis: a positive relationship with celiac disease.** _J Pediatr_ 1994, **124**:57–62.
Of 245 consecutive children with dyspeptic symptoms undergoing upper endoscopy, 60 were found to have chronic gastritis and 25 to have coeliac disease. A total of nine children were found to have lymphocytic gastritis, all of whom had coeliac disease and none of whom had any evidence of _H. pylori_ infection, contrary to the experience in adults.

27. Garau P, Orenstein SR, Neigut DA, Putnam PE, Reyes J. Tzakis AG, _et al._:
• **Role of endoscopy following small intestinal transplantation in children.** _Transplant Proc_ 1994, **26**:136–137.
Infection or rejection were documented on small-bowel biopsy in a series of children who had undergone small intestinal transplants.

28. Ruuska T, Vaajalahti P, Arajarvi P, Maki M: **Prospective evaluation of**
• **upper gastrointestinal mucosal lesions in children with ulcerative colitis and Crohn's disease.** _J Pediatr Gastroenterol Nutr_ 1994, **19**:181–186.
A prospective study looked at the upper gastrointestinal mucosal lesions in 88 consecutive children diagnosed with Crohn's disease (41 patients) and ulcerative colitis (47 patients). Upper gastrointestinal findings were seen in 80% of children with Crohn's disease. In addition, 75% of those children with ulcerative colitis also had lesions.

29. Holcomb GW, Sharp KW, Neblett WW, Morgan WM, Pietsch JB: **Laparoscopic cholecystectomy in infants and children: modifications and cost analysis.** _J Pediatr Surg_ 1994, **29**:900–904.
The course of 26 children undergoing laparoscopic cholecystectomy were reviewed for indications, complications, length of stay and costs. The actual operating costs were less for open cholecystectomies as some of the instruments used in the laparoscopic procedure are disposable. The length of stay and overall costs were more favourable for the laparoscopic procedures.

30. Smith BM, Schropp KP, Lobe TE, Rogers DA, Presbury GJ, Wilimas JA, _et al._: **Laparoscopic splenectomy in childhood.** _J Pediatr Surg_ 1994, **29**:975–977.
The technique for laparoscopic splenectomy was described in seven patients, where tissue morcellation was used along with five separate trocar sites.

31. Curran TJ, Raffensperger JG: **The feasibility of laparoscopic Swenson pull-through.** _J Pediatr Surg_ 1994, **29**:1273–1275.
The Swenson pull-through procedure, which originally was developed on a dog model, was performed successfully by laparoscope on 13 mongrel dogs.

32. Machida HM, Catto Smith AG, Gall DG, Trevenen C, Scott RB: **Allergic**
•• **colitis in infancy: clinical and pathologic aspects.** _J Pediatr Gastroenterol Nutr_ 1994, **19**:22–26.
Thirty-five consecutive infants seen over a period of 3 years with blood mixed in the stools at the mean age of 4 weeks were studied with laboratory investigations and colonoscopy. This revealed 25 with macroscopic colitis and 31 with histologic inflammation with the principle finding of more than 20 eosinophils per high power field or nodular lymphoid hyperplasia. There was a significant difference in the mean haemoglobin, albumin and eosinophil count in the group with allergic colitis. When viewed individually, however, laboratory values were only 48%, 81% and 10% sensitive, respectively. Twenty-one infants with both low haemoglobin and albumin had a feeding change, with cessation of bleeding immediately in 19 and gradually in two.

33. Foy TM, Hawkins EP, Peters KR, Shearer WT, Ferry GD: **Colonic ulcers and lower GI bleeding due to disseminated aspergillosis.** _J Pediatr Gastroenterol Nutr_ 1994, **18**:399–403.
An immunosuppressed infant with severe combined immune deficiency after bone marrow transplant developed bloody diarrhoea and was found to have multiple discrete ulcers on colonoscopy, later diagnosed as disseminated aspergillus.

34. Sachdevaa RS, Jaeger A, Norton K, Raucher H, Norton K, Dolgin SE, _et al._: **Intramural hematoma of the transverse colon in battered child syndrome.** _J Pediatr Gastroenterol Nutr_ 1994, **18**:111–113.
An intramural haematoma of the transverse colon was demonstrated on colonoscopy in a preschool child who was abused.

35. Orloff MJ, Orloff MS Rambotti M: **Treatment of bleeding esophagogastric varices due to extrahepatic portal hypertension: results of portal–systemic shunts during 35 years.** _J Pediatr Surg_ 1994, **29**:142–154.
A 35-year experience with portal–systemic shunts for extrahepatic portal hypertension in 162 children and young adults was presented where prior treatments had failed, including only 68 who had received sclerotherapy. The 5- and 10-year survival rates were 99% and 96%, respectively.

36. Debray D, Pariente D, Urvoas E, Hadchouel M, Bernard O: **Sclerosing cholangitis in children.** _J Pediatr_ 1994, **124**:49–56.
Fifty-six children with sclerosing cholangitis were studies over a 20-year period at a major centre in France, with only four having endoscopic retrograde cholangiography, while 40 had percutaneous transhepatic cholangiography, and 12 had operative cholangiography.

37. Grosfeld JL, Rescorla FJ, Skinner MA, West KW, Scherer LR: **The spectrum of biliary tract disorders in infants and children.** _Arch Surg_ 1994, **129**:513–520.
Three hundred children were evaluated over 22 years, including 102 with biliary atresia, 29 with choledochal cyst and 169 with cholelithiasis. ERCP was performed only in a handful of children with gallstones.

38. Guelrud M, Mujica C, Jaen D, Plaz J, Arias J: **The role of ERCP in the**
•• **diagnosis and the treatment of idiopathic recurrent pancreatitis.** _Gastrointest Endosc_ 1994, **40**:428–436.
Fifty-one children were evaluated for recurrent pancreatitis for diagnosis or intervention. ERCP was successful in all but one patient and an aetiology for the chronic pancreatitis was found in 74%. Biliary anomalies were found in almost 25%, pancreatic anomalies were found in another 25%, and chronic pancreatitis or pseudocysts were found in 20%. Endoscopic treatment was performed in 18 patients and was successful in 83% including sphincterectomy for stones, sphincter of Oddi dysfunction and pseudocysts.

39. Mohan P, Holcomb GW, Ziegler MM: **Recurrent jaundice and pancreatitis in a child with pancreatobiliary duct anomalies.** _J Pediatr Gastroenterol Nutr_ 1994, **18**:386–390.
An ERCP proved unsuccessful in a 3-year-old patient with chronic pancreatitis causing obstructive jaundice; surgical sphincteroplasty was required.

40. Lang T, Berquist W, Rich E, Cox K, De Vries P, Cahill J, *et al*.: **Treatment of recurrent pancreatitis by endoscopic drainage of a duodenal duplication.** *J Pediatr Gastroenterol Nutr* 1994, **18**:494–496.
A side-viewing ERCP endoscope was used in a 4-year-old boy with relapsing pancreatitis to drain a duodenal duplication near the ampulla of Vater.

41. Guelrud M, Daoud G, Mendoza S, Gordils A, Gelrud A: **Endoscopic sphincterectomy in a 6-month old infant with choledocholithiasis and double gall bladder.** *Am J Gastroenterol* 1994, **89**:1587–1589.

A successful sphincterotomy was performed by ERCP in a 6-month-old patient with a stone obstructing the common duct in addition to the finding of a double gallbladder that was not detected on sonogram.

Dr Keith J. Benkov, Division of Pediatric Gastroenterology and Nutrition, Mount Sinai Medical Center, Box 1198 1 Gustave Levy Place, New York, NY 10029, USA.

# Colonoscopy and sigmoidoscopy

## Rainer Sander

1st Department of Internal Medicine, Municipal Hospital Harlaching, Munich, Germany

## Introduction

The main thrust of relevant publications in 1994 concerned the areas of preparation, sedation, colonoscopic surveillance and patient comfort during colonoscopy. Some studies produced significant and noteworthy results, while others merely confirmed known facts.

## Preparation

Bowel cleansing prior to colonoscopy again proved to be one of the major topics dealt with in the literature. Once more, oral polyethylene glycol-based electrolyte lavage solution (PEG-ELS) proved to be the standard against which all other methods were evaluated.

In a prospective and randomized study involving 450 patients, Cohen et al. [1••] compared three different bowel cleansing methods, namely polyethylene glycol solution (PEG; GoLYTELY, Braintree Labs. Inc., Braintree, MA, USA), sulphate-free PEG (PEG-SF; NuLYTELY, Braintree Labs. Inc., Braintree, MA, USA), 4 litres of each being taken orally, and a sodium phosphate solution (fleet phospho-soda, C.B. Fleet Co., Lynchburg, VA, USA), administered in two fractions of 45 ml each, one at 16.00 h on the day before the examination and the second at 06.00 h on the day of the examination. The three groups showed no differences in terms of number or nature of side effects, such as insomnia, abdominal cramps, nausea, vomiting, asthenia and/or anal irritation, or in body weight or biochemical parameters. The only notable finding was intermittent asymptomatic hyperphosphataemia in the sodium phosphate group. The examination times were also comparable for each of the cleansing methods. The endoscopists judged cleansing in the sodium phosphate groups to be appreciably superior to that in the other two groups (90% versus 70% and 73%). The acceptance by patients of the smaller amounts of the sodium phosphate solution employed was also significantly better than in the other two groups (83% were prepared, if necessary, to repeat the process, as compared with 19% and 33% for PEG and PEG-SF, respectively). The clearly favoured sodium phosphate is thus recommended as the standard method for pre-colonoscopy bowel cleansing, although extreme caution must be exercised in patients with impaired renal function.

According to other reports, the obvious superiority of administering sodium phosphate in two fractions is dependent on the time and the fractionation of the administration. Thus, in another, admittedly small, prospective randomized trial involving 52 patients, it was reported that single-dose administration of 90 ml sodium phosphate solution provided inferior cleansing compared with PEG lavage [2].

While the addition of 120 mg simethicone to PEG-ELS resulted in an appreciable reduction in the formation of bubbles within the bowel, no significant differences were found in terms of the quality of colonoscopy [3•]. The main advantage of adding simethicone appears to be improved acceptance by the patient. The authors observed a lower level of illness and fewer sleep disorders during the preparation phase, and they surmised a positive effect on patient comfort due to a reduction in the production of gas bubbles coupled with speedier emptying of the bowel on termination of the examination. The study showed that patients with inflammatory bowel disease (IBD; ulcerative colitis and Crohn's disease) appeared to tolerate PEG-ELS with added simethicone particularly well.

Bowel cleansing in elderly, hospitalized patients is known to be considerably more difficult than in young, mobile outpatients, mainly because bowel motility depends on the physical activity of the patient. One study therefore adopted the logical approach of adding a motility-promoting substance to improve the effectiveness of standard precolonoscopy bowel cleansing methods [4•]. A total of 120 outpatients aged < 60 years, and 73 patients aged > 60 years were given either 10 ml cisapride or placebo, 30 min prior to lavage with

---

### Abbreviations

CT—computed tomography; **IBD**—inflammatory bowel disease; **MRI**—magnetic resonance imaging; **Nd:YAG**—neodymium yttrium aluminium garnet; **PEG**—polyethylene glycol solution; **PEG-ELS**—polyethylene glycol-based electrolyte lavage solution; **PEG-SF**—sulphate-free polyethylene glycol solution.

magnesium citrate solution. Although patient acceptance and quality of cleansing were equal in both groups, preparation in the group receiving cisapride proved to be significantly shorter in patients aged > 60 years [4•]. Furthermore, the amount of fluid that needed to be suctioned off during colonoscopy was clearly smaller in this group. It is worth deciding whether, in addition, cisapride has an optimizing effect on other peroral cleansing methods.

Of the above-mentioned cleansing measures, sodium phosphate appears to be the least expensive [5]. According to Berry and DiPalma [5], preparation with the sodium phosphate costs $1.76 compared with $20.72 for GoLYTELY. The economic aspect is, of course, only one of many other points that need to be taken into account.

In our own patients, we obtain good cleansing with X-Prep, a liquid extract of senna, which is given on the day before the examination. In addition, our patients also receive 1 litre GoLYTELY solution to drink in the afternoon on the same day as the X-Prep, as well as a further 1 litre 2 h prior to the examination. Patient toleration and acceptance of this combination (or 'compromise') solution are good.

## Sedation

Colonoscopy has the reputation of being a particularly painful examination. As a result, many patients expect to receive a general anaesthetic, or at least heavy sedation, prior to the procedure. There is also a tendency among many examiners to administer medication prior to an endoscopic examination, with the aim, among others, of preserving the patient's willingness to undergo a repeat procedure if necessary. On the other hand, it is known that most relevant (including fatal) complications are due not to the endoscopy itself, but to side effects of the medication. It should therefore be our aim to medicate only those patients who have a real need, especially in view of the fact that some 30% of all non-medicated patients experience no, and 55% only minimal, pain during the examination [6]. Only in 23% of all patients undergoing colonoscopy was intravenous sedation required. Accordingly, by adopting an appropriate selective approach to sedation, experienced colonoscopists found that, on completion of an examination, 92% of the patients, mainly of Oriental origin, declared themselves ready to undergo a necessary re-colonoscopy without prior sedation. Seow-Choen *et al.* from Singapore [6] found a further advantage of such an approach. Non-sedated patients are better able to cope with information and/or instructions during the procedure, and are more capable of understanding what the examiner is doing. In premedicated patients, the administration of an antidote (flumazenil) once the caecum has been intubated may help the patient undergoing video colonoscopy consciously to experience and understand the inspection of the bowel during withdrawal of the instrument and any therapeutic operative interventions that might be needed.

Observations made by the group headed by Saunders [7••] may ease the situation prevailing, in particular, in endoscopy units that are cramped for space and/or have a large outpatient throughput. In a double-blind, randomized, placebo-controlled study, these authors compared inhalation of nitrous oxide/oxygen with conventional intravenous sedation (50 mg pethidine, 2.5 mg midazolam). Both methods were equally effective in comparison with placebo. With the exception of a higher incidence of headache following the use of nitrous oxide/oxygen, both groups had a similar side-effect profile. The great advantage of the nitrous oxide/oxygen inhalation method was a substantial reduction in the recovery period after the procedure (32 min versus 60 min with pethidine/midazolam). With both forms of sedation, patients with severe chronic obstructive lung disease pose a problem. A theoretical point still to be clarified is the long-term risk to the medical staff associated with exposure to nitrous oxide. Here, an impairment of the vitamin B12-dependent enzyme, methionine synthetase, may result, possibly leading in turn to bone marrow depression, megaloblastic changes or neurological dysfunction. A gas scavenging system, as used in operating suites, would answer this problem.

Experienced endoscopists are aware of the beneficial effect of a reassuring talk with the patient about to be examined. There is no doubt that calm confidence on the part of the physician reduces the number of patients requiring pre-procedure medication. In this context, a novel approach is described by a French working group who performed colonoscopy under hypnosis, and is of some interest [8•]. In a group of 24 patients, 12 were able to be hypnotized. None of the members of this subgroup required medication prior to a complete examination of the bowel, while in the (non-hypnotizable) control group, 50% did so. All hypnotized patients declared their readiness to undergo a re-colonoscopy under the same conditions. This compares with only two out of the 12 patients in the control group. This study thus describes a form of relaxation completely free from side effects. It must, however, be noted that only one-half of the total number of patients proved capable of being hypnotized. Also, the shortage of personnel able to perform hypnosis, together with the time factor involved (especially in a busy endoscopy unit) will limit the use of this technique.

## Comfort and quality

Now that total colonoscopy has become a routine examination, more attention is being directed to the question of quality. The criteria for this are patient comfort, the completeness of the examination, the time requirement and the risk of possible complications. An editorial by Williams [9••] looks at these points. The psychological situation of a feeling of helplessness and a fear of pain from the procedure and/or the results of the examination on the part of the patient can be tempered by the understanding and reassuring manner of the physician when explaining the procedure immediately prior to, or during, its execution. The question of medication needs to be dealt with in a flexible manner, for only a small percentage of patients really need it. Thus, in view of the well-known side effects and possible complications associated with sedatives and analgesics, primary medication cannot be justified for all patients. Nor is there any justification for always denying such medication on principle, as unnecessary pain will be experienced by some patients, or a compromise may have to be made limiting the completeness of the examination. Evidence for the quality of an endoscopic unit is that at least 95% of all colonoscopies performed (in the cleansed bowel in which there are no strictures) should be able to be properly completed. Although the time needed to achieve intubation to the caecum is also a factor contributing to quality, our aim should not be to complete the examination in record time. In other words, the time factor is secondary to risk reduction, patient comfort and completeness of the colonoscopic examination.

An important aspect of patient acceptance of the method, or patient compliance in regard to repeat examinations, is customer satisfaction with the intervention and how this can be established and improved. This question has been investigated in a study by Salmon *et al.* [10], who designed a 31-item questionnaire to be completed by the patient immediately following colonoscopy. A basic analysis of the answers given revealed three components relating to the patient's acceptance of colonoscopy: satisfaction, physical discomfort and emotional distress. It is obvious from this study, however, that it is difficult to distinguish clearly between these terms. I therefore personally consider a painless examination to contribute to patient satisfaction, while, conversely, optimal patient satisfaction is difficult to reconcile with pain felt during the procedure. Nevertheless, any attempt to deal with the multidimensionality of the way in which patients experience colonoscopy certainly makes good sense.

In its widest sense, patient comfort may be extended to include optimal information for the patient, which is mandatory not only for legal reasons but also because it can help promote a relationship of trust between the patient and the physician and thus promote patient well-being and co-operation. A significant improvement may be the additional use of an explanatory video tape by the physician [11].

## Technique

The level of technical perfection of modern endoscopes and of present-day examination techniques are such that a total colonoscopy can now be performed in more than 95% of cases. Nevertheless, new strategies and variations capable of more rapidly overcoming difficult situations in individual cases continue to be described. One report [12], for example, describes the use of forceps to help negotiate a difficult passage. The passage of the colonoscope 'over the forceps', however, was already described in 1977 by Gabrielson and Granquist who in this way facilitated intubation of the ileocaecal valve. In this report, the biopsy forceps are passed approximately 10 cm beyond the endoscope to a fold and, using gentle tension on the forceps, the colonoscope is jiggled with a forward motion over the forceps.

If the endoscopist allows himself sufficient time, the terminal ileum can be intubated in 79% of cases. According to Kundrotas *et al.* [13•], the average time requirement is 3.5 min, range 0.5–10 min. On account of the time needed, these authors recommend intubation of the terminal ileum only on a case-by-case basis. Our own experience shows that the ileocaecal valve can be negotiated in under 3 min in more than 90% of cases.

## Complications

Ignoring respiratory and cardiovascular reactions to intravenous sedatives and analgesics, the typical complications of colonoscopy itself are perforation and, more rarely, haemorrhage. These occur for the most part during therapeutic procedures. In individual cases, however, mechanical injuries of neighbouring organs of the colorectum may occur. An Austrian working group [14•] reported observing a small bowel ileus following diagnostic colonoscopy which revealed no remarkable findings. Two hours after the procedure, severe attacks of colic occurred in the right lower quadrant of the abdomen, followed by the clinical picture of an acute abdomen with guarding. During subsequent surgical intervention, a necrotic, adhesion-induced strangulated segment of ileum was resected. The authors consider the entry of air via the incompetent ileocaecal valve to have been implicated in the strangulation of the small bowel segment, and they recommended that severe postendoscopic, colicky abdominal pain should prompt us to consider not merely a perforation, but also the extremely rare possibility of strangulation of the small bowel.

As has been reported on a number of occasions, mechanical compression or withdrawal-related trauma may result in splenic rupture during colonoscopy. For the most part, the treatment of choice in such cases has been immediate surgery. Heath *et al.* [15] reported on the case of a 66-year-old male presenting with pain in the left upper abdomen radiating to the back and left shoulder. He developed circulatory collapse states on days 1–5 following colonoscopy. The computed tomography (CT) scan revealed a subcapsular haematoma. Since the patient carried an increased surgical risk, he was treated (successfully) by conservative means. The authors recommend that conservative treatment should be considered in cases in which patients do not lose any appreciable amounts of blood, do not bleed into the peritoneum and have no evidence of a subcapsular haematoma on the CT image. In all other cases, a splenectomy is mandatory.

In association with colonoscopy, acute pancreatitis has also been observed [16]. Despite the fact that the authors consider trauma to be likely in the aetiopathogenesis, probably because of compression of the pancreas by the colonoscope occurring during the examination, I believe that intermittent spasm of the sphincter of Oddi induced by meperidine (50 mg) should also be considered. In the case described, the patient's pancreatitis (which cleared up completely) was treated by conservative means.

## Inflammatory bowel disease

In view of the risk of perforation, some experienced endoscopists strenuously advise against passing the colonoscope beyond the rectum when there is severe acute colitis. If we follow the conclusions of a study by the French authors Carbonnel *et al.* [17•], however, this fear of complication would appear to be less than fully justified, at least when the examiner has plenty of experience. The authors performed colonoscopy in 85 consecutive patients with severe acute ulcerative colitis, passing the instrument at least up to the caecum in 74% of the cases. With the exception of a single case of postendoscopic bowel dilatation, no complications were observed, in particular no perforations. At least 46 patients, however, presented with severe, deeply ulcerated inflammation of the colon. Although the study aimed to demonstrate the safety, accuracy and usefulness of colonoscopy in the management of these patients, some of the statements and conclusions of the authors do not appear quite convincing. They state that, in patients with known ulcerative colitis, total colonoscopy is possibly not necessary. Apart from the exclusion of a malignancy associated with the chronic bowel inflammation, a knowledge of the distribution pattern of the disease is certainly of decisive importance for its management; for example, patients with ulcera-

tive colitis involving mainly the left hemicolon can be given local medication in addition to the systemic medication. Furthermore, the statement that Crohn's disease responds better to drug treatment than does ulcerative colitis is not generally accepted. Also worth noting is the report by the authors that about 50% of the 85 consecutive patients with ulcerative colitis had to be submitted to surgery because of the failure of conservative treatment. This is an unusually high rate for a large and respected gastrointestinal department.

Of practical importance is the re-confirmation that in a very high percentage of cases a rectal biopsy provides definitive information about the type of inflammatory disease presenting in the colorectum. A study dealing with this point [18] documented the fact that rectal biopsies are useful for distinguishing between acute self-limiting colitis and idiopathic IBD, even when tissue specimens cannot be obtained within the first few days of the disease. Seven histological features were found to be highly predictive of IBD: distorted crypt architecture, crypt atrophy, a villous surface, mixed lamina propria inflammation, basal lymphoid aggregates, basally located isolated giant cells and epithelioid granulomas. In this study as well, however, it was pointed out that biopsy alone does not permit an overall assessment of the disease status, with macroscopic findings and all the other clinical data being required in addition.

When the primary diagnosis is acute colitis, consideration should also be given to the possibility of an infective cause; it is not sufficient merely to investigate the patient's stools. Matsumoto *et al.* [19•] showed that cultures obtained from forceps biopsy material removed from the inflamed parts of the bowel are more likely to contain pathogenic bacteria than cultures of stools. The importance of the difference (50% versus 20%, $P < 0.05$) is difficult to determine in this small study (n = 20). Nevertheless, the information is very useful for daily practice, since suitable targeted treatment can be selected only when the pathogens (and their sensitivities) have been reliably determined. The most commonly found micro-organisms in this study were *Campylobacter*, *Salmonella* and *Yersinia*.

The importance in the endoscopic unit of routine magnetic resonance imaging (MRI) for the differential diagnosis of ulcerative colitis and Crohn's disease, and also for determining the severity of the inflammation, has yet to be established. This imaging procedure is very expensive and is not capable of replacing an endoscopic biopsy examination of the colon, for example, in endoscopic surveillance to exclude a carcinoma or dysplasia in patients with chronic ulcerative colitis. Nevertheless, a recent study involving 20 patients showed that the information about the extent and severity of the inflammatory changes in ulcerative colitis and Crohn's disease obtained with MRI, using T1-weighted fat-suppressed, spin-echo and gadolinium enhancement, can be equally as reliable as that provided by colonoscopy with biopsy [20•].

In 3% of all patients with intestinal amoebiasis caused by *Entamoeba histolytica*, a life-threatening fulminant colitis develops. In a case report [21], the fate of four patients with such severe bowel disease was described. All four patients presented with an acute abdomen, and were submitted to surgery on account of signs of ischaemia or perforation; two patients died during the postoperative phase. On the basis of their experience, with the aim of lowering the morbidity and mortality rates of fulminant amoebic colitis, the authors urgently recommend prompt detection of *Entamoeba histolytica*. They also recommend that, following confirmation of the diagnosis, surgery be carried out as early as possible in combination with selective pathogen-directed chemotherapy.

## Operative endoscopy

Savides and Jensen [22] described three cases in which they identified the source of diverticular bleeding as being visible vessels in the margin of the diverticulum, which they then successfully treated using bipolar electrocauterization. What is remarkable about this case report is not so much the successful haemostasis as the identification of bleeding vessels in the diverticular margin. None of these lesions have been observed in our own department, where our working group has carried out emergency colonoscopies on more than 500 bleeding patients over the last 20 years. In the vast majority of cases of diverticular haemorrhage, it is not even possible to accurately identify the bleeding diverticulum itself. Thus, the authors recommendation that a prospective, randomized, controlled study be performed to investigate the significance of such visible blood vessels in diverticular haemorrhage must be considered purely theoretical. Moreover, as the authors themselves confirm, most bleeds from diverticula stop spontaneously. Furthermore, it may be noted that in addition to bipolar electrocoagulation, other reliable endoscopic therapeutic alternatives are available, with the proviso, however, that in cases of bleeding from the base of a diverticulum great care must be exercised during treatment.

In many cases, successful treatment of strictures of the gastrointestinal tract affected by Crohn's disease simply means prolonging the time between operations. If drug treatment elicits no response, and if resection of the stricture is not desirable, all that remains for the physician is to try the endoscopic approach. Despite a considerable number of relapses, some follow-up observations after endoscopic procedures show at least partial successes. Rolney [23•] reported on the results obtained, mainly with endoscopic balloon dilatation, in 45 patients from two centres (Leuven and Örebro). Although he observed two perforations and two massive afterbleeds, he also noted that 27 patients experienced a lengthy symptom-free period. The main problem with dilatation of Crohn's strictures is the tendency towards recurrence, which makes frequent repeat procedures necessary.

The possibilities and effectiveness of tattooing with India ink are well known. Two studies [24,25•] confirmed this in 14 and 20 patients, respectively. A new approach was attempted by the working group headed by Salomon [25•], who, by means of suitable sterilization and preparation of the India ink, sought to avoid the risks caused by infection or hypersensitivity reactions to particles of the dye. The authors recommended that 3–4 depots, each about 1 ml in volume, of India ink (Koh-I-Noor, Bloomsbury, NJ, USA) in a dilution of 1 : 100 be injected submucosally around the lesion to be marked, but only after prior autoclaving of the ink for 20 min at a temperature of 110–121°C and a pressure of 27.6 kPa (4 psi), and then injecting the ink through a Millex-CV 0.22-micron filter (Millipore, Bedford, MA, USA). In this way, malignant or pre-malignant lesions can be marked for the duration of the time interval to scheduled surgery, even when this is several months.

## Laser applications

In general, the main use of the laser in the field of gastrointestinal endoscopy is the treatment, in particular palliative, of tumours (Fig. 1). The neodymium yttrium aluminium garnet (Nd:YAG) laser, the most commonly used therapeutic laser, is now routinely employed for the adjunctive treatment of villous adenomas, especially in the colorectum, that cannot be completely removed with the diathermy snare. This technique, developed by our group in the early 1980s, is justifiable, however, only when it is absolutely certain that the lesion concerned is a pure benign neoplasia. A Portuguese working group headed by Maciel [26] reported on their experience with the use of the laser to treat 31 patients with villous adenomas in the rectum, the histopathological investigation being performed mainly on multiple forceps biopsies (additionally in snare biopsies in only some cases). The initial success reported for this treatment was 100%, only one carcinoma and two recurrent adenomas being observed in the follow-up period. This study has a number of shortcomings, however. The exact size of the lesions treated was not stated, nor was any clear indication of the definitive follow-up time given. Furthermore, in order to make a representative statement as to the

(a)                       (b)                       (c)

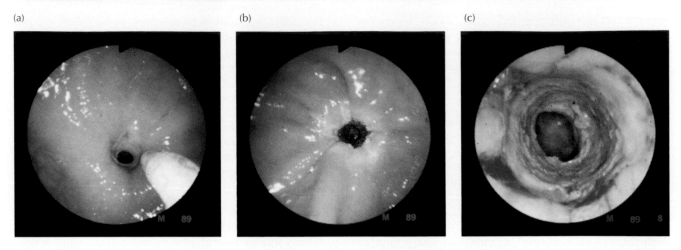

**Fig. 1.** Palliation of a stenotic recurrent rectal carcinoma with the Nd:YAG laser. (a) A 4-cm long stenosis can be seen in the rectum, together with the light transmission system of the Nd:YAG laser visible in the foreground on the right. The lumen of the stricture measures only about 3 mm. (b) The situation immediately after treatment. A centrally vaporized stricture with the luminal surface showing signs of carbonization. The surrounding tissue appears whitish and oedematous. Intubation with the endoscope is not yet possible. (c) Five days after the procedure, the 13-mm colonoscope can now be inserted without the need for further photocoagulation or vaporization.

biological significance of the lesions, at least 90–95% of the tumour mass would have to be removed with the snare, which was not so in this case. In operable patients, laser therapy can only be justified as an adjunctive treatment for non-removable residual polyp tissue. Only in the case of inoperable patients with large villous tumours can primary laser therapy be considered acceptable.

## Colonoscopic surveillance

In any discussion of the usefulness or otherwise of colonoscopic surveillance of patients carrying an increased risk of cancer, we very quickly encounter the cost factor. Only secondary consideration is given to other constraining issues, such as patient mental stress or the risk of complications. In the literature of 1993 and 1994, the focus of colonoscopic surveillance was on patients with ulcerative colitis. Calculations made by a working group from Stockholm showed that the cost of annual surveillance of a patient with ulcerative colitis with total involvement of the colon was $223 (colonoscopy including biopsy) [27•]. On the basis of the number of carcinomas detected in ulcerative colitis patients and the total number of colonoscopies performed, the group calculated the cost of detecting a carcinoma to be about $7270, and declared themselves in favour of regular colonoscopic biopsy surveillance of patients with long-standing ulcerative pancolitis.

In contrast, the authors of another Swedish study [28] came to the conclusion that, in view of the comparatively low rate of malignancies observed among 131 patients with ulcerative colitis (58 with total colitis for more than 10 years), namely four colorectal carcinomas

and four high-grade dysplasias, the cost–benefit question needs further consideration.

After reviewing 10 prospective studies involving 1225 patients, Bernstein *et al.* [29••] pointed out the need for more differentiated information about the patient, and greater involvement of ulcerative colitis patients in the management of their disease. While their recommendation of immediate colectomy in patients with confirmed high-grade dysplasia is generally accepted (see also [28,30,31•]), it is considered that, for patients with low-grade dysplasia, different strategies ranging from colectomy [29••] to regular surveillance [27•] can be applied. Corman [30], in a comment on Bernstein's paper, drew attention to the study by Choi *et al.* [32] which demonstrated that a colonoscopic surveillance significantly lowered the carcinoma mortality rate of ulcerative colitis patients. Out of 41 patients with ulcerative colitis in whom a carcinoma developed, 19 had been on colonoscopic surveillance, while 22 had not. The carcinomas in the surveillance group were detected at an earlier stage, and the carcinoma-related mortality in the surveillance group was four compared with 11 cases in the other group, a statistically significant difference.

In view of all this, the conclusions drawn by Axon [31•] cannot be accepted. This author recommended a first follow-up colonoscopy 8–10 years after the initial diagnosis of ulcerative colitis, counselling of patients with total colonic involvement with respect to their risk and a further colonoscopic examination only when symptoms occur.

Furthermore, studying postoperative endoscopic surveillance programmes in patients who have undergone resection of a colorectal carcinoma, Eckardt *et al.* [33**] reported a significantly higher 5-year survival rate in patients showing good, as opposed to poor, compliance (80% versus 59%, $P < 0.0002$). In this study, 212 patients were investigated; 88 had participated fully in the follow-up programme while 124 had not. The reason for the superior survival rate in the surveillance group was the discovery of recurrent tumours at an early stage.

## References and recommended reading

Papers of particular interest, published within the annual period of review, have been highlighted as:

- •    of special interest
- ••   of outstanding interest

1.   Cohen SM, Wexner SD, Binderow SR, Nogueras JJ, Daniel NRN, Ehrenpreis
••   ED, *et al.*: **Prospective, randomized, endoscopic-blinded trial comparing precolonoscopy bowel cleansing methods.** *Dis Colon Rectum* 1994, **37**:689–696.
The pre-colonoscopy bowel cleansing effects of GoLYTELY (PEG), NuLYTELY (PEG-SF) and a sodium phosphate solution (fleet phospho-soda) were compared. Sodium phosphate proved superior in terms of acceptance and effectiveness, with no more side effects than the other methods.

2.   Marshall JB, Barthel JS, King PD: **Short report: prospective, randomized trial comparing a single dose sodium phosphate regimen with PEG-electrolyte lavage for colonoscopy preparation.** *Aliment Pharmacol Ther* 1993, **7**:679–682.
PEG electrolyte lavage proved to be more effective in bowel cleansing when compared with single-dose sodium phosphate (90 ml the day before colonoscopy).

3.   Lazzoroni M, Petrillo M, Desideri S, Bianchi Porro G: **Efficacy and toler-**
•   **ability of polyethylene-glycol-electrolyte lavage solution with and without simethicone in the preparation of patients with inflammatory bowel disease for colonoscopy.** *Aliment Pharmacol Ther* 1993, **7**:655–659.
In this study PEG-ELS proved an effective means of bowel cleansing. The addition of 120 mg simethicone improved tolerability and acceptance.

4.   Ueda S, Iishi H, Tatsuta M, Oda K, Osaka S: **Addition of cisapride shortens**
•   **colonoscopy preparation with lavage in elderly patients.** *Aliment Pharmacol Ther* 1994, **8**:209–214.
This study encourages attempts to improve pre-colonoscopy bowel cleansing by stimulating motility with 10 mg cisapride. Hospitalized patients could also benefit, in addition to elderly patients.

5.   Berry MA, DiPalma JA: **Review article: orthograde gut lavage for colonoscopy.** *Aliment Pharmacol Ther* 1994, **8**:391–395.
The authors provide an overview of safety, tolerance and efficacy of peroral bowel preparation.

6.   Seow-Choen F, Leong A, Tsang C: **Selective sedation for colonoscopy.** *Gastrointest Endosc* 1994, **40**:661–664.
Primary medication is replaced by situation-adapted secondary medication together with improved patient information and co-operation. Complementary use of flumazenil is recommended.

7.   Saunders BP, Fukumoto M, Halligan S, Masaki T, Love S, Williams CB:
••   **Patient administered nitrous oxide/oxygen inhalation provides effective sedation and analgesia for colonoscopy.** *Gastrointest Endosc* 1994, **40**:418–421.
Inhaled nitrous oxide/oxygen was as effective as intravenous sedation with pethidine/midazolam. This double-blind, randomized study identifies an interesting alternative to colonoscopy medication, especially in outpatients in view of the short recovery phase.

8.   Cadranel JF, Benhamou Y, Zylberberg P, Novello P, Luciani F, Valla D, *et*
•   *al.*: **Hypnotic relaxation: a new sedative tool for colonoscopy.** *J Clin Gastroenterol* 1994, **18**:127–129.
An interesting approach to sedation without drugs. In hypnotizable patients, hypnotic relaxation was effective.

9.   Williams CB: **Comfort and quality in colonoscopy.** *Gastrointest Endosc*
••   1994, **40**:769–770.
This editorial clearly defines the two main criteria for colonoscopy: patient comfort and quality of the examination. Preconditions are experience, sensitivity and flexibility on the part of the examiner.

10.   Salmon P, Shah R, Berg S, Williams CB: **Evaluating customer satisfaction with colonoscopy.** *Endoscopy* 1994, **26**:342–346.
An attempt to improve the satisfaction of the customer with the aid of a questionnaire.

11.   Agre P, Kurtz RC, Krauss BJ: **A randomized trial using videotape to present consent information for colonoscopy.** *Gastrointest Endosc* 1994, **40**:271–276.
Video tapes used adjunctively or as an alternative information medium saved time and proved more effective than oral information given by the doctor on its own.

12.   Kasmin FE, Cohen SA, Siegel JH: **Passage of the colonoscope 'over the forceps' to achieve total colonoscopy in difficult cases.** *Endoscopy* 1994, **26**:330–331.
The title says it all.

13.   Kundrotas LW, Clement DJ, Kubik C, Robinson AB, Phillip AW: **A pro-**
•   **spective evaluation of successful terminal ileum intubation during routine colonoscopy.** *Gastrointest Endosc* 1994, **40**:544–546.
This study shows a 79% success rate for intubation of the ileum, with no difference being found between various levels of endoscopic skill.

14.   Wallner M, Allinger S, Wiesinger H, Prischl FC, Kramar R, Knoflauch P:
•   **Small bowel ileus after diagnostic colonoscopy.** *Endoscopy* 1994, **26**:329.
Insufflation of air through a non-competent ileocaecal valve with subsequent strangulation of a small bowel segment is suspected to be the cause of small bowel ileus following diagnostic colonoscopy.

15.   Heath B, Rodgers A, Taylor A, Lavergne J: **Splenic rupture: an unusual complication of colonoscopy.** *Am J Gastroenterol* 1994, **89**:449–450.
The title says it all.

16.   Thomas A, Mitre R: **Acute pancreatitis as a complication of colonoscopy.** *J Clin Gastroenterol* 1994, **19**:177–179.
Description of a very rare complication of the endoscopic examination of the colorectum.

17.   Carbonnel F, Lavergne A, Lemann M, Bitoun A, Valleur P, Haute Feulle P,
•   *et al.*: **Colonoscopy of acute colitis.** *Dig Dis Sci* 1994, **39**:1550–1557.
Colonoscopy is demonstrated as a safe and accurate method of determining the severity of colitis in 85 consecutive patients with florid ulcerative colitis, of whom 42 non-responders to drug therapy had to be submitted to colon resection.

18.   Surawicz CM, Haggitt RC, Hussemann M, McFarland L: **Mucosal biopsy diagnosis of colitis: acute self-limited colitis and idiopathic inflammatory bowel disease.** *Gastroenterology* 1994, **107**:755–763.
This study once more draws attention to the importance of mucosal biopsy (in particular from the rectum) for the differential diagnosis of acute self-limiting colitis and IBD.

19.   Matsumoto T, Iida M, Kimura Y, Masatoshi F: **Culture of colonoscopically**
•   **obtained biopsy specimens in acute infectious colitis.** *Gastrointest Endosc* 1994, **40**:184–187.
In the comparatively small number of 20 patients, this Japanese group found that cultures of biopsy specimens obtained during colonoscopy may be more diagnostically sensitive than cultures of faecal samples. These results differ from those of other studies.

20.   Shoenut PJ, Semelka RC, Magro CM, Silverman R, Yafffe CS, Micflikier
•   AB: **Comparison of magnetic resonance imaging and endoscopy in distinguishing the type and severity of inflammatory bowel disease.** *J Clin Gastroenterol* 1994, **19**:31–35.
Twenty consecutive patients with IBD underwent colonoscopy plus biopsy and MRI. Both methods proved to be equally effective in differentiating ulcerative colitis from Crohn's disease and determining the severity of the disease.

21.   Chun D, Chandrasoma P, Kiyabu M: **Fulminant amebic colitis.** *Dis Colon Rectum* 1994, **37**:535–539.
Four cases of life-threatening manifestation of intestinal amoebiasis are presented. Early therapy is urgently recommended.

22.   Savides TJ, Jensen DM: **Colonoscopic hemostasis for recurrent diverticular hemorrhage associated with a visible vessel: a report of three cases.** *Gastrointest Endosc* 1994, **40**:70–71.

Three case reports on colonoscopic hemostasis for recurrent diverticular hemorrhage associated with a visible vessel.

23.   Rolney P: **Anastomotic strictures in Crohn's disease: a new field for**
•     **therapeutic endoscopy.** *Gastrointest Endosc* 1993, **39**:862–864.
Another attempt to prove the value of endoscopic treatment of strictures in Crohn's disease. Forty-five patients were treated at two centres, with varying results.

24.   Botoman VA, Pietro M, Thirlby RC: **Localization of colonic lesions with endoscopic tattoo.** *Dis Colon Rectum* 1994, **37**:775–777.
Indian ink tattooing is a reliable method of marking malignant or premalignant lesions.

25.   Salomon P, Berner JS, Waye JD: **Endoscopic India ink injection: a method**
•     **for preparation, sterilization and administration.** *Gastrointest Endosc* 1993, **39**:803–805.
Inflammatory and hypertensive reactions following ink injection can be avoided by filtration and sterilization. The outcome of 20 patients treated showed no complications when using the techniques recommended.

26.   Maciel J, Barbosa J, Junior A: **Endoscopic Nd:YAG laser surgery in the treatment of villous adenomas of the rectum.** *Hepatogastroenterology* 1994, **41**:58–60.
A report of 31 patients with villous adenomas successfully treated with the laser.

27.   Rubio CA, Slezak P, Befrits R: **The costs of colonoscopy in patients with**
•     **ulcerative pancolitis in Sweden.** *Endoscopy* 1994, **26**:228–230.
This study shows that colonoscopy including biopsy for the surveillance of patients with chronic ulcerative colitis is not as expensive as is generally maintained: an annual colonoscopy costs $223, and the authors continue to recommend periodic endoscopic examinations.

28.   Jonsson B, Ahsgren L, Andersson LO, Stenling R, Rutegard J: **Colorectal cancer surveillance in patients with ulcerative colitis.** *Br J Surg* 1994, **81**:689–691.
A total of 131 patients with ulcerative colitis were followed up in a prospective study.

29.   Bernstein C, Shanahan F, Weinstein WM: **Are we telling the truth about**
••    **surveillance colonoscopy in ulcerative colitis?** *Lancet* 1994, **343**:71–74.
This article offers a review of 10 prospective studies involving 1225 patients undergoing surveillance for dysplasia. It concludes that both high-grade and low-grade dysplasias are indications for colectomy, and that patients with indefinite or negative dysplasia findings should undergo regular colonoscopic surveillance, especially if the disease has been present for many years.

30.   Corman ML: **Understanding surveillance colonoscopy.** *Lancet* 1994, **343**:556–557.
This is a comment on Bernstein's article [29••].

31.   Axon ATR: **Cancer surveillance in ulcerative colitis — a time for reap-**
•     **praisal.** *Gut* 1994, **35**:587–589.
The author of this leading review article is not convinced of the value of endoscopic surveillance of patients with ulcerative colitis. A critical analysis of 12 studies is presented.

32.   Choi PM, Nugent FW, Schoetz DJ Jr, Silverman ML, Haggitt RC: **Colonoscopic surveillance reduces mortality from colorectal cancer in ulcerative colitis.** *Gastroenterology* 1993, **105**:418–424.

33.   Eckardt VF, Stamm H, Kanzler G, Bernhard G: **Improved survival after**
••    **colorectal cancer in patients complying with a postoperative endoscopic surveillance program.** *Endoscopy* 1994, **26**:523–527.
Of 212 patients receiving a resection for colorectal cancer, 88 participated in an endoscopic surveillance programme, while 124 did not. The overall 5-year survival rate was significantly higher *(P < 0.0002) in the surveillance group (80 versus 59%).*

Rainer R. Sander, Internist — Gastroenterologe, Oberarzt der 1. Med. Abteilung, Städt. Krankenhaus Harlaching, Akademisches Lehrkrankenhaus der LM-Universität München, Sanatoriumsplatz 2, D-81545 München.

# Colon polyps and cancer

## Douglas K. Rex

Division of Gastroenterology/Hepatology, Indiana University Medical Center,
Indianapolis, USA

## Trends in colorectal cancer incidence and risk factors

Chu et al. [1••] reviewed trends in colorectal cancer incidence and mortality in the United States from 1950–1990. The incidence was similar in both sexes in 1950 but has risen steadily in men since 1950 while declining slightly in women (Fig. 1). The result is that the incidence of colorectal cancer is now about 1.6 times greater in men than in women. Chu et al. were uncertain of the cause, but suggested that the shift in incidence has resulted from increased smoking rates in men in the first half of this century, with a very long induction period. Increased smoking rates in women did not occur until much later (the late 1940s), which is why increased colorectal cancer incidence rates have not yet been seen in women. In two related studies, Giovannucci et al. [2•,3•] suggested that a basis for this hypothesis does exist. Using data from the ongoing Health Professional's Follow-up Study and the Nurse's Health Study, they found that, in both sexes, a history of smoking for less than 20 years was associated with an increased risk of small adenomas (risk ratio 1.45 in women and 2.96 in men) but not of large adenomas (> 1 cm in size). Smoking for more than 20 years was associated with an increased risk of large adenomas but not small adenomas. Cigarette smoking was unrelated to colorectal cancer until 35 years after smoking began, and then the risk increased with the number of years of smoking. The results suggest that an increased risk in women may only now be beginning to show up, and suggest a basis for more intensive screening in long-term smokers.

Chu et al. [1••] found that mortality in men in the United States remained stable over the period 1950–1990 with the increased incidence being offset by a 29% improvement in survival since 1950 (Fig. 2). In women, mortality decreased dramatically as a result of both decreased incidence and improved survival (Fig. 2). One other dramatic finding was noted in this paper. In 1985, incidence of colorectal cancer and mortality

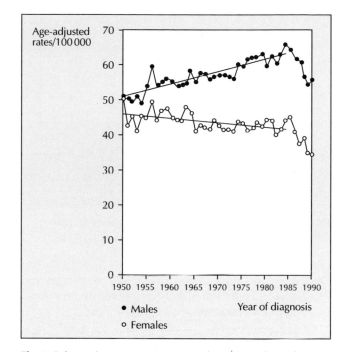

**Fig. 1.** Colorectal cancer incidence rates for white males and females in Connecticut, USA, from 1950 to 1990.

began to decline in both sexes in the United States at a rate of 2–3% per year. Detailed evaluation revealed that initially there was a peak followed by a decline in the incidence of metastatic disease beginning in 1975. This was followed by sequential peaks and subsequent declines of regional, local and in situ carcinomas, respectively. Chu et al. argued convincingly that these trends were the result of widespread application of colonic imaging studies first to symptomatic and then to progressively more asymptomatic persons. Indeed, in 1985 Medicare began to record sharp rises in the number of colonoscopies and sigmoidoscopies performed in the United States, presumably corresponding to the diagnosis of President Reagan's colon cancer. England and Canada, which have no national screening guidelines similar to those proposed by the American Cancer Society (ACS), have not recorded similar de-

---

### Abbreviations

ACS—American Cancer Society; APC—adenomatous polyposis coli; ASCRS—American Society of Colon and Rectal Surgeons; CHRPE—congenital hypertrophy of retinal pigment epithelium; CT—computed tomography; DCBE—double-contrast barium enema; DCC—deleted in colon cancer; FAP—familial adenomatous polyposis; HNPCC—hereditary non-polyposis colorectal cancers; TNM—tumour node metastasis.

© Current Science Ltd ISBN 1-85922-187-4 ISSN 0952-6293

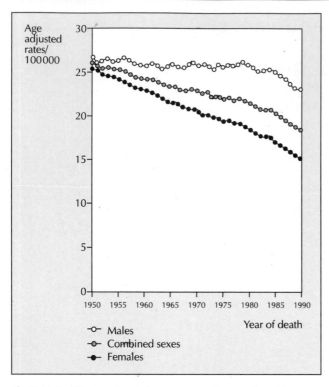

**Fig. 2.** United States colorectal cancer mortality rates for white males and females from 1950 to 1990.

clines in colorectal cancer incidence. Apparently the aggressive and widespread diagnostic, screening and surveillance approach jointly adopted by American physicians and patients is an effective one.

A prospective study of health professionals in the Nurse's Health Study and the Health Professional's Follow-up Study [4•] revealed an overall relative risk of colorectal cancer in people with a positive family history of colorectal cancer of 1.64 for men and 1.77 for women. For participants younger than 45 years of age, the relative risk was 5.37 which had fallen by the age of 65 years to 1.09. Thus, in older people, a positive family history is of little significance. Two or more affected relatives increased the risk in women to 3.79. The authors concluded that for the majority of people with a family history of colorectal cancer, particularly those aged 60 years or older, the increased risk in not large. However, the increased risk among younger people supports the ACS recommendations for early colonoscopic screening in this group.

Textbooks typically list breast cancer as a risk factor for colorectal cancer. However, two case–control studies published in 1994 [5•,6•] found that the relative risk of colorectal cancer was only 1.1. Furthermore, a screening colonoscopy study [7•] in asymptomatic women with breast cancer found that the prevalence of adenomas was identical to that in a group of asymptomatic, average-risk women (18%). Thus, women with breast cancer should receive the same colorectal cancer screening measures as an average-risk women. In one meta-analysis, endometrial cancer and ovarian cancer were associated with relative risks of 1.4 and 1.6, respectively [5•]. Whether more intensive screening is justified for women with these risk factors remains undecided.

Workers at the University of Kansas identified 6642 patients undergoing autopsy over a 34-year period who had no pre-mortem diagnosis of either gallstones or colorectal cancer [8•]. Although there was no overall association, subgroup analysis did reveal an association between asymptomatic gallstones and asymptomatic right-sided colorectal cancer in women (odds ratio 6.79, 95% confidence interval 1.14–46.47). The discussion in this paper contains a nice review of the extensive literature on the association of cholecystectomy in colorectal cancer, although some important papers have been published since this paper was submitted. The authors suggest that the true association may involve the reason for cholecystectomy (gallstones) and not the cholecystectomy itself. My overall assessment of some very complicated literature is that women with cholecystectomy (and possibly those with asymptomatic gallstones?) have a relative risk for right-sided colon cancer of about 2.0, many years after the cholecystectomy. Critically, it is still not certain whether interval screening colonoscopy is justified in such patients.

In 1988, an excess of colorectal cancer incidence was linked to manufacturing polypropylene [9]. In an incidence study, polypropylene manufacturing workers who were negative at the initial screen were re-screened by flexible sigmoidoscopy. There were modest and non-statistically significant excesses in polyp incidence, but there were so many confounding factors and poorly controlled variables that the issue is likely to remain unsettled. In a case–control study, body iron stores (serum ferritin levels) were shown to be associated with adenomatous polyps [10]. However, the results vary from those of three previous case–control studies. Verification and considerable clarification will be needed before this finding can be considered of any clinical significance.

## Chemoprevention of colorectal neoplasia

Aspirin now appears to be the most promising general chemopreventive agent for colorectal cancer. Early suspicions that its effect was related primarily to increased bleeding from colorectal cancers, and thus earlier detection, have been shown to be incorrect by studies indicating that aspirin also prevents adenomas [11•]; even a few doses per week appears to be effective. Low doses of aspirin are also associated with up to a ten-fold increased risk of hospitalization for complicated peptic ulcer, however, and may have other serious long-term toxicities. A general recommendation for colorectal cancer chemoprevention with aspirin must, therefore, await positive cost-effectiveness analyses and, preferably, additional prospective trials. A sensible review of the association of aspirin and colorectal cancer prevention was published [12•]. Additional support for a theoretical basis for the preventive effect of aspirin was obtained from basic research studies of colonoscopically or surgically resected tissue. In one study [13], increased prostaglandin $E_2$ levels were found in colorectal cancers as well as background mucosa of patients with cancer. In the other study [14•], cyclo-oxygenase-1 and cyclo-oxygenase-2 messenger (m)RNA levels were studied in colorectal cancer, adenomas and background mucosa. Cyclo-oxygenase-2 expression was upregulated by 1.5- to 50-fold in 12 out of 14 cancers, and was increased in half of the adenomas. Thus, this enzyme may be a target for chemoprevention.

Sulindac is known to decrease the number and the size of colorectal polyps in patients with familial polyposis, although it does not result in their complete disappearance. Its use is popular in certain areas to suppress rectal polyps after subtotal colectomy. A group with extensive experience suggested using 100 mg twice daily until the polyps disappeared and then attempting tapering [15]. Successful maintenance doses varied from 100 to 300 mg daily with 200 mg/day being the average. The authors suggested that long-term failures to suppress polyps usually result from inadequate dosing. Indomethacin suppositories also caused regression of rectal polyps in two patients after subtotal colectomy [16]. Two studies this year, however, suggest that reliance on sulindac for prevention of cancer in familial polyposis is inappropriate. In one [17•], sulindac did not influence the labelling index (a measure of cell proliferation), despite decreasing the size and the number of polyps. In the other study [18], a 68-year-old woman was started on oral sulindac 35 years after an ileorectal anastomosis, after being found to have over 100 rectal polyps. Her polyps promptly disappeared but, during every 3-month observation by sigmoidoscopy, she developed a '1–2 cm flat ulcerated lesion' in the rectum, subsequently shown to be adenocarcinoma extending to the perirectal fat and involving six lymph nodes. The best treatment for familial polyposis surely remains carefully timed total proctocolectomy.

A 4-year clinical trial in 864 adenoma patients whose colons had been cleared of adenomas by colonoscopy studied whether β-carotene (25 mg daily), vitamin C (1 g daily) and vitamin E (400 mg daily), or β-carotene plus vitamin C and E, were superior to placebo in preventing recurrent adenomas [19]. No protective effect was observed during 1- and 4-year follow-up colonoscopies.

Considerable epidemiologic data links high intakes of dietary fibre, particularly wheat fibre, to a decreased risk of colorectal cancer. Reddy et al. [20] showed that wheat but not oat or corn bran was associated with decreased faecal excretion of diacylglycerols, which have been implicated in experimental colon carcinogenesis. From the perspective of colorectal cancer, it appears that (at least for now) advice to patients regarding increased dietary fibre should focus on wheat fibre.

## Polypectomy

Shirai et al. [21] performed injection polypectomy using a mixture of 4.7% sodium chloride and 0.05% epinephrine in 645 polyps, while the technique was not used in 430 polyps. No randomization was performed. Remarkably, there was no post-polypectomy bleeding in either group. This post-polypectomy bleeding rate is so low compared with previously reported series that the extent of follow-up must be questioned. Two perforations occurred in the non-injected group. Both polyps were < 1 cm in size and the perforations occurred from inclusion of normal tissue. Thus, the difference in complications must be attributed to bad technique. The study does not, therefore, prove that injection therapy is safer than non-injection therapy. Regardless of the solution used, I see no reason to use injection therapy unless it facilitates mechanical removal of the polyp, or there is a need to make a wide cautery burn (particularly in the right colon). The technique can be very useful in broad, flat sessile polyps, as pointed out in an excellent accompanying editorial by Waye [22].

'Tiny' monopolar oval and hexagonal snares were used to perform efficient polypectomy of 183 polyps ≤ 7 mm in size [23•] (Fig. 3). The authors report that these snares have essentially replaced hot biopsy forceps in their practice, and I concur as they have all but replaced hot forceps in my own practice. They are almost as efficient as hot forceps, provide a more controlled burn, probably a more complete polypectomy and may well be safer, although these claims should be proven in a randomized prospective trial.

A feasibility study of a new bipolar polypectomy device has been reported [24]. The device was claimed to be useful for removing small polyps behind folds in the splenic and hepatic flexures, which may be hard to reach with forceps or polypectomy snares. The device deploys a hook (Fig. 4) which grabs the tip of the polyp, allowing it to be lifted. The hook is then pulled into a

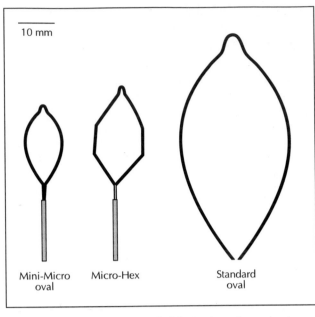

**Fig. 3.** Tiny snares for the removal of diminutive colorectal polyps. Fully opened Mini-Micro oval (left) and Micro-Hex loop (centre) snares, displayed next to standard oval snare.

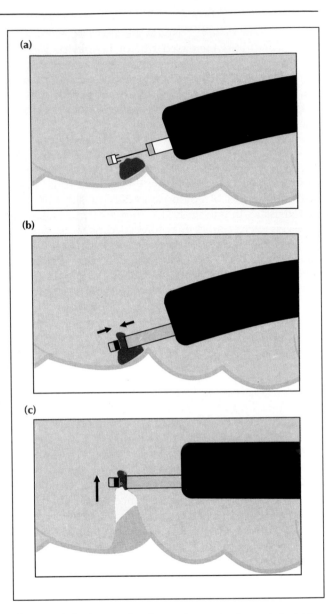

**Fig. 4.** (a) Difficult to reach polyp on the proximal aspect of a fold. (b) The polyp is drawn into the cutting cup of the device by simultaneous closure of the grasping tip and closure of the sheath. (c) Application of bipolar current with the polyp 'tented' until a rim of desiccation is evident.

sheath which allows retrieval of a specimen for histology, while bipolar current destroys the rest of the polyp. The paper [24] is a very preliminary report, which does not establish whether this device is easier to use than current technologies, or whether it provides adequate histologic specimens or adequate destruction of polyps.

Use of the Olympus (Olympus Corporation, Lake Success, New York, USA) HX-3L clipping device for polypectomy has been previously reported. Iida *et al.* [25] in Japan reported the use of the device (Fig. 5) for the removal of 42 polyps, ranging in size from 4 to 23 mm, of which only 14% were sessile. They experienced no complications but the number of patients studied is too small to justify claims of improved safety. At this time, polyp clipping followed by snare resection does not appear to be a substantive addition to the polypectomy armamentarium.

Another study of endoscopic estimates of polyp size showed that endoscopists at all levels of training consistently underestimate polyp size [26]. This particular study used ball bearings and a latex colon model. Problems in polyp size estimation would appear to be of greatest relevance to research studies, which should now clearly state how polyp size was estimated. One technique for accurate estimation of polyp size, which uses a polyp measuring probe (Fig. 6), was shown to be accurate when used with either video or fibreoptic endoscopes [27]. Retrieval of polyps < 1 cm in size by placing a 4 × 4 inch gauze pad between the suction tubing and the colonoscope was reported to be more efficient, less expensive and faster than the use of

suction traps (Fig. 7) [28]. Another method for retrieving polyps involved pulling the snare a few centimetres into the channel, suctioning the polyp, withdrawing the scope from the patient and pushing the snare out to expel the polyp [29]. This could be convenient for polyps in the rectum or distal colon.

Endoscopic band ligation was used to control delayed post-polypectomy haemorrhage from multiple polypectomy sites in an anticoagulated patient who had failed other methods of endoscopic therapy to control the bleeding [30]. Three different bleeding stalks were banded. A standard polypectomy snare passed through the colonoscope was used to grasp the L-locking slot of the inner cylinder and pull the cylinder into the friction adapter for releasing the band (Fig. 8).

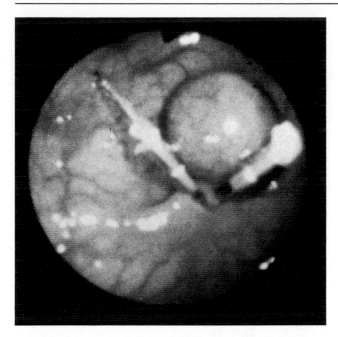

**Fig. 5.** Two clips were applied at the base of a sessile polyp which subsequently became cyanotic. Published with permission [25].

## Incident polyps after negative examinations

Hixson *et al.* [31] reported the incidence of new adenomas 2 years after their well known 'tandem colonoscopy' study, in which patients underwent colonoscopy twice in the same day by different examiners. Presumably these patients had very 'clean' colons. Nevertheless, when 58 were followed up with colonoscopy 2 years later, adenomas were found in 52%, and 38% were judged to have 'new' lesions. New lesions were defined as those occurring in a colon segment which was free of polyps at the time of the initial tandem colonoscopy. All 'new' lesions were tubular adenomas, and 25 out of 31 were ≤ 5 mm in size. However, three new lesions were 10, 12 and 20 mm in size (three were sessile). This substantial incidence is somewhat unexpected, and partly reflects the older male population studied. Certainly factors which predict the presence of polyps on the initial examination (such as male gender and old age) are also predictors of polyp recurrence. Nevertheless, the study shows that even after the most meticulous clearing colonoscopy imaginable there can be a substantial recurrence rate of adenomas.

Three papers addressed the incidence of polyps in individuals who had an initial negative flexible sigmoidoscopy. In a prospective study [32•] performed largely in male business executives, 259 asymptomatic, average-risk men who had had a negative flexible sigmoidoscopy while aged 50 years or older underwent a second examination at least 2 years after the first (mean 3.4 years). Six per cent had adenomas at the

(a)  (b)

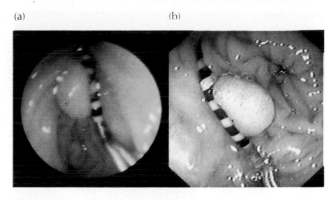

**Fig. 6.** (a) Fibreoptic and (b) video photographs of a polyp measuring device adjacent to the same polyp (1 mm divisions).

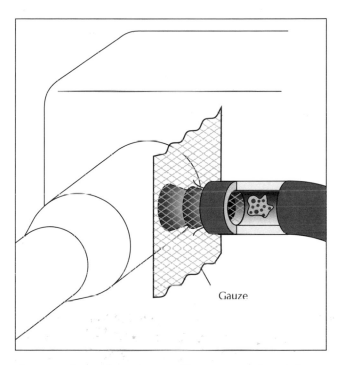

**Fig. 7.** Use of a 4 × 4 gauze to trap polyps suctioned through the colonoscope

second examination, but there were no cancers or adenomas ≥ 1 cm in size. An age greater than 60 years predicted a greater likelihood of adenomas (10% compared with 3% in those under 60 years of age). The authors concluded that the ACS could safely expand its recommended interval to 5 years in people who are initially negative. In a similarly negative study [33•], 116 patients aged 45 years or older had an 8.6% presence of adenomas at flexible sigmoidoscopy, but only 1 out of 101 (1%) had an adenoma at a 1-year follow-up examination. The authors stated the findings support the recent recommendations of the ACS to drop the initial follow-up flexible sigmoidoscopy 1 year after an initial negative examination. On the other hand, a re-screening study [34] in 64 male chemical factory workers found polyps in five (7.2%). The percentage

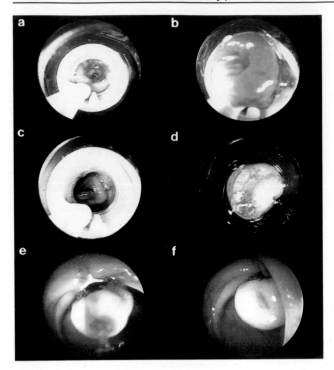

**Fig. 8.** Two separate polypectomy stalks (a–c and d–f) with visible vessels which are sequentially visualized (a, d), suctioned into the friction fit adaptor (b, e) and banded (c, f)

of these that were adenomas was uncertain, as only two of them were colonoscoped. The authors actually recommended a return to the old ACS guidelines of two consecutive negative examinations 1 year apart. However, the population studied may be atypical (32% had polyps on the initial examination), there was incomplete data on the pathology, and the sample size was small. Furthermore there were no cancers or mention of large or dysplastic adenomas. It seems that returning to two examinations, 1 year apart, is the wrong direction to be heading.

Twenty-nine patients aged 50–80 years in a Veterans Administration Hospital who had a negative colonoscopy at least 5 years previously were recruited for a follow-up colonoscopy [35]. Forty-one per cent of these patients had an adenoma, but the largest was a 1 cm tubulovillous lesion in the rectum. Thus, retrospectively identified normal colonoscopies do not predict a polyp-free status for life, although they may predict an absence of 'bad' adenomas for at least 5 years.

Previous colonoscopic screening studies have shown a high prevalence of adenomas and cancers in Lynch syndrome patients. Lanspa *et al.* [36•] reported six Lynch syndrome patients identified by case review who developed colorectal cancer 31–53 months after a negative colonoscopy. Several of the patients had multiple negative colonoscopies. Until genetic tests for the Lynch syndromes are available and their use is fully

understood, all potentially affected family members should undergo colonoscopy at the age of 25 years and every 2–3 years thereafter indefinitely. Extension of the interval to 5 years after a negative examination is unsafe in these people.

## Polyps — general

Flat adenomas in early colon cancers continue to be reported, primarily in the Japanese literature. A morphologic study of 17 early non-polypoid 'superficial-type' adenomas and nine adenocarcinomas or adenomas with severe dysplasia found that the adenomas and adenocarcinomas were very similar in size and gross endoscopic appearance [37•]. The tumours could, however, be distinguished by the surface appearance of the unsectioned tumours using a dissecting microscope. Adenomas with mild or moderate dysplasia had neoplastic crypts with a large diameter, whereas those with severe dysplasia or adenocarcinoma had neoplastic crypts that were gathered tightly together. Adenocarcinomas and adenomas with severe dysplasia had no residual focus of less dysplastic adenomas. Two out of the five adenocarcinomas were associated with lymph node metastases. The authors felt that the non-polypoid growth pattern, absence of associated adenoma of mild or moderate dysplasia, and a tendency towards submucosal invasion and even lymph node metastases with small lesions, was compatible with several potential growth mechanisms. These would include *de novo* carcinogenesis, tumours arising from small superficial-type adenomas with severe dysplasia that is rapidly displaced by expanding carcinoma, or cancers arising from so-called 'aberrant crypts'. Aberrant crypts are minute lesions which have been described in animal models of carcinogenesis and in normal regions of colorectal mucosa in patients with advanced cancers. They are presumed to be pre-cancerous lesions. The prevalence of flat adenomas and early flat colon cancers in Western countries remains uncertain. Flat adenomas occur in the hereditary flat adenoma syndrome and have been described by Lanspa in Western people at average risk. However, Lanspa did not report high-grade dysplasia in flat adenomas and his lesions may not be the same as those frequently reported by Japanese workers.

Evidence for varied development of flat and polypoid type cancers was shown in a Japanese study which found that the ras p21 product was not expressed in flat lesions, whereas the p53 gene is expressed in both flat and polypoid neoplasms [38].

Japanese reports on the prevalence of flat or depressed early colon cancers in colorectal cancer series are quite variable, ranging from 0 to 16%. A series of seven flat or depressed colonic lesions was evaluated blindly by two experienced pathologists in different Japanese institutions [39•]. One pathologist designated five of the seven lesions as cancer, and the remainder as 'borderline cancer'. The other pathologist called only one of the seven lesions cancer. The authors reasonably concluded that discrepancies in the prevalence of flat or depressed early colon cancers in Japan are dependent primarily on the lack of standards for determination of criteria for invasion. This is an obviously important issue which hopefully will be promptly addressed.

In a well-controlled study, Hofstad et al. from Norway [40••] reported 1-year colonoscopy findings in 103 patients in whom 222 polyps ≤ 10 mm in size had been left in place. They were able to find 85% of the original 222 polyps. Sizes larger than 5 mm and locations in the sigmoid and rectum were significant predictors of recovery. No change in polyp size was found in 78 polyps, and a maximal change of ± 1 mm in size occurred in 156 polyps. For unclear reasons, polyps with an initially recorded diameter of ≤ 5 mm increased significantly ($P = 0.05$) whereas polyps between 5 and 9 mm initially decreased significantly ($P = 0.04$). The overall size at 1 year did not change significantly. Only one polyp grew to a size ≥ 10 mm. Another two polyps ≥ 10 mm detected at 1 year in the controls were not seen at the initial investigation. The investigators used a number of very plausible controls on size, appearance and location of the original polyps to make certain that they were dealing with recovered versus new polyps. Half of the patients had new polyps, with most of them being small, more likely to be proximal and associated with multiplicity of polyps at the initial colonoscopy. All of these features have been previously shown to predict recurrent adenomas in post-polypectomy studies. The plan is to repeat the colonoscopies twice more at yearly intervals, and the study should provide important data on the growth rate of polyps.

Zarchy and Ershoff [41••] identified 226 asymptomatic and symptomatic patients without anaemia or positive faecal occult blood tests but with adenomas on flexible sigmoidoscopy. Adenomas were classified as advanced if they were > 1 cm in size or had villous histology or severe dysplasia. All patients underwent colonoscopy, and predictors of advanced lesions in the proximal colon were advanced lesions on flexible sigmoidoscopy (11.8% versus < 1% if no advanced lesions on flexible sigmoidoscopy) and male sex (8.2% versus 1.3%). The investigators suggested that colonoscopy is unnecessary when flexible sigmoidoscopy shows only tubular adenomas ≤ 1 cm in size. However, professional societies should advocate this position before it is followed in the United States.

A follow-up series of 54 malignant polyps removed colonoscopically found that vascular invasion in four cases did not predict an adverse outcome [42•]. Positive margins predicted an adverse outcome in only one out of 11 cases if the endoscopist recorded macroscopic complete resection, but in three out of three cases in which endoscopic complete resection was not achieved. This confirms that cautery destroys all residual tumour in many patients with completely resected polyps and positive margins. However, surgery is still appropriate for good candidates with positive margins.

A patient with familial juvenile polyposis associated with arteriovenous malformations in the lungs and liver was reported [43]. Several previous cases of generalized juvenile polyposis, occurring either sporadically or on a familial basis, have been associated with arteriovenous malformations in the lungs, liver or brain.

A patient developed multiple large hyperplastic polyps coincident with adenocarcinoma arising in an adenoma [44]. The 16 hyperplastic polyps that were 1–2 cm in size were scattered throughout the colon. Despite these occasional cases, there are still no data that hyperplastic polyps can themselves transform into cancer. Similarly, distal hyperplastic polyps cannot be considered markers for important proximal colon neoplasia.

## Follow-up after polypectomy; cancer resection

The American Society of Colon and Rectal Surgeons (ASCRS) surveyed its 1663 members regarding their follow-up strategies after resection of colon (not rectal) cancer [45•]. The results showed little variation in follow-up strategy with tumour node metastasis (TNM) stage. Most surgeons performed some sort of follow-up rather than taking a totally nihilistic approach, and most (94%) do it themselves rather than returning patients to their primary physicians for surveillance. Only 45% used a computed tomography (CT) scan at any interval and only 15% used a bone scan. Eighty per cent performed regular chest X-rays and, of these, half ordered them annually. Liver injury tests and complete blood counts were utilized by 75%, but there was wide variation in the utilized intervals. Carcinoembryonic antigen was utilized consistently, usually at 3-month intervals for the first year or two, then dropping to every 6 months for the next couple of years and eventually to yearly tests. Colonoscopy was performed annually for the first 5 years by more than half. Thus, overuse of post-cancer resection surveillance colonoscopy has persisted in the United States despite recommendations from the American Gastroenterological Association and the Standards Task Force of the ASCRS. The optimal approach is a clearing colonoscopy in the pre- or perioperative period, followed by a 1-year examination. If this examination is negative or shows only small tubular adenomas, the next examination can be done 3 years later.

An Australian surgeon reported his experience in 231 post-cancer resection patients undergoing surveillance colonoscopy between 1972 and 1990 [46•]. Examinations were generally done annually until the colon was clear of neoplasia. Patients with synchronous adenomas at the time of initial resection were more likely (73%) to develop metachronous adenomas than those without synchronous adenomas (52%). Four patients developed metachronous cancers, all in the proximal colon and at a mean interval of 7.75 years after initial resection. The authors pointed out that all four cancers arose in a group of 22 patients who had both synchronous adenomas and recurrent metachronous adenomas. This observation deserves additional attention, since it supports an increasingly popular idea that patients with previous neoplasia can be stratified for intensity of surveillance based on features such as number, size and degree of villous and dysplastic components in previous adenomas.

The same Australian surgeon estimated a two-thirds reduction in colorectal cancer incidence in his own colonoscopy practice [47•], utilizing observed versus expected incidence data in a fashion similar to that previously utilized by the National Polyp Study and the Funen Adenoma Follow-up Study. In this study the expected incidence was calculated from Australian epidemiologic data and adenoma-bearing reference populations in the medical literature.

A case–controlled study showed that extensive smoking history was associated with a greater chance of incident polyps 3 years after clearing colonoscopy [48•].

A study performed in Hawaii found a several-fold higher incidence of recurrent polyps in Caucasians compared to Japanese patients 1 year after a clearing colonoscopy, after correction for other predictors of recurrence [49]. No explanation is apparent and the observation requires confirmation.

In a series of 212 patients undergoing surveillance following cancer resection [50], patients were divided into 'compliant and non-compliant' groups. Compliant patients were those who regularly attended for surveillance examination, including yearly colonoscopy, for 5 years. The compliant patients had better overall survival than non-compliant patients ($P < 0.002$), but the difference could not be accounted for by detection of resectable recurrences of cancer. The results are therefore difficult to understand, and contrast with previous studies showing that detection of anastomotic recurrences that are surgically curable are very uncommon.

## Advances in genetics

Colorectal cancer is a genetic disease. Sporadic cancers are associated with progressive accumulation of mutations in the adenomatous polyposis coli (APC) gene, k-ras oncogene, the p53 gene, and the 'deleted in colon cancer' (DCC) gene. As with previous studies, APC gene mutations were commonly found (25 out of 59 cases) in sporadic adenomas but not hyperplastic polyps [51]. APC mutations were present in all regions with different degrees of dysplasia in the same adenoma. This is compatible with the commonly advocated position that APC mutations represent a very early step in the development of an adenoma. However, APC mutations were more common (odds ratio 6.67) in villous than in tubular adenomas and in large adenomas, suggesting that APC mutations can occur early or late in tumorigenesis. Thus, although a preferred order of mutations seems to generally exist, this order is not invariant and perhaps accumulation rather than order is most important in progression to late adenoma stages.

### Familial adenomatous polyposis

Germ-line mutations in the APC locus underlie familial adenomatous polyposis (FAP), Gardner's syndrome and Turcot's syndrome — now recognized to be variants of the same disease. The APC gene is a very large gene, containing 8538 nucleotides and 15 exons or coding regions. Variations in clinical presentation such as number of polyps, age of cancer development, retinal pigment hypertrophy, etc. are partly related to the location of the mutation in a given kindred. However, kindreds with the same APC mutation also demonstrate phenotype variability, indicating that environmental or other genetic influences modify the expression of FAP. This was shown by examining 11 kindreds with a common APC mutation (which affects approximately 20% of kindreds), a five base pair deletion at codon 1309 [52•]. These 11 unrelated kindreds included 74 patients with FAP, and there was intra- and interfamily variability in polyp density and distribution, age at onset of cancer and extra colonic manifestations.

The majority of APC mutations occur in the middle portion of the gene, and are point mutations or frameshifts that result in stop codons. The resultant protein product is shortened or 'truncated'. The normal APC protein is a cytosolic protein that appears to associate with cytoskeletal proteins. Truncation somehow results in disruption of normal cell growth and survival. The characteristic lesion of FAP is a diffusely hyperproliferative epithelium, which serves as the background for development of adenomas and cancers.

Synthesis of truncated proteins is the basis for the current commercial 'genetic test' for FAP. This test involves *in vitro* transcription of the APC protein, and identification of its length by gel electrophoresis [53**]. This test is currently available from Hoffman-LaRoche (Research Park Triangle, NC, USA) and costs approximately $700 for the initial assay on the proband. The test is not perfectly sensitive as only 80% of affected kindreds have a positive test. This less than perfect sensitivity reflects the fact that the responsible mutation does not result in a truncated APC protein in every kindred. However, if the proband has a positive test, then the test will be essentially 100% accurate in identifying affected relatives (and the cost of testing relatives is reduced to about $200 per person because the assay is simpler once the mutation has been identified). If the proband has a negative test, then more tedious genetic tests, for example, linkage analysis, must be used or traditional sigmoidoscopic screening must be relied on.

Petersen [54*] recently summarized recommendations for use of the APC gene test. When the test is positive, no change in conventional screening guidelines is recommended. People who are test positive undergo annual colon examinations beginning at the age of 10 years, together with counselling to prepare for an eventual prophylactic colectomy, and genetic counselling. Surgery should not be considered until polyps have developed. If the APC gene test is negative then patients are screened by flexible sigmoidoscopy at the ages of 18, 25 and 35 years. These screenings are selected to accommodate for false-negative laboratory error and phenomena such as tissue mosaicism or *de novo* mutations. APC gene tests can have both positive and negative consequences (Fig. 9) [54*], and should always be administered in the context of genetic counselling.

Total proctocolectomy and ileoanal anastomosis is not always accompanied by complete resection of the rectal mucosa, a point emphasized by the first report of invasive adenocarcinoma following prophylactic proctocolectomy with ileoanal anastomosis [55].

Desmoid tumours are second only to metastatic cancer as a cause of death in FAP (Gardner's syndrome). Desmoids occur in 10% of FAP patients and are more common after abdominal surgery, that is, after colectomy [56*,57*]. There is familial aggregation, with a risk of 25% in first-degree relatives of patients with desmoids versus 8% in third-degree relatives. However, desmoids are not limited to specific APC mutations. Long-term survival is common in patients with unresectable desmoids. Palliative resection can be attempted for symptomatic desmoids but the procedure has substantial morbidity and mortality. Curative resec-

| If result is APC positive |
|---|
| *Positive consequences* |
| Removal of uncertainty and doubt |
| Earlier detection of polyps and prevention of cancer |
| Able to plan and be emotionally prepared for the future |
| Increased compliance with colon examination routine |
| Greater choice of surgical (or other intervention) options |
| |
| *Negative consequences* |
| Denial, anger, depression, chronic anxiety |
| For children, upset and worry about what family of friends might think of them, increased worry about death, increased fear about surgery |
| Interference with work or school |
| Worry about children and their future |
| Loss of insurability |
| Eventual colon surgery and possible change in lifestyle |
| **Is result is APC negative** |
| *Positive consequences* |
| Removal of uncertainty and doubt; relief |
| Can select a less secure, but more appealing career |
| Can assume that children will not develop familial adenomatous polyposis |
| Fewer medical costs related to familial adenomatous polyposis |
| Better potential for insurability |
| |
| *Negative consequences* |
| Feeling bad about not having it when other family members do have it |

**Fig. 9.** Potential consequences of APC testing

tions are usually followed by recurrence but should be undertaken when small mesenteric desmoids are encountered incidentally during laparotomy.

The Italian Registry of familial polyposis reviewed causes of death in 350 deceased patients with FAP [58*]. Deaths were due to colorectal cancer in 78.1% of cases, extra colonic cancer in 9.5% of cases, desmoid tumours in 3.6% and 8.8% from other causes. Colectomy was clearly associated with improved survival. Interestingly there was no difference in survival between total colectomy and ileorectal anastomosis versus total proctocolectomy in the first 10 years after diagnosis. However, there were very few patients with ileoanal anastomosis who had over 10 years of follow-up. The risk of cancer in the rectal stump after ileorectal anastomosis was 14.5% after 15 years and 25.2% after 25 years, with corresponding risks of death from rectal cancer of 4.3% and 9.3%, respectively. In the discussion, the authors make a case for ileorectal anastomosis, based on the overall low risk of cancer death from subsequent rectal cancer and the improved quality-of-life. In fact about half of FAP patients in Italy are still operated on with ileorectal anastomosis. The quality-of-life of FAP patients after total proctocolectomy is, however, generally excellent, and the burden of many proctoscopic examinations for surveillance should not be underestimated. As mentioned earlier, surgery appears to provoke the appearance of desmoid tumours, and the authors suggested it is important to avoid early surgery, particularly in patients with a family history of desmoid tumours.

A group of Canadian workers studied molecular linkage analysis and congenital hypertrophy of retinal pigment epithelium (CHRPE) for pre-symptomatic diagnosis of FAP [59•]. With the availability of truncation assays, molecular linkage analysis is, of course, unlikely to enter widespread clinical use. Examinations for CHRPE were scored as one small lesion (< 500 microns), score 1; one or more large retinal lesions (> 500 microns), score 3. A score of 4 or more was considered to be a positive diagnostic indicator for FAP. Among 166 affected and 31 clinically unaffected (> 35 years of age) patients from FAP families, CHRPE screening had a sensitivity of 55%, a specificity of 93.5%, a positive predictive value of 97% and a negative predictive value of 28%. Thus, in FAP families who manifest CHRPE, CHRPE screening is highly predictive when positive. However, the role of CHRPE screening in an era of effective genetic screening is uncertain.

### Hereditary non-polyposis colorectal cancer

Hereditary non-polyposis colorectal cancers (HNPCC; Lynch syndromes) constitute the most common inherited cancer syndromes, and account for about 5% of all colorectal cancers. Molecular biologists have been rapidly characterizing the gene mutations that account for HNPCC. Since December 1993, when the first gene was linked and cloned, a total of four genes associated with HNPCC have been cloned. Any affected kindred has a germ-line mutation in only one of the four genes, but the clinical syndromes appear to be identical or very similar regardless of which mutated gene the kindred carries. Thus, HNPCC is a heterogeneic disease. Each of the four genes codes for an enzyme that associates with DNA, proofreads newly synthesized strands for errors, and repairs errors. The HNPCC genes (like the APC gene) behave as classic tumour suppressor genes. Thus, an affected person has a germ-line mutation in one allele. When the second allele becomes inactivated by somatic mutation, DNA repair no longer occurs normally. This results in accumulation of mutations elsewhere in the genome and eventually emergence of neoplastic cell lines. The widespread genetic damage that has occurred in HNPCC tumours is readily recognized in areas of short repeating sequences of DNA called 'microsatellite DNA'. Thus, HNPCC tumours exhibit the 'microsatellite instability' phenotype, which is likely to be essentially synonymous with inactivation of one of the HNPCC mutation repair genes.

The first two HNPCC genes identified show homology to two bacterial DNA mismatch repair genes called mut S and mut L. The two human genes are designated hMSH2 (second mut S homologue in the human genome) and hMLH1 (first mut L homologue in the human genome), and they are located on chromosomes 2 and 3, respectively [60•–62•]. The last two human HNPCC genes discovered show greatest homology to a yeast mismatch repair gene (which itself bears homology to mut L). The yeast gene carries the name 'PMS1'. Thus, the two human genes are designated hPMS1 and hPMS2, and are located on chromosomes 2 and 7, respectively [63••]. It is not yet clear what percentage of Lynch kindreds each of the four genes accounts for, but in one study 40% of classic HNPCC kindreds were associated with germ-line mutations in hMSH2 [64•]. Undoubtedly, additional HNPCC genes will be identified.

Commercial genetic tests for HNPCC are not yet available. Many of the mutations in HNPCC genes lead to truncated proteins. Thus, truncation assays, similar to those used commercially in FAP, could identify some HNPCC kindreds. You can be certain that many groups are scrambling to develop commercially usable assays, which will have much wider applicability than the current FAP assays.

Interestingly, 13% of sporadic colorectal cancers have the microsatellite instability phenotype, indicating that somatic mutation in both alleles of an HNPCC gene is a component of the development of a subset of sporadic colorectal cancer.

A Dutch group investigated 49 families with at least three relatives affected with colorectal cancer in two successive generations [65]. Forty-one families satisfied the Amsterdam criteria for HNPCC (more than three relatives with verified colorectal cancer, one of them being a first-degree relative of the other two, at least successive generations affected, and one relative diagnosed before the age of 50 years). Eight families did not meet the criteria of a relative affected before the age of 50 years. Those with classic HNPCC by Amsterdam criteria were clearly distinct from the other group (right colon cancers in 58% versus 13%, synchronous cancers in 23% versus 3%, associated adenomas in 14.5% versus 30%, associated extracolonic cancers in 66% versus 0%). In the classic HNPCC cases, 92% of the cancers had occurred by the age of 60 years. The age of diagnosis in successive generations of HNPCC patients decreased, and the finding could not be accounted for by screening for asymptomatic cancers, although it could have resulted from ascertainment bias. The authors concluded that the Amsterdam criteria, and particularly the age at diagnosis criterion, defines a clinically distinct group of familial cancers. They suggested that screening intervals could be decreased after the age of 60 years in HNPCC kindreds, since the risk of developing colorectal cancer appears to drop. They suggested that screening should begin at a substantially earlier age than the youngest case in the previous generation. No explanation was evident for the phenomenon of decreasing age of diagnosis in successive generations. In the eight kindreds with 'late onset' familial colorectal cancer, it was not clear whether the cancers represented chance clustering, shared environmental influences, or a different (and as yet undefined) gene defect. Of course, clinical genetic screening for HNPCC genes (when it becomes available) will substantially alter screening protocols.

## Non-endoscopic colonic imaging

Several series of barium enema were reported, but nothing novel appeared. Iron deficiency anaemia predicted cancer by barium enema in one series [66]. Two series for combined flexible sigmoidoscopy and double contrast barium enema were reported, one claiming that extensive sigmoid diverticulosis portends a poor sensitivity of DCBE for polyps [67], and the other finding no effect of diverticulosis at all [68]. Hough *et al.* [69] reported a diagnostic algorithm for evaluating symptomatic patients, and the associated results in 66 patients with rectal bleeding. They begin with flexible sigmoidoscopy and, if neoplasms are found, they proceed to colonoscopy. If the sigmoidoscopy is negative they performed a modified double-contrast barium enema (DCBE), designed to focus attention on the colon proximal to the sigmoid. They believed this approach would be as sensitive as colonoscopy, and twice as safe. Although it may be safe, it certainly is not as sensitive as colonoscopy.

Thirty-nine Japanese children aged 2–8 years with rectal bleeding were evaluated for juvenile polyps by ultrasonography after saline enema [70]. They were given glycerine enemas as preparation and chloral hydrate as sedation. Twenty-five had polyps detected, all of which were left-sided and all were confirmed by colonoscopy, polypectomy and histology. Of the 14 children with negative ultrasound, none had recurrent bleeding, although five underwent colonoscopy at their parent's request, each of which was negative. Thus the ultrasound was 100% accurate in diagnosing juvenile polyps. It appears that the authors are extremely good at percutaneous colonic ultrasonography. This apparently has merit in the population, although the system is so predictive (64%) of juvenile polyps that proceeding directly to colonoscopy might also have merit.

On the other hand, hydrocolonic ultrasonography performed dismally in 52 patients in whom the procedure was performed prior to blinded colonoscopy [71]. The technique missed three out of three cancers and had an overall sensitivity of 6.9% for polyps. The reasons for these dramatic discrepancies between studies are not yet clear.

## Screening

Lang and Ransohoff [72*] examined the previously published Minnesota randomized trial of faecal occult blood testing for the effect of false-positive faecal occult blood testing. As many will recall, the Minnesota study found a 33% reduction in colorectal cancer mortality in a group screened annually by faecal occult blood testing, with positive tests evaluated by colonoscopy. Remarkably, rehydration resulted in 9.8% of all tests performed being positive in the Minnesota trial. In turn, 38% of the annually screened group had at least one colonoscopy during the trial. Lang and Ransohoff calculated that one-third to one-half of the mortality reduction resulted from colonoscopy on 'false-positive' faecal occult blood testing, and concluded that 'annual faecal occult blood test screening with rehydration is a haphazard method of selecting people for colonoscopy'.

The Swedish faecal occult blood testing study of Kewenter *et al.* has some unique features [73*]. First, although the slides are rehydrated, positive tests are only evaluated if they are positive on a second, repeat testing. Kewenter *et al.* have previously shown that this improves the positive predictive value of testing with only a small loss of sensitivity. The practice of retesting was made necessary because the initial positive rate for rehydrated slides of 5.8% in 1983 had risen to a remarkable 14.3% by 1992, despite dietary and medication controls. The phenomenon of increasing positivity rate was also observed in the Minnesota trial, and suggests that the slides have changed, although the manufacturer denies this [73*]. Second, Kewenter *et al.* used flexible sigmoidoscopy and DCBE to evaluate positives, whereas other trials have essentially all used colonoscopy. I find the failure to use colonoscopy hard to accept when several trials have reported phenomenal miss rates for cancers by barium enema in patients with positive faecal occult blood tests, although Kewenter *et al.* continue to argue that very few cancers have been missed in their trial and they are apparently constrained from using colonoscopy by financial considerations. Their report contains the results of an initial screening, rescreening 16–24 months later, and follow-up. Compliance for screening and rescreening was 63% and 60%, respectively. The positive predictive value (using the above methodology of only evaluating positives on repeat testing) was 5% for cancer and 13.6% for adenomas ≥ 1.0 cm in size on the initial screen and 3.3% and 11.9%, respectively, on the rescreening. As expected, the screened group had earlier Dukes' stages but mortality data are not yet available. At this stage I find the most important data from the trial to be the shockingly high rate of positive rehydrated slides on the first testing.

A survey of 875 gastroenterologists age 40 years or above and 261 gastroenterologists under the age of 40 years was conducted to determine their attitudes toward the ACS guidelines for colorectal cancer screening and whether or not those over the age of 40 years had themselves undergone screening [74•]. Overall, the response rate to the survey was 46%. Sixty-eight per cent of respondents felt the ACS recommendations were adequate; 32% did not. Of those disagreeing, 58% preferred screening colonoscopy, and 22% preferred flexible sigmoidoscopy without faecal occult blood testing. Of those aged 40 years and over, only 38% strictly followed the ACS guidelines themselves, 39% partially, and 23% did not follow them (note that revised guidelines do not recommend average-risk screening until the age of 50 years). Reasons cited for failure to comply themselves were lack of time, inconvenience, and procrastination. The authors noted that if a knowledgeable group of physicians do not themselves follow colorectal cancer screening guidelines, it should not be overly surprising that primary care physicians are not aggressive in screening their eligible patients, even if they agree in principle with the guidelines.

Yet another study [75] showed that nurses can perform competent and safe screening flexible sigmoidoscopy.

A private practice group in the United States offered screening colonoscopy in the office for a total charge of $150 [76•]. Patients were billed the usual charges if colonoscopy and polypectomy were performed. This charge is probably unrealistic for widespread application, since it does not cover the actual costs of colonoscopy. Nevertheless, charge reduction is one route to utilizing screening colonoscopy on a more widespread basis.

A Los Angeles family practice group reported that, among 414 consecutive asymptomatic persons aged ≥ 50 years undergoing flexible sigmoidoscopy with 60-cm scopes (after GoLYTELY preparation!), they found adenomas in only 10 people (2.4%) [77]. This is a very low prevalence rate compared with other reports, and is very difficulty to explain. Among 452 persons having previous negative examination and undergoing repeat screening (at intervals ranging from 5 to 21 years), only two (0.4%) had incident polyps, which was lower than the initial prevalence rate ($P = 0.017$). This would support not rescreening, but the numbers are so low compared with other reports that the data are hard to evaluate. Interestingly, six out of the 12 patients with polyps underwent colonoscopy, which detected 16 additional synchronous lesions, only five of which were beyond the range of a 60-cm sigmoidoscope. Thus, operator skill is one potential explanation for the very low prevalence and incidence rates.

Fifty positive faecal occult blood tests obtained in hospitalized patients by digital rectal examination were found to have a positive predictive value of 8% for cancer (two colon cancers and two upper gastrointestinal tract cancers) [78]. However, the patients with cancer all had other indications (symptoms) for evaluation. There still remains a remarkable paucity of data on the value of occult blood testing of stools obtained by digital examination in either asymptomatic inpatients or outpatients, and prospective studies are sorely needed.

A study of the acceptance of screening flexible sigmoidoscopy was performed in a group of patients at a German rehabilitation centre [79]. Over a 20-month interval, there were 1166 patients aged 50–60 years who were considered eligible for screening. The authors managed to complete faecal occult blood testing on all of them and 667 (57%) accepted a sigmoidoscopy. The authors justifiably concluded that patients in clinical rehabilitation centres provide an important opportunity for colorectal cancer screening. This would appear to be particularly useful in Germany, where 700 000–800 000 individuals undergo clinical rehabilitation for chronic illnesses yearly.

An English group studied the relationship of gastrointestinal symptoms in colorectal carcinoma with respect to controls and to age [80]. There were 273 patients and an equal number of controls. Among the controls, abdominal pain (11.2% versus 4%), mucous drainage, (10.4% versus 2%) faecal incontinence (6.4% versus 0%), and altered flatus frequency (16.8% versus 8.1%) were more common in those aged 70 years or older compared with those who were younger. A variety of symptoms were quite prevalent in the general population. Virtually every symptom studied was more common in the cases than in the controls. The authors stated that, in people above the age of 70 years, a change in bowel habit, anorexia, weight loss, abdominal pain and rectal bleeding were particularly predictive of cancer. The presentation of the data may be somewhat misleading, as several colonoscopy studies have shown that abdominal symptoms in the absence of bleeding are poor predictors of colorectal cancer.

Dinning *et al.* [81••] retrospectively identified 112 patients with colon cancers proximal to the splenic flexure who had undergone complete colonoscopy. They found that the colon was devoid of 'sentinel' neoplasia distal to the splenic flexure and distal to the descending colon–sigmoid junction in 69% and 72% of patients, respectively. By multiplying these numbers by the percentage of colon cancers that are proximal to the splenic flexure, they calculated that screening flexible sigmoidoscopy will be negative for sentinel neoplasia in at least 25% of persons with prevalent colon cancers.

These results support the findings of two other abstracted, but not yet published, studies.

## Gastrin and colorectal cancer

Hypergastrinaemia as a factor in the pathogenesis of colorectal cancer has been the subject of many studies. The association of hypergastrinaemia and colon cancer is, however, extremely tenuous, as was pointed out in a nice review of the literature [82]. In the most serious blow to the gastrin hypothesis, Penman *et al.* [83•] measured preoperative and meal-stimulated gastrin levels in 42 patients with colorectal tumours and 34 matched controls. *Helicobacter pylori* status was also controlled for, as it is known to be associated with hypergastrinaemia. There was no difference in gastrin levels between the cancer patients and controls, and resection did not cause gastrin levels to decrease, except in five patients who became *H. pylori* negative. The authors suggested that previously noted decreases in gastrin levels after tumour resection could be attributed to eradication of *H. pylori* infection as a result of perioperative antibiotics. The issue of gastrin causing colorectal cancer is now all but dead. From the perspective of colorectal cancer there is no reason to obtain or respond to a serum gastrin level.

## General reviews

Two excellent long reviews appeared. One was on epidemiology and contained 304 references [84•]. The other was an excellent synopsis of clinical papers on colon polyps and cancer appearing in the 1992 and 1993 literature and summarizing 159 references [85•]. Another good review appeared on polyposis syndromes [86•] and two by distinguished authors were written on screening [87,88].

## References and recommended reading

Papers of particular interest, published within the annual period of review, have been highlighted as:

* of special interest
** of outstanding interest

1. Chu KC, Tarone RE, Chow W-H, Hankey BF, Gloeckler Ries LA: **Temporal**
** **patterns in colorectal cancer incidence, survival, and mortality from 1950 through 1990.** *J Natl Cancer Inst* 1994, **86**:997–1006.
The incidence of colorectal cancer is now greater in white males than females in the United States. However, in 1985, the incidence and mortality from colorectal cancer began dropping at a rate of 2–3% per year in both sexes, probably related to the widespread use of sigmoidoscopy and colonoscopy.

2. Giovannucci E, Rimm EB, Stampfer MJ, Colditz GA, Ascherio A, Kearney
• J, *et al.*: **A prospective study of cigarette smoking and risk of colorectal adenoma and colorectal cancer in U.S. men.** *J Natl Cancer Inst* 1994, **86**:183–191.
Smoking for less than 20 years had a strong correlation with small colorectal adenomas. Smoking for more than 20 years was correlated to large adenomas, and for more than 35 years was correlated with cancer.

3. Giovannucci E, Colditz GA, Stampfer MJ, Hunter D, Rosner BA, Willett
• WC, *et al.*: **A prospective study of cigarette smoking and risk of colorectal adenoma and colorectal cancer in U.S. women.** *J Natl Cancer Inst* 1994, **86**:192–199.
A relationship between smoking and colorectal cancer, similar to that seen above in men, was also documented in women.

4. Fuchs CS, Giovannucci EL, Colditz GA, Hunter DJ, Speizer FE, Willett WC:
• **A prospective study of family history and the risk of colorectal cancer.** *N Engl J Med* 1994, **331**:1669–1674.
Evaluation of a large group of health professionals found an overall relative risk of developing cancer of 1.72 in people with a positive family history of cancer. The risk was increased in those with multiple relatives, and decreased dramatically for persons over the age of 60 years with a positive family history.

5. Schoen RE, Weissfeld JL, Kuller LH: **Are women with breast, endometrial,**
• **or ovarian cancer at increased risk for colorectal cancer?** *Am J Gastroenterol* 1994, **89**:835–842.
A meta-analysis found age-adjusted relative risks of developing colorectal cancer in women with breast cancer, endometrial cancer, and ovarian cancer of 1.1, 1.4, and 1.6, respectively.

6. Eisen GM, Sandler RS: **Are women with breast cancer more likely to**
• **develop colorectal cancer?** *J Clin Gastroenterol* 1994, **19**:57–63.
A meta-analysis found that there is no significant increase in colorectal cancer in women with a history of breast cancer.

7. Rex DK, Sledge GW, Harper PA, Ulbright TM, Loehrer PJ, Helper DJ, *et*
• *al.*: **Colonic adenomas in asymptomatic women with a history of breast cancer.** *Am J Gastroenterol* 1993, **88**:2009–2014.
A screening colonoscopy study found that women over the age of 50 years had an 18% chance of harbouring adenomas in the colon, whether or not they had a personal history of breast cancer.

8. McFarlane MJ, Welch KE: **Gallstones, cholecystectomy, and colorectal**
• **cancer.** *Am J Gastroenterol* 1994, **88**:1994–1999.
An autopsy study found that asymptomatic gallstones were associated with asymptomatic colorectal cancer, particularly right-sided cancer.

9. Lewis RJ, Lerman SE, Schnatter AR, Hughes JI, Vernon SW: **Colorectal polyp incidence among polypropylene manufacturing workers.** *J Med* 1994, **36**:174–181.
An incidence study of polyps in polypropylene manufacturing workers showed non-statistically significant and modest increases in adenomatous polyps.

10. Nelson RL, Davis FG, Sutter E, Sobin LH, Kikendall JW, Bowen P: **Body iron stores and risk of colonic neoplasia.** *J Natl Cancer Inst* 1994, **86**:455–460.
A case–control study of serum ferritin levels in patients undergoing colonoscopy suggested that iron exposure may be related to adenoma formation. Overall not very convincing.

11. Giovannucci E, Rimm EB, Stampfer MJ, Colditz GA, Ascherio A, Willett
• WC: **Aspirin use and the risk for colorectal cancer and adenoma in male health professionals.** *Ann Intern Med* 1994, **121**:241–246.
Among male health professionals in the United States, regular aspirin use (≥ 2 times per week) was associated with a relative risk of 0.68 for colorectal cancer, 0.51 for advanced colorectal cancer and 0.77 for adenomas, with all reductions statistically significant.

12. Paganini-Hill A: **Aspirin and the prevention of colorectal cancer: A**
• **review of the evidence.** *Semin Surg Oncol* 1994, **10**:158–164.
A clinically oriented and readable review of the aspirin–colorectal cancer connection.

13. Pugh S, Thomas GAO: **Patients with adenomatous polyps and carcinomas have increased colonic mucosal prostaglandin E₂.** *Gut* 1994, **35**:675–678.
Increased prostaglandin $E_2$ levels were found in colorectal cancers, as well as the background mucosa of patients with cancer.

14. Eberhart CE, Coffey RJ, Radhika A, Giardiello FM, Ferrenbach S, Dubois
• RN: **Up-regulation of cyclooxygenase 2 gene expression in human colorectal adenomas and adenocarcinomas.** *Gastroenterology* 1994, **107**: 1183–1188.
Cyclo-oxygenase-2 may be a target for chemoprevention.

15. Labayle D, Boyer J, Drouhin F, Zarka Y, Fischer D: **Sulindac in familial adenomatous polyposis.** *Lancet* 1994, **343**:417–418.
From an experienced group, this paper contains dosing recommendations for sulindac in patients with FAP.

16.    Hirata K, Hideaki I, Ohsato K: **Regression of rectal polyps by indomethacin suppository in familial adenomatous polyposis. Report of two cases.** *Dis Colon Rectum* 1994, **37**:943–946.
Indomethacin was effective in causing regression of rectal polyps.

17.    Spagnesi MT, Tonelli F, Dolara P, Caderni G, Valanzano R, Anastasi A, *et al.*: **Rectal proliferation and polyp occurrence in patients with familial adenomatous polyposis after sulindac treatment.** *Gastroenterology* 1994, **106**:362–366.
Despite a reduction in polyp occurrence, abnormal mucosal proliferation persisted after sulindac therapy in patients with FAP.

18.    Thorson AG, Lynch HT, Smyrk TC: **Rectal cancer in an FAP patient after sulindac.** *Lancet* 1994, **343**:180.
Despite regression of rectal polyps, a Dukes' C cancer developed in the rectum of an FAP patient on sulindac.

19.    Greenberg ER, Baron JA, Tosteson TD, Freeman DH Jr, Beck GJ, Bond JH, *et al.*: **A clinical trial of antioxidant vitamins to prevent colorectal cancer adenoma.** *N Engl J Med* 1994, **331**:141–147.
In a 4-year study utilizing colonoscopy, β-carotene and vitamins C and E were ineffective in preventing recurrent colorectal adenomas. Several critical letters appeared later in the journal.

20.    Reddy BS, Simi B, Engle A: **Biochemical epidemiology of colon cancer: effect of types of dietary fiber on colonic diacylglycerols in woman.** *Gastroenterology* 1994, **106**:883–889.
Wheat bran was associated with decreased faecal excretion of diacylglycerols, which have been implicated in experimental colon carcinogenesis.

21.    Shirai M, Nakamura T, Matsuura A, Ito Y, Kobayashi S: **Safer colonoscopic polypectomy with local submucosal injection of hypertonic saline–epinephrine solution.** *Am J Gastroenterol* 1994, **89**:334–338.
In a non-randomized study, the authors claim that injection polypectomy is easier and safer than non-injection. It may be true, but this study does not prove it.

22.    Waye JD: **Saline injection colonoscopic polypectomy.** *Am J Gastroenterol* 1994, **89**:305–306.
Some sound advice regarding injection polypectomy.

23.    McAfee JH, Katon RM: **Tiny snares prove safe and effective for removal of diminutive colorectal polyps.** *Gastrointest Endosc* 1994, **40**:301–303.
Tiny snares have replaced hot forceps in these authors' practice.

24.    McNally PR, DeAngelis SA, Rison DR, Sudduth RH: **Bipolar polypectomy device for removal of colon polyps.** *Gastrointest Endosc* 1994, **40**:489–491.
This is a feasibility study for a bipolar polypectomy device for removal of polyps on the proximal sides of folds.

25.    Iida Y, Miura S, Munemoto Y, Kasahara Y, Asada Y, Toya D, Fujisawa M: **Endoscopic resection of large colorectal polyps using a clipping method.** *Dis Colon Rectum* 1994, **37**:179–180.
The authors conclude that endoscopic clipping of polyps has many advantages, but they are a long way from proving it.

26.    Margulies C, Krevsky B, Catalano MF: **How accurate are endoscopic estimates of size.** *Gastrointest Endosc* 1994, **40**:174–177.
This is the second paper suggesting that endoscopists regularly underestimate polyp size.

27.    Hofstad B, Vatn M, Larsen S, Huitfeldt HS, Osnes M: **In site measurement of colorectal polyps to compare video and fiberoptic endoscopes.** *Endoscopy* 1994, **26**:461–465.
The authors report that video and fibreoptic endoscopes are equally reliable in measuring polyps, provided that the polyps are measured with their measuring probe.

28.    Khanduja KS, Pons R: **Efficient technique for retrieving small polyps from the colon and rectum following snare polypectomy.** *Dis Colon Rectum* 1994, **37**:190.
The authors report a poor man's substitute for a suction trap (for retrieving polyps) after suctioning them through the colonoscope.

29.    Black HM, Schechter S, Thornton S, Eisenstat TE: **Simple method for polyp retrieval during colonoscopy.** *Dis Colon Rectum* 1994, **37**:949.
Another little trick for polyp retrieval; pull the snare back in the channel a few centimetres, suction the polyp, withdraw the scope and push the polyp out with the snare. Of course, how often do you want to remove the colonoscope from the patient to retrieve a polyp?

30.    Slivka A, Parsons WG, Carr-Locke DC: **Endoscopic band ligation for treatment of post-polypectomy hemorrhage.** *Gastrointest Endosc* 1994, **40**:230–232.
A patient with coagulopathy-related bleeding from multiple colonic polypectomy sites was treated by band ligation of the bleeding sites.

31.    Hixson LJ, Fennerty B, Sampliner RE, McGee DL, Garewal H: **Two-year incidence of colon adenomas developing after tandem colonoscopy.** *Am J Gastroenterol* 1994, **89**:687–691.
Even after two thorough clearing colonoscopies on the same day (tandem colonoscopy), there is a substantial recurrence rate of adenomas in older men.

32.    Rex DK, Lehman GA, Ulbright TM, Smith JJ, Hawes RH: **The yield of a second screening flexible sigmoidoscopy in average-risk persons after one negative examination.** *Gastroenterology* 1994, **106**:593–595.
A flexible sigmoidoscopy in average-risk people 3 years after a negative examination had only a 6% yield of adenomas, with no adenomas > 1 cm. The authors recommend expanding the screening interval to every 5 years.

33.    Brint SL, DiPalma JA, Herrera JL: **Colorectal cancer screening: is one-year surveillance sigmoidoscopy necessary?** *Am J Gastroenterol* 1993, **88**: 2019–2021.
One year after a negative flexible sigmoidoscopy, only one out of 101 people had an adenoma on repeat flexible sigmoidoscopy.

34.    Krevsky B, Fisher RS: **Yield of rescreening for colonic polyps using flexible sigmoidoscopy.** *Am J Gastroenterol* 1994, **89**:1165–1168.
In a study of only 64 screenees, 7.2% had polyps on flexible sigmoidoscopy 1 year after a negative examination. However, the histology of the polyps was uncertain.

35.    Squillace S, Berggreen P, Jaffe P, Fennerty MG, Hixson L, Garweal H, *et al.*: **A normal initial colonoscopy after age 50 does not predict a polyp-free status for life.** *Am J Gastroenterol* 1994, **89**:1156–1159.
Among 29 patients (largely male) aged 50–70 years, retrospectively identified as having a normal colonoscopy 5 years previously, 41.4% had an adenoma on repeat colonoscopy. However, only one lesion was 1 cm in size.

36.    Lanspa SJ, Jenkins JX, Cavalieri RJ, Smyrk TC, Watson P, Lynch J, *et al.*: **Surveillance in Lynch syndrome: how aggressive?** *Am J Gastroenterol* 1994, **89**:1978–1980.
Among 225 HNPCC patients, 10.2% had colorectal cancer within 5 years of colonoscopy or colon resection. Thus expanding the screening interval beyond 2–3 years in these patients is inappropriate.

37.    Minamoto T, Sawaguchi K, Ohta T, Itoh T, Mai M: **Superficial-type adenomas and adenocarcinomas of the colon and rectum: a comparative morphological study.** *Gastroenterology* 1994, **106**:1436–1443.
Flat early colon cancers and severely dysplastic adenomas were shown to have distinct surface morphology when examined with a dissecting microscope. They could not be distinguished from mild or moderately dysplastic adenomas by size or gross appearance. Flat early colon cancers invade early and spread aggressively.

38.    Yukawa M, Fujimori T, Maeda S, Tabuchi M, Nagasako K: **Comparative clinicopathological and immunohistochemical study of ras and p53 in flat and polypoid type colorectal tumours.** *Gut* 1994, **35**:1258–1261.
There are some molecular differences between flat and polypoid tumours, as p53 was expressed in both, whereas ras p21 was expressed only in polypoid tumours.

39.    Uno Y, Munakata A, Tanaka M: **The discrepancy of histologic diagnosis between flat early colon cancers and flat adenomas.** *Gastrointest Endosc* 1994, **40**:1–5.
Two experienced Japanese pathologists varied greatly in their identification of cancer among seven flat colonic neoplasms.

40.    Hofstad B, Vatn M, Larsen S, Osnes M: **Growth of colorectal polyps: recovery and evaluation of unresected polyps of less than 10 mm, 1 year after detection.** *Scand J Gastroenterol* 1994, **29**:640–645.
A nicely performed study showed that polyps under 10 mm in size change very little in size over 1 year.

41.    Zarchy TM, Ershoff D: **Do characteristics of adenomas on flexible sigmoidoscopy predict advanced lesions on baseline colonoscopy?** *Gastroenterology* 1994, **106**:1501–1504.
Patients with only small ≤ 1 cm tubular adenomas on sigmoidoscopy had a < 1% prevalence of advanced adenomas in the proximal colon.

42.    Moore JW, Hoffmann DC, Rowland R: **Management of the malignant colorectal polyp: the importance of clinicopathological correlation.** *Aust N Z J Surg* 1994, **64**:242–246.

Another series evaluating pathologic features of malignant colon polyps. For patients with involvement of the margin, evidence of complete endoscopic resection still predicted cure of the lesion, and incomplete endoscopic resection predicted recurrence.

43. Radin DR: **Hereditary generalized juvenile polyposis: association with arteriovenous malformations and risk of malignancy.** *Abdom Imaging* 1994, **19**:140–142.
Generalized juvenile polyposis, whether sporadic or familial, can be associated with arteriovenous malformations in the lung, liver, or brain.

44. Warner AS, Glick ME, Fogt F: **Multiple large hyperplastic polyps of the colon coincident with adenocarcinoma.** *Am J Gastroenterol* 1993, **89**:123–125.
Multiple large hyperplastic polyps rarely co-exist with adenocarcinomas, although the cancers still arise in adenomatous polyps.

45. Vernava III AM, Longo WE, Virgo KS, Coplin MA, Wade TP, Johnson FE:
• **Current follow-up strategies after resection of colon cancer.** *Dis Colon Rectum* 1994, **37**:573–583.
Surgeons are in general over utilizing colonoscopy for post-cancer resection surveillance.

46. Chen F, Stuart M: **Colonoscopic follow-up of colorectal carcinoma.** *Dis*
• *Colon Rectum* 1994, **37**:568–572.
In a single surgeon's practice, metachronous cancer occurred only in the proximal colon at a mean interval of 7.75 years after initial resection. A small subset of patients with synchronous adenomas at initial resection and recurrent metachronous adenomas appeared to be at substantially greater risk of developing cancer.

47. Meagher AP, Stuart M: **Does colonoscopic polypectomy reduce the inci-**
• **dence of colorectal carcinoma?** *Aust N Z J Surg* 1994, **64**:400–404.
In a single surgeon's colonoscopy practice, the observed incidence of cancer developing during post-polypectomy surveillance was less than expected.

48. Jacobson JS, Neugut AI, Murray T, Garbowski GC, Forde KA, Treat MR, et
• al.: **Cigarette smoking and other behavioral risk factors for recurrence of colorectal adenomatous polyps (New York City, NY, USA).** *Cancer Causes Control* 1994, **5**:215–220.
Cigarette smoking was associated with an increase risk of recurrent adenomas after clearing colonoscopy.

49. Phillips DL, Okamura D, Tokumine T: **Ethnic differences in the recurrence of adenomatous polyps after colonoscopic polypectomy.** *Hawaii Med J* 1994, **53**:16–18.
Recurrent polyps in Hawaii were more likely in Caucasians compared to Japanese. No explanation was apparent.

50. Eckardt VG, Stamm H, Kanzller G, Bernhard G: **Improved survival after colorectal cancer in patients complying with a postoperative endoscopic surveillance program.** *Endoscopy* 1994, **26**:523–527.
Compliance with postoperative colonoscopy was associated with improved survival. However, indifferences in mortality could not be accounted for by detection of surgically curable recurrences.

51. De Benedetti L, Sciallero S, Gismondi V, James R, Bafico A, Biticchi R, et al.: **Association of APC gene mutations and histological characteristics of colorectal adenomas.** *Cancer Res* 1994, **54**:3553–3556.
APC gene mutations were found in 25 out of 59 sporadic adenomas, but not in hyperplastic polyps. APC mutations were present in all regions of the adenoma, despite the degree of dysplasia, indicating that they are an early step in adenoma development.

52. Giardiello FM, Krush AJ, Petersen GM, Booker SV, Kerr M, Tong LL, et
• al.: **Phenotypic variability of familial adenomatous polyposis in 11 unrelated families with identical APC gene mutation.** *Gastroenterology* 1994, **106**:1542–1547.
Eleven unrelated families with the same APC gene mutation demonstrated variability in polyp density, diameter, distribution and extra colonic lesions, indicating that environmental or other genetic factors influence the phenotypic expression of FAP.

53. Powell SM, Petersen GM, Krush AJ, Booker S, Jen J, Giardiello FM, et al.:
•• **Molecular diagnosis of familial adenomatous polyposis.** *N Engl J Med* 1993, **329**:1982–1987.
APC mutations usually result in truncated proteins. This paper describes the 'truncation assay' which is the basis of the current commercial assay. The assay was positive in 82% of FAP kindreds.

54. Petersen GM: **Knowledge of the adenomatous polyposis coli gene and its**
• **clinical application.** *Ann Med* 1994, **26**:205–208.
Good advice on the use of APC gene testing and genetic counselling.

55. Hoehner JC, Metcalf AM: **Development of invasive adenocarcinoma following colectomy with ileoanal anastomosis for familial polyposis coli.** *Dis Colon Rectum* 1994, **37**:824–828.
Invasive adenocarcinoma developed in residual rectal mucosa following total proctocolectomy and ileoanal anastomosis.

56. Rodriguez-Bigas MA, Mahoney MC, Karakousis CP, Petrelli NJ: **Desmoid**
• **tumors in patients with familial adenomatous polyposis.** *Cancer* 1994, **74**:1270–1274.
Interesting study of 24 FAP patients with desmoid tumours.

57. Gurbuz AK, Giardiello FM, Petersen GM, Krush AJ, Offerhaus GJ, Booker
• SV, et al.: **Desmoid tumours in familiar adenomatous polyposis.** *Gut* 1994, **34**:377–381.
Interesting study of frequency of clinical features of desmoid tumours in FAP patients.

58. Bertario L, Presciuttini S, Sala P, Rossetti C, Pietroiusti M: **Causes of death**
• **and postsurgical survival in familial adenomatous polyposis: results from the Italian Registry.** *Sem Surg Oncol* 1994, **10**:225–234.
Colorectal cancer accounted for 78% of deaths among 350 FAP patients. Extracolonic cancers accounted for 9.5% and desmoids 3.6%. The risk of dying from rectal cancer after ileorectal anastomosis was 4.3% and 9.3% at 15 and 25 years, respectively.

59. Bapat BV, Parker JA, Berk T, Cohen Z, McLeod RS, Ray PN, et al.:
• **Combined use of molecular and biomarkers for presymptomatic carrier risk assessment in familial adenomatous polyposis: implications for screening guidelines.** *Dis Colon Rectum* 1994, **37**:165–171.
Screening for congenital hypertrophy of the retinal pigment epithelium had a positive predictive value for FAP of 97%, but a sensitivity of only 55%.

60. Nyström-Lahti M, Sistonen P, Mecklin JP, Pylkkänen L, Aaltonen LA,
• Järvinen H, et al.: **Close linkage to chromosome 3p and conservation of ancestral founding haplotype in hereditary nonpolyposis colorectal cancer families.** *Proc Natl Acad Sci USA* 1994, **91**:6054–6058.
Mapping of hMLH1 to chromosome 3p.

61. Bronner CE, Baker SM, Morrison PT, Warren G, Smith LG, Lescoe MK, et
• al.: **Mutation in the DNA mismatch repair gene homologue hMLH1 is associated with hereditary non-polyposis colon cancer.** *Nature* 1994, **368**:258–261.
Cloning and sequencing of hMLH1.

62. Papadopoulos N, Nicolades NC, Wei YF, Ruben SM, Carter KC, Rosen CA,
• et al.: **Mutation of mutL homolog in hereditary colon cancer.** *Science* 1994, **263**:1625–1629.
Identification of mutations of hMLH1 in HNPCC kindreds.

63. Nicolaides NC, Papadopoulos N, Liu B, Wei YF, Carter FC, Ruben SM, et
•• al.: **Mutations of two PMS homologues in hereditary nonpolyposis colon cancer.** *Nature* 1994, **371**:75–80.
Cloning, sequencing, chromosome localization and mutational analysis of hPMS1 and hPMS2.

64. Liu B, Parsons RE, Hamilton SR, Petersen GM, Lynch HT, Watson P, et al.:
• **hMSH2 mutations in hereditary nonpolyposis colorectal cancer kindreds.** *Cancer Res* 1994, **54**:4590–4594.
Forty per cent of classic HNPCC kindreds were associated with germ-line mutations in hMSH2.

65. Vasen HFA, Friffioen G, Nagengast FM, Cats A, Menko FH, Oskam W, et
• al.: **Clinical heterogeneity of familial colorectal cancer and its influence on screening protocols.** *Gut* 1994, **35**:1262–1266.
Families meeting the Amsterdam criteria for HNPCC form a clinically distinct group from families with clustering of colorectal cancer but no cases diagnosed before the age of 50 years. In HNPCC families the age of cancer diagnosis was younger with successive generations.

66. Guthrie JA, Saifuddin A, Simpkins KC, de Dombal FT: **It is worth doing barium enemas on patients with unexplained iron deficiency anaemia?** *Clin Radiol* 1994, **49**:375–478.
A high yield was described for barium enema in patients with iron deficiency anaemia.

67. Stefánsson T, Bergman A, Ekbom A, Nyman R, Påhlman L: **Accuracy of double contrast barium enema and sigmoidoscopy in the detection of polyps in patients with diverticulosis.** *Acta Radiol* 1994, **35**:442–446.

Diverticulosis impeded the sensitivity of DCBE for polyps in the sigmoid colon.

68.    Brewster NT, Grieve DC, Saunders JH: **Double-contrast barium enema and flexible sigmoidoscopy for routine colonic investigation.** *Br J Surg* 1994, **81**:445–447.

A report of same-day flexible sigmoidoscopy and DCBE. Sigmoidoscopy was superior in polyp detection and inflammatory bowel disease while barium enema was more sensitive for diverticular disease; nothing new. Diverticular disease did not reduce the sensitivity of barium enema for polyp detection.

69.    Hough DM, Malone DE, Rawlinson J, De Gara CJ, Moote DJ, Irvine EJ, *et al.*: **Colon cancer detection: an algorithm using endoscopy and barium enema.** *Clin Radiol* 1994, **48**:170–175.

The authors report their experience in 66 patients with rectal bleeding, who underwent a flexible sigmoidoscopy, followed by colonoscopy if polyps were detected and modified DCBE if flexible sigmoidoscopy was normal.

70.    Nagita A, Amemoto K, Yoden A, Yamazaki T, Mino M, Miyoshi H: **Ultrasonographic diagnosis of juvenile colon polyps.** *J Pediatr* 1994, **124**:535–540.

Percutaneous colonic ultrasonography was extremely sensitive in the detection of juvenile colon polyps.

71.    Chui DW, Gooding GAW, McQuaid KR, Griswold V, Grendell JH: **Hydrocolonic ultrasonography in the detection of colonic polyps and tumors.** *N Engl J Med* 1994, **331**:1685–1688.

Percutaneous colonic ultrasonography was essentially useless in the detection of colon polyps and cancer. Reasons for the differences are not certain.

72.    Lang CA, Ransohoff DF: **Fecal occult blood screening for colorectal**
•      **cancer.** *JAMA* 1994, **271**:1011–1013.

Calculation that one-third to one-half of the colorectal cancer mortality reduction in the Minnesota faecal occult blood testing trial resulted from haphazard selection for colonoscopy through false-positive occult blood tests.

73.    Kewenter J, Breveinge H, Engarås B, Haglind E, Åhrén C: **Results of**
•      **screening, rescreening, and follow-up in a prospective randomized study for detection of colorectal cancer by fecal occult blood testing.** *Scand J Gastroenterol* 1994, **29**:468–473.

Another report of the large Swedish faecal occult blood testing trials. Interesting features are slide rehydration, evaluation only if positive on retesting and evaluation of positives by flexible sigmoidoscopy and DCBE rather than colonoscopy

74.    Afridi SA, Jafri SF, Marshall JB: **Do gastroenterologists themselves follow**
•      **the American Cancer Society recommendation for colorectal cancer screening?** *Am J Gastroenterol* 1994, **89**:2184–2187.

Sixty-eight per cent of gastroenterologists felt the ACS guidelines for colorectal screening were adequate. Of the 32% who did not, 58% preferred screening colonoscopy. Only 38% of adult gastroenterologists themselves followed ACS guidelines strictly.

75.    Maule WF: **Screening for colorectal cancer by nurse endoscopists.** *N Engl J Med* 1994, **330**:183–187.

Nurses can do competent and safe screening colonoscopy.

76.    Rogge JD, Elmore MF, Mahoney SJ, Brown ED, Troiano FP, Wagner DR,
•      *et al.*: **Low-cost, office-based, screening colonoscopy.** *Am J Gastroenterol* 1994, **89**:1775–1780.

Screening colonoscopy for $150 if no polyps found.

77.    Sakamoto MS, Hara JH, Schlumpberger JM: **Screening flexible sigmoidoscopy in a low-risk, highly screened population.** *J Fam Pract* 1994, **38**:245–248.

Family doctors performing screening flexible sigmoidoscopy identified polyps in only 2.4% of prevalence examinations and 0.4% of rescreening examinations.

78.    Pochapin MB, Fine SN, Eisorfer RM, Rigas B: **Fecal occult blood testing in hospitalized patients.** *J Clin Gastroenterol* 1994, **19**:274–277.

Positive faecal occult blood tests on stools obtained by digital examination in hospitalized patients were unlikely to predict colonic neoplasia unless there were other symptomatic indications. An important topic, but the study was small and additional data are surely needed.

79.    Armbrecht U, Manus B, Brägelmann R, Stockbrügger RW, Stolte M: **Acceptance and outcome of endoscopic screening for colonic neoplasia in patients undergoing clinical rehabilitation for gastrointestinal and metabolic diseases.** *Z Gastroenterol* 1994, **32**:3–7.

Acceptance for flexible sigmoidoscopy was extremely good in patients visiting a clinical rehabilitation centre.

80.    Curless R, French J, Williams GV, Jams OFW: **Comparison of gastrointestinal symptoms in colorectal carcinoma patients and community controls with respect to age.** *Gut* 1994, **35**:1267–1270

Symptoms compatible with colorectal cancer are common in the general population, and symptoms are more common in people older than 70 years.

81.    Dinning JP, Hixson LJ, Clark LC: **Prevalence of distal colonic neoplasia**
••     **associated with proximal colon cancers.** *Arch Intern Med* 1994, **154**:853–856.

Most proximal colon cancer are not associated with distal 'sentinel neoplasia', detection of which at flexible sigmoidoscopy would lead to colonoscopy and detection of the cancer. Thus, screening flexible sigmoidoscopy will fail to detect a sizable fraction of prevalent colon cancer.

82.    Begos DG, Modlin IM: **Gastrin and colon cancer [editorial].** *J Clin Gastroenterol* 1994, **18**:189–193.

A nice review; largely suggests that no role for gastrin in colon carcinogenesis is established.

83.    Penman ID, El-Omar E, Ardill JES, McGregor JR, Galloway DJ, O'Wyer
•      PJ, *et al.*: **Plasma gastrin concentrations are normal in patients with colorectal neoplasia and unaltered following tumor resection.** *Gastroenterology* 1994, **106**:1263–1270.

This study found no association of hypergastrinaemia with colon cancer after controlling for confounding factors such as *H. pylori* infection.

84.    Potter JD, Slattery ML, Bostick RM, Gapstur SM: **Colon cancer: a review**
•      **of the epidemiology.** *Colon Cancer* 1993, **15**:499–545.

Extensive review of the epidemiology of colorectal cancer.

85.    McGahan RP, Gilinsky NH: **Colonic tumors.** *Endoscopy* 1994, **26**:70–87.
•
Excellent review of 1992 and 1993 papers on clinical and endoscopic topics with regard to colonic tumours.

86.    Rustgi AK: **Hereditary gastrointestinal polyposis and nonpolyposis syn-**
•      **dromes.** *N Engl J Med* 1994, **331**:1694–1701.

Nice review of polyposis syndromes and HNPCC.

87.    Bennett DH, Hardcastle JD: **Screening for colorectal cancer.** *Postgrad Med J* 1994, **70**:469–474.

Review of cancer screening

88.    Ransohoff DF: **The case for colorectal cancer screening.** *Hosp Pract* 1994, **29**:25–32.

Review of cancer screening.

Douglas K. Rex, Division of Gastroenterology/Hepatology, Indiana University Medical Center, Indianapolis, Indiana, USA.

# General topics

## Christopher B. Williams

St Mark's Hospital for Colorectal and Intestinal Disorders, London, UK

### Training and performance in gastrointestinal endoscopy

Peter Cotton, describing himself as an 'aggressive gastroenterologist' (an internist practising endoscopic surgery), throws down a gauntlet suggesting that there should be a new look at the potentially chaotic future of gastrointestinal training and practice [1••]. He gives a characteristically pithy view of the past situation in gastroenterology, when the physician gastroenterologist could be 'leisurely and contemplative' and his surgeon colleague 'authoritative, unscientific and risky'. Cotton foresees, however, a new generation of young academics with a long-term scientific interest in endoscopy now that 'outcome evaluation research is becoming fundable as well as fashionable'. One of his suggestions is that gastrointestinal clinical practice would be enhanced by adopting a multidisciplinary team approach and that gastrointestinal trainees might start with a 2–3 year 'core curriculum' before branching out into their preferred area(s) of special expertise. This might result, in addition to traditional medical gastroenterologists and 'cutting surgeons', in a third intermediate grouping with particular aptitude for cross-border interventional skills (including high-level endoscopy, minimal invasive therapy and aspects of radiology or other forms of imaging) (Fig. 1).

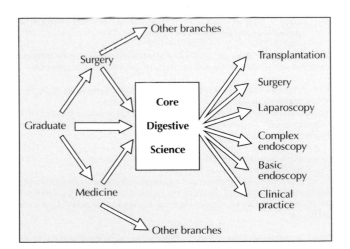

**Fig. 1.** A suggested 2–3 year 'core curriculum' for all gastrointestinal trainees. Published with permission [1••]

What Cotton describes, and is putting into action in a new academic centre, is happening to some extent around the world, but in a piecemeal and individualized fashion. Formalizing or popularizing the idea would bring new respectability to gastrointestinal technical activities and teaching. It should also help to fend off the unwholesome and counterproductive interprofessional 'turf' skirmishes that otherwise threaten the developing gastrointestinal scene. An accompanying editorial by the respected Mayo Clinic clinicians, however, suggests that radical restructuring may be generally impracticable, but that fostering of close medical–surgical relationships is probably the most workable answer [2].

### Consent, preparation and medication

Obtaining informed consent before an endoscopic procedure is an integral but problematic matter. There is an onus on the physician personally to provide the patient with the facts necessary to make an informed decision, including awareness of the risks and possible alternative strategies. Since the physician is under some time pressure, but the patient must not be put under duress, the demonstration that a videotape can add to informed consent gives a welcome lead [3]. An editorial speculates that interactive video programmes for informed consent should perform even better, allowing skilled presentation and provide tailoring of in-depth information available to meet the concerns of the individual [4]. A further bonus of the electronic approach would be the ability to document the items considered by the patient, including responses to the interactive process. This 'consent database' should be easy to organize and would be potentially useful if any dispute arose after the event.

Another editorial considers the numerous components which contribute to safe performance of gastrointestinal endoscopy [5]. These components include not only the clinical assessment of the patient, proper training of the endoscopist and the nurse–assistant support team, but also the new attitude to slow titration of medication (if any) at low dosage, rather than the 'knockout' approach

**Abbreviations**

ERCP—endoscopic retrograde cholangiopancreatography.

| Procedure | Healthy | Prosthetic joints/grafts | Valvular heart disease | Prosthetic heart valves | Previous endocarditis | Immune compromised* | Ascites* |
|---|---|---|---|---|---|---|---|
| Upper gastrointestinal endoscopy | No | No | Optional | Yes | Yes | Optional | Optional |
| Colonoscopy/sigmoidoscopy | No | No | Optional | Yes | Yes | Optional | Optional |
| Oesophageal dilatation | No | No | Yes | Yes | Yes | Optional | Optional |
| Oesophageal sclerotherapy | No | No | Yes | Yes | Yes | Optional | Optional |
| ERCP (without obstruction) | No | No | Optional | Yes | Yes | Optional | Optional |
| ERCP (with obstruction)* | Yes | Yes | Yes | Yes | Yes | Yes | Yes |
| Percutaneous gastrostomy* | Yes | Yes | Yes | Yes | Yes | Yes | Yes |

*Prophylaxis for endoscopic retrograde cholangiopancreatography (ERCP) with obstruction, percutaneous gastrostomy and immunocompromised patients may vary according to suspected pathogens.

**Fig. 2.** Schematic representation of antibiotic prophylaxis requirements for gastrointestinal endoscopy, in relation to individual risk status. High-risk: Gentamycin 1.5 mg/kg plus ampicillin 2 g i.v. or i.m. either repeated at 8 h or followed by amoxycillin 1.5 g orally (Vancomycin 1 g i.v. over 1 h instead of ampicillin if penicillin allergic). At risk: Amoxycillin 3 g orally 1 h before procedure and 1.5 g, 6 h later (Erythromycin ethylsuccinate 800 mg, 2 h before and 400 mg, 6 h later if penicillin sensitive). Published with permission [8••].

of old. One of the end-of-year literature reviews published in *Endoscopy* gives a valuable compendium of articles in the 1990–1993 period relating mainly to medication for endoscopy, but touches also on other issues such as oxygenation monitoring, psychological aspects and bowel preparation [6•]. A short review covering the use of benzodiazepine/opiate sedation in teaching hospitals in the Netherlands (whose patients are renowned for their stoicism) shows that sedation is not generally used for upper gastrointestinal endoscopy and frequently not used for colonoscopy. It is used for endoscopic retrograde cholangiopancreatography (ERCP), however, primarily because of the benefits to the endoscopist during long-lasting procedures or the amnesic benefits for those that may need repeating [7]. Whether short-term heroism is a virtue in civilized society, or (avoidable) unpleasant memories can be considered acceptable, are basic questions about which any humane endoscopist needs a viewpoint, but one capable of being adapted to the wishes of the patient before him.

An excellently clear and wide-ranging literature review on endoscopy-related infections highlights the relative rarity of serious clinical sequelae, even though most endoscopic procedures may occasionally produce bacteraemia [8••]. The worst offenders are oesophageal sclerotherapy (which can cause peritonitis), dilatation and lasering, and any ERCP procedure in the presence of biliary obstruction. The recommendations for antibiotic prophylaxis have become less stringent over the years. Only patients with previous endocarditis or prosthetic heart valves are mandated to have antibiotics but it is thought wise to protect others predisposed to risk by immunodepression, ascites or an obstructed biliary system. A useful tabular summary and detailed antibiotic suggestions are reproduced in Figure 2.

## References and recommended reading

Papers of particular interest, published within the annual period of review, have been highlighted as:

- • of special interest
- •• of outstanding interest

1. Cotton PB: **Interventional gastroenterology (endoscopy) at the crossroads: a plea for restructuring in digestive diseases.** *Gastroenterology* 1994, **107**:294–299.
•• A pithy commentary on the changing face of gastroenterology, which needs a new, more multidisciplinary approach, and also revised training arrangements. Trainees might start with a 2–3 year 'core curriculum' before branching out, whether into medical gastroenterology, gastrointestinal surgery or possibly a new grouping with cross-border interventional skills. Without a new framework for training and practice, counterproductive 'turf' issues are likely to damage prospects for gastrointestinal endoscopy.

2. McGill DB, Moody FG: **Invasive endoscopy and the medical/surgical divide.** *Gastroenterology* 1994, **107**:306–308.
An editorial commenting on Cotton's hopes for radical restructuring in gastroenterology; the authors feel that fostering close medical–surgical relationships is probably the most workable answer.

3. Agre P, Kurtz RC, Krauss BJ: **A randomised trial using videotape to present consent information for colonoscopy.** *Gastrointest Endosc* 1994, **40**:271–276.
Viewing a videotape alone was as effective in presenting information for informed consent as viewing the tape and also discussing the procedure with the physician.

4. Plumeri PA: **Informed consent for gastrointestinal endoscopy in the 90's and beyond.** *Gastrointest Endosc* 1994, **40**:379–382.
An editorial (accompanying the article by Agre *et al.* [3]) speculating that interactive video programmes could improve the quality of informed consent and also document the patients responses for medico-legal reasons.

5. Keefe EB: **Determinants of safe endoscopy.** *Gastrointest Endosc* 1994, **40**:379–382.
An editorial considering the numerous components contributing to safe performance of gastrointestinal endoscopy, including assessment of the patient, proper training of the endoscopist and nurse–assistant team, and titrated administration of low-dose medication.

6. Lazzaroni M, Bianchi Porro G: **Preparation, premedication and surveillance in gastrointestinal endoscopy.** *Endoscopy* 1994, **26**:3–8.
• End-of-year literature review covering articles from 1990–1993 relating mainly to medication, but touching on other issues such as oxygenation monitoring, psychological aspects and bowel preparation.

7. Nagengast FM: **Sedation and monitoring in gastrointestinal endoscopy.** *Scand J Gastroenterol* 1993, **28** (suppl 200):28–32.

A short review of usage of benzodiazepine/opiate sedation for gastrointestinal endoscopy finds that teaching hospitals in the Netherlands generally use no sedation for upper gastrointestinal endoscopy and frequently none for colonoscopy, but they do sedate for ERCP.

8. Schembre D, Bjorkman DJ: **Review article: endoscopy-related infections.**
•• *Aliment Pharmacol Ther* 1993, **7**:347–355.
Clear, wide-ranging literature review highlights the rarity of serious clinical sequelae in spite of the fact that most endoscopic procedures occasionally produce bacteraemia. Oesophageal procedures such as sclerotherapy, dilatation or laser and ERCP involving biliary obstruction are high risk. Only patients with previous endocarditis or a heart valve prosthesis mandate antibiotic prophylaxis (often oral amoxycillin 3 g before and 1.5 g after) but it is wise to protect others with ascites, immunodepression or an obstructed biliary system.

Christopher B. Williams, St Mark's Hospital for Colorectal and Intestinal Disorders, London, UK.

# Bibliography of the current world literature

This bibliography is compiled by gastrointestinal endoscopists from the journals listed at the end of this publication. It is based on literature entered into our database between 1st January 1994 and 31st December 1994 (articles are generally added to the database about two and a half months after publication). In addition, the bibliography contains every paper annotated by reviewers; these references were obtained from a variety of bibliographic databases and published between the beginning of the review period and the time of going to press. The bibliography has been grouped into topics that relate to the reviews in this issue.

- • Papers considered by the reviewers to be of special interest.
- •• Papers considered by the reviewers to be of outstanding interest.

The number in square brackets following a selected paper, e.g. **[7]**, refers to its number in the annotated references of the corresponding review.

## Contents

## Endoscopy of the oesophagus

Abid S, Champion G, Richter JE, McElvein R, Slaughter RL, Koehler RE: **Treatment of**
• **Achalasia: the Best of Both Worlds [see Comments].** *Am J Gastroenterol* 1994, **89**:979–985. **[45]**.

Adachi Y, Kitamura K, Tsutsui S, Ikeda Y, Matsuda H, Sugimachi K: **How to Detect Early Carcinoma of the Esophagus.** *Hepatogastroenterology* 1993, **40**:207–211.

Anon: **Cancer Surveillance in Barrett's Esophagus: what is the End Point? [Letter].** *Gastroenterology* 1994, **106**:275–276.

Armstrong D: **The Oesophagus.** In *Annual of Gastrointestinal Endoscopy.* Edited by
• Cotton PB, Tytgat GNJ, Williams CB. London: Current Science Ltd, 1994:15–28. **[4]**.

Bataller R, Llach J, Salmeron JM, Elizalde JI, Mas A, Pique JM, *et al.*: **Endoscopic**
• **Sclerotherapy in Upper Gastrointestinal Bleeding Due to Mallory–Weiss Syndrome.** *Am J Gastroenterol* 1994, **89**:2147–2150. **[36]**.

Beck PL, Blustein PK, Andersen MA: **Aphthous Esophageal Ulceration: a Novel**
• **Presentation of Crohn's Disease?** *Can J Gastroenterol* 1994, **8**:101–104. **[29]**.

Bennett JR, Dakkak M: **An Improved Method for Oesophageal Intubation [Letter;**
• **Comment].** *Ann R Coll Surg Engl* 1993, **75**:449–450. **[56]**.

Berggreen PJ, Harrison ME, Sanowski RA, Ingebo K, Noland B, Zierer S: **Techniques and Complications of Esophageal Foreign Body Extraction in Children and Adults.** *Gastrointest Endosc* 1993, **39**:626–630.

Bernstein D, Barkin JS: **Pneumatic Dilation of a Sigmoid Esophagus in Achalasia Using an Overtube.** *Gastrointest Endosc* 1993, **39**:549–550.

Bonelli L: **Barretts Esophagus — Results of a Multicentric Survey.** *Endoscopy* 1993, **25**:652–654.

Bosch O, Gonzalez Campos C, Jurado A, Guijo I, Miro C, Renedo G, *et al.*: **Esophageal**
• **Inflammatory Fibroid Polyp. Endoscopic and Radiologic Features.** *Dig Dis Sci* 1994, **39**:2561–2566. **[25]**.

Boyce HW Jr: **Stents for Palliation of Dysphagia Due to Esophageal Cancer.** *N Engl J Med* 1993, **329**:1345.

Bramhall SR, Veitch PS, Gourevitch D, Wicks AC: **An Improved Method for Oesophageal Intubation.** *Ann R Coll Surg Engl* 1993, **75**:189–192.

Broor SL, Raju GS, Bose PP, Lahoti D, Ramesh GN, Kuma A, Sood GK: **Long Term Results of Endoscopic Dilatation for Corrosive Oesophageal Strictures.** *Gut* 1993, **34**:1498–1501.

Cantero D, Yoshida T, Ito T, Suzumi M, Tada M, Okita K: **Esophageal Hemangioma:**
• **Endoscopic Diagnosis and Treatment.** *Endoscopy* 1994, **26**:250–253. **[20]**.

Chan ACW, Leong HT, Chung SSC, Li AKC: **Lipiodal as a Reliable Marker for Stenting**
• **in Malignant Esophageal Stricture [Letter].** *Gastrointest Endosc* 1994, **40**:520–521. **[64]**.

Chaves DM, Sakai P, Mester M, Spinosa SR, Tomishige T, Ishioka S: **A New Endoscopic**
• **Technique for the Resection of Flat Polypoid Lesions.** *Gastrointest Endosc* 1994, **40**:224–226. **[38]**.

Chawla SK, Ramani K, Chawla K, LoPresti P, Mahadevia P: **Giant Esophageal Ulcers of**
• **AIDS: Ultrastructural Study.** *Am J Gastroenterol* 1994, **89**:411–415. **[30]**.

Chung SCS, Leong HT, Leung JWC, Li AKC: **Palliation of Malignant Oesophageal**
• **Obstruction by Endoscopic Alcohol Injection.** *Endoscopy* 1994, **26**:275–277. **[65]**.

Ciarolla DA, Traube M: **Short-Term Clinical Monitoring after Pneumatic Dilation.** *Dig Dis Sci* 1993, **38**:1905–1908.

Clark GW, Smyrk TC, Burdiles P, Hoeft SF, Peters JH, Kiyabu M, *et al.*: **Is Barrett's**
• **Metaplasia the Source of Adenocarcinomas of the Cardia?** *Arch Surg* 1994, **129**:609–614. **[14]**.

Collard JM, Otte JB, Kestens PJ: **Endoscopic Stapling Technique of Esophagodiverticulostomy for Zenker Diverticulum.** *Ann Thorac Surg* 1993, **25**:642–644.

Conio M: **Endoscopic Features of Barretts Esophagus.** *Endoscopy* 1993, **25**:642–644.

Cox JGC, Winter RK, Maslin SC, Dakkak M, Jones R, Buckton GK, Hoare RC, Dyet JF,
•• Bennett JR: **Balloon or Bougie for Dilatation of Benign Esophageal Stricture?** *Dig Dis Sci* 1994, **39**:776–781. **[42]**.

Dawsey SM, Lewin KJ, Wang GQ, Liu F-S, Nieberg RK, Yu Y, *et al.*: **Squamous**
• **Esophageal Histology and Subsequent Risk of Squamous Cell Carcinoma of the Esophagus. A Prospective Follow-up Study from Linxian, China.** *Cancer* 1994, **74**:1686–1692. **[15]**.

Devhire J, Quarre JP, Love J, Cremer M: **Self-expandable Stent and Injection of**
• **Tissure Adhesive for Malignant Bronchoesophageal Fistula.** *Gastrointest Endosc* 1994, **40**:508–510. **[59]**.

D'Haens G, Rutgeerts P, Geboes K, Vantrappen G: **The Natural History of Esophageal**
•• **Crohn's Disease: Three Patterns of Evolution.** *Gastrointest Endosc* 1994, **40**:296–300. **[27]**.

Ell C, Hochberger J, Fietkau R, Schneider T, Schmitt M, Hahn EG: **New Bougie Applicator System for Intraluminal High Dose Rate Afterloading Radiotherapy of Esophageal Carcinoma.** *Endoscopy* 1993, **25**:236–239.

Ell C, Hochberger J, May A, Fleig WE, Hahn FG: **Coated and Uncoated Self-expanding**
• **Metal Stents for Malignant Stenosis in the Upper GI Tract: Preliminary Clinical Experiences with Wallstents.** *Am J Gastroenterol* 1994, **89**:1496–1500. **[58]**.

Fruhwirth H, Rabl L, Hauser H, Schmid C, Beham A, Klein GE: **Endoscopic Findings of**
• **Pseudoxanthoma Elasticum.** *Endoscopy* 1994, **26**:507. **[24]**.

Gelfand GAJ, Finley RJ: **Quality of Life with Carcinoma of the Esophagus.** *World J*
• *Surg* 1994, **18**:399–405. **[62]**.

Glover JR, Sargeant IR, Bown SG, Lees WR: **Non-optic Endosonography in Advanced Carcinoma of the Esophagus.** *Gastrointest Endosc* 1994, **40**:194–198.

Gore S, Healey CJ, Sutton R, Eyrebrook IA, Gear MWL, Shepherd NA, Wilkinson SP: **Regression of Columnar Lined (Barrett) Oesophagus with Continuous Omeprazole Therapy.** *Aliment Pharmacol Ther* 1993, **7**:623–628.

Greager JA, Donahue PE, Reichard K, Kucich V, Lubienski M, Barker W, Reyes HM: **Endoscopically Defined Treatment Strategies in Patients with Locally Advanced Esophageal Cancer.** *Surg Endosc* 1994, **8**:384–388.

Gschossmann JM, Bonner JA, Foote RL, Shaw EG, Martenson JA, Su J: **Malignant Tracheoesophageal Fistula in Patients with Esophageal Cancer.** *Cancer* 1993, **72**:1513–1521.

Hashizume M, Ohta M, Ueno K, Tomikawa M, Kitano S, Sugimachi K: **A Transparent Endoscopic Elastic Band Ligating Device.** *Gastrointest Endosc* 1993, **39**:686–688.

Hassall E: **Invited Review — Barrett's Esophagus — New Definitions and Approaches in Children.** *J Pediatr Gastroenterol Nutr* 1993, **16**:345–364.

Hassall E: **Barrett's Esophagus — Congenital or Acquired [Review].** *Am J Gastroenterol* 1993, **88**:819–824.

Hintze RE, Binmoeller KF, Adler A, Veltzke W, Thonke F, Soehendra N: **Improved**
• **Endoscopic Management of Severe Upper Gastrointestinal Haemorrhage Using a New Wide-channel Endoscope.** *Endoscopy* 1994, **26**:613–616. **[35]**.

Hizawa K, Iida M, Matsumoto T, Kohrogi N, Suekane H, Yao T, *et al.*: **Gastrointestinal**
• **Manifestations of Cowden's Disease. Report of Four Cases.** *J Clin Gastroenterol* 1994, **18**:13–18. **[5].**
Horan TA, Urschel JD, MacEachern NA, Shulman B, Crowson AN, Magro C: **Esophageal**
• **Perforation in Recessive Dystrophic Epidermolysis Bullosa.** *Ann Thorac Surg* 1994, **57**:1027–1029. **[21].**
Horwitz B, Krevsky B, Buckman RF, Fisher RS, Dabezies MA: **Endoscopic Evaluation of Penetrating Esophageal Injuries.** *Am J Gastroenterol* 1993, **88**:1249–1253.
Inoue H, Noguchi O, Saito N, Takeshita K, Endo M: **Endoscopic Mucosectomy**
• **for Early Cancer Using a pre-looped Plastic Cap [Letter].** *Gastrointest Endosc* 1994, **40**:263–264. **[37].**
Jaakkola A, Reinikainen P, Ovaska J, Isolauri J: **Barrett's Esophagus after**
• **Cardiomyotomy for Esophageal Achalasia.** *Am J Gastroenterol* 1994, **89**:165–169. **[13].**
Jaspersen D, Kvrner T, Schorr W, Brennenstuhl M, Hammar C-H: **Extragastric**
• **Dieulafoy's Disease as Unusual Source of Intestinal Bleeding. Esophageal Visible Vessel.** *Dig Dis Sci* 1994, **39**:2558–2560. **[23].**
Jerome-Zapadka KM, Clarke MR, Sekas G: **Recurrent Upper Esophageal Webs in**
• **Association with Heterotopic Gastric Mucosa: Case Report and Literature Review.** *Am J Gastroenterol* 1994, **89**:421–424. **[18].**
Jonsson P, Hogstrom H: **Non-Operative Treatment of Benign Oesophageal Strictures — Results after Endoscopic Balloon Dilatation and $H_2$-Antagonists.** *Eur J Surg* 1993, **159**:405–407.
Kadakia SC, Parker A, Carrougher JG, Shaffer RT: **Esophageal Dilation with Polyvinyl Bougies, Using a Marked Guidewire Without the Aid of Fluoroscopy — an Update.** *Am J Gastroenterol* 1993, **88**:1381–1386.
Karita M, Tada M: **Endoscopic and Histologic Diagnosis of Submucosal Tumors**
• **of the Gastrointestinal Tract Using Combined Strip Biopsy and Bite Biopsy.** *Gastrointest Endosc* 1994, **40**:749–753. **[39].**
Kim CH, Cameron AJ, Hsu JJ, Talley NJ, Trastek VF, Pairolero PC, *et al.*: **Achalasia:**
• **Prospective Evaluation of Relationship Between Lower Esophageal Sphincter Pressure, Esophageal Transit, and Esophageal Diameter and Symptoms in Response to Pneumatic Dilation.** *Mayo Clin Proc* 1993, **68**:1067–1073. **[46].**
Kim SL, Waring JP, Spechler SJ, Sampliner RE, Doos WG, Krol WF, *et al.*: **Diagnostic**
•• **Inconsistencies in Barrett's Esophagus.** *Gastroenterology* 1994, **107**:945–949. **[9].**
Lambert R: **Palliation of Carcinoma of the Esophagus: is There a Hope for Cure?** *Am J Gastroenterol* 1994, **89** (suppl):S27–S40.
Leong S, Kortan P, Gray R, Marcon N, Haber G: **Transgastric Esophagoscopy with**
• **Antegrade Dilation [Case Report].** *Endoscopy* 1994, **26**:622–624. **[43].**
Lerut TE, Deleyn P, Coosemans W, Vanraemdonck D, Cuypers P, Vancleynenbreughel B: **Advanced Esophageal Carcinoma.** *World J Surg* 1994, **18**:379–387.
Levine DS, Haggitt RC, Blount PL, Rabinovitch PS, Rusch VW, Reid BJ: **An Endoscopic Biopsy Protocol can Differentiate High-Grade Dysplasia from Early Adenocarcinoma in Barrett's Esophagus.** *Gastroenterology* 1993, **105**:40–50.
Levine ML: **Endoscopic Appearance of the Lower Esophageal Sphincter in**
• **Achalasia: a Diagnostic Sign [Letter].** *Gastrointest Endosc* 1994, **40**:124–125. **[17].**
Lim CT, Quah RF, Loh LE: **A Prospective Study of Ingested Foreign Bodies in**
• **Singapore.** *Arch Otolaryngol Head Neck Surg* 1994, **120**:96–101. **[70].**
Liu SF, Shen Q, Dawsey SM, Wang GQ, Nieberg RK, Wang ZY, *et al.*: **Esophageal**
• **Balloon Cytology and Subsequent Risk of Esophageal and Gastric-cardia Cancer in a High-risk Chinese Population.** *Int J Cancer* 1994, **57**:775–780. **[16].**
Marcial M, Villafaqa M: **Esophageal Ectopic Sebaceous Glands: Endoscopic and**
• **Histologic Findings.** *Gastrointest Endosc* 1994, **40**:630–632. **[6].**
Marks RD, Richter JE: **Peptic Strictures of the Esophagus [Review].** *Am J Gastroenterol* 1993, **88**:1160–1173.
Marks RD, Richter JE, Koehler RE, Spenney JG, Mills TP, Champion G: **Omeprazole**
•• **Versus $H_2$-receptor Antagonists in Treating Patients with Peptic Stricture and Esophagitis.** *Gastroenterology* 1994, **106**:907–915. **[40].**
Mathis G, Sutterlutti G, Dirschmid K, Feurstein M, Zimmermann G: **Crohn's Disease of**
• **the Esophagus Dilation of Stricture and Fibrin Sealing of Fistulas.** *Endoscopy* 1994, **26**:508. **[26].**
McLean DM: **Esophageal Ulcers as Presenting Features of Human Immunodeficiency Virus Disease [Letter].** *J Infect Dis* 1993, **168**:1596.
Mearin F, Armengol JR, Chicharro L, Papo M, Balboa A, Malagelada JR: **Forceful**
• **Dilatation Under Endoscopic Control in the Treatment of Achalasia: a Randomised Trial of Pneumatic Versus Metallic Dilator.** *Gut* 1994, **35**:1360–1362. **[47].**
Menke-Pluymers MBE, Mulder AH, Hop WCJ, Van Blankenstein M, Tilanus HW, the
• Rotterdam Oesophageal Tumour Study Group: **Dysplasia and Aneuploidy as Markers of Malignant Degeneration in Barrett's Oesophagus.** *Gut* 1994, **35**:1348–1351. **[12].**
Mion F, Bernard G, Valette P-J, Lambert R: **Spontaneous Esophageal Haematoma:**
• **Diagnostic Contribution of Echoendoscopy.** *Gastrointest Endosc* 1994, **40**:503–505. **[22].**
Moreira LS, Coelho RCL, Sadala RU, Dani R: **The use of Ethanol Injection Under**
• **Endoscopic Control to Palliate Dysphagia Caused by Esophagogastric Cancer.** *Endoscopy* 1994, **26**:311–314. **[66].**
Nabeya K, Hanaoka T, Li S, Nyumura T: **What is the Ideal Treatment for Early Esophageal Cancer.** *Endoscopy* 1993, **25**:670–671.
Nair LA, Reynolds JC, Parkman HP, Ouyang A, Strom BL, Rosato EF, *et al.*:
•• **Complications During Pneumatic Dilation for Achalasia or Diffuse Esophageal Spasm. Analysis of Risk Factors, Early Clinical Characteristics, and Outcome.** *Dig Dis Sci* 1993, **38**:1893–1904. **[48].**
Naveau S, Ratziu V, Chaput JC: **Palliative Endoscopic Therapy of Malignant Esophageal and Cardial Strictures.** *Gastroenterol Clin Biol* 1993, **17**:740–746.
Nelson DB, Silvis SE, Ansel HJ: **Management of a Tracheoesophageal Fistula with**
• **a Silicone-covered Self-expanding Metal Stent.** *Gastrointest Endosc* 1994, **40**:497–499. **[34].**
Okuda K: **Intratumor Ethanol Injection.** *J Surg Oncol* 1993, (suppl 3):97–99.
Orlowska J, Jarosz D, Gugulski A, Pachlewski J, Butruk E: **Squamous Cell Papillomas**
• **of the Esophagus: Report of 20 Cases and Literature Review.** *Am J Gastroenterol* 1994, **89**:434–437. **[7].**
Panzini L, Burrell MI, Traube M: **Instrumental Esophageal Perforation Chest Film**
• **Findings.** *Am J Gastroenterol* 1994, **89**:367–370. **[52].**
Papsin BC, Friedberg J: **Aerodigestive-tract Foreign Bodies in Children: Pitfalls in**
• **Management.** *J Otolaryngol* 1994, **23**:102–108. **[68].**
Parkman HP, Ogorek CP, Harris AD, Cohen S: **Nonoperative Management of**
• **Esophageal Strictures Following Esophagomyotomy for Achalasia.** *Dig Dis Sci* 1994, **39**:2102–2108. **[50].**
Pasricha PJ, Fleischer DE, Kalloo AN: **Endoscopic Perforations of the Upper**
•• **Digestive Tract: a Review of Their Pathogenesis, Prevention, and Management.** *Gastroenterology* 1994, **106**:787–802. **[1].**
Pasricha PJ, Ravich WJ, Hendrix TR, Sostre S, Jones B, Kalloo AN: **Treatment of**
•• **Achalasia with Intrasphincteric Injection of Botulinum Toxin. A Pilot Trial.** *Ann Intern Med* 1994, **121**:590–591. **[44].**
Pezzi JS, Shiau Y-F: **A Method for Removing Meat Impactions from the Esophagus.**
• *Gastrointest Endosc* 1994, **40**:634–636. **[71].**
Provenzale D, Kemp JA, Arora S, Wong JB: **A Guide for Surveillance of Patients with**
•• **Barrett's Esophagus.** *Am J Gastroenterol* 1994, **89**:670–680. **[11].**
Przemioslo RT, Mee AS: **Omeprazole in Possible Esophageal Crohn's Disease**
• **[Letter].** *Dig Dis Sci* 1994, **39**:1594–1595. **[28].**
Pugliese V: **The Role of Endoscopy in Esophageal Cancer — Summary of a Videoendoscopy Session.** *Endoscopy* 1993, **25**:645–647.
Rai AS, Steer H: **Lesson of the Week: the First 15cm are Important in Upper Gastrointestinal Endoscopy.** *BMJ* 1993, **306**:1742.
Raijman I, Kortan P, Haber GB, Marcon NE: **Contrast Injection to Identify Tumor**
• **Margins During Esophageal Stent Placement.** *Gastrointest Endosc* 1994, **40**:222–224. **[63].**
Raijman I, Walden D, Kortan P, Haber GB, Fuchs E, Siemens M, Kandel G, Marcon NE:
• **Expandable Esophageal Stents: Initial Experience with a New Nitinol Stent.** *Gastrointest Endosc* 1994, **40**:614–621. **[60].**
Reissman P, Fich A, Eid A, Rivkind A: **Esophageal Phytobezoar Causing Acute**
• **Dysphagia: a Rare Complication of Gastric Bezoar.** *J Clin Gastroenterol* 1994, **18**:159–160. **[67].**
Robbins MI, Shortsleeve MJ: **Treatment of Acute Esophageal Food Impaction**
• **with Glucagon, an Effervescent Agent, and Water.** *AJR Am J Roentgenol* 1994, **162**:325–328. **[69].**
Sampliner RE: **High-Grade Dysplasia in Barretts Esophagus — an Evolving Clinical Dilemma.** *Am J Gastroenterol* 1993, **88**:1811–1812.
Saraswat VA, Dhiman RK, Mishra A, Naik SR: **Correlation of 24-hr Esophageal pH**
•• **Patterns with Clinical Features and Endoscopy in Gastroesophageal Reflux Disease.** *Dig Dis Sci* 1994, **39**:199–205. **[3].**
Schwartz HM, Cahow CE, Traube M: **Outcome after Perforation Sustained During Pneumatic Dilatation for Achalasia.** *Dig Dis Sci* 1993, **38**:1409–1413.
Sen A, Lea RE: **Spontaneous Oesophageal Haematoma — a Review of the Difficult Diagnosis.** *Ann R Coll Surg Engl* 1993, **75**:293–295.
Shaker R: **Unsedated Trans-nasal Pharyngoesophagogastroduodenoscopy (T-EGD):**
• **Technique.** *Gastrointest Endosc* 1994, **40**:346–348. **[2].**
Shukla NK, Goel AK, Seenu V, Nanda R, Deo SV, Kriplani AK: **Endoscopically Guided Placement of Nasogastric Tubes in Patients with Esophageal Carcinoma with Absolute Dysphagia — Report of a 3-Year Experience.** *J Surg Oncol* 1994, **56**:217–220.
Sibille A, Lambert R, Lapeyre B, Souquet J-C, Descos F, Ponchon T: **Survival Following**
• **Non-surgical Multimodal Treatment for Oesophageal Squamous Cell Carcinoma.** *Eur J Gastroenterol Hepatol* 1994, **6**:287–292. **[53].**
Smith PM, Kerr GD, Cockel R, Ross BA, Bate CM, Brown P, *et al.*: **A Comparison**
•• **of Omeprazole and Ranitidine in the Prevention of Recurrence of Benign Esophageal Stricture.** *Gastroenterology* 1994, **107**:1312–1318. **[41].**
Spinelli P, Cerrai FG, Ciuffi M, Ignomirelli O, Meroni E, Pizzetti P: **Endoscopic**
• **Stent Placement for Cancer of the Lower Esophagus and Gastric Cardia.** *Gastrointest Endosc* 1994, **40**:455–457. **[55].**
Stevens PD, Lightdale CJ, Green PHR, Siegel LM, Garcia-Carrasquillo RJ, Rotterdam
• H: **Combined Magnification Endoscopy with Chromendoscopy for the Evaluation of Barrett's Esophagus.** *Gastrointest Endosc* 1994, **40**:747–749. **[10].**
Swaroop VS, Desai D, Mohandas KM, Dhir V, Dave UR, Gulla RI, *et al.*: **Dilation of**
• **Esophageal Strictures Induced by Radiation Therapy for Cancer of the Esophagus.** *Gastrointest Endosc* 1994, **40**:311–315. **[54].**
Tarnasky PR, Brazer SR, Leung JWC: **Esophageal Perforation During Achalasia**
• **Dilation Complicated by Esophageal Diverticula.** *Am J Gastroenterol* 1994, **89**:1583–1585. **[49].**
Tsang T-K, Chodash HB: **Perforation after Catheter-guided Endoscopic Intubation**
• **[Letter].** *Gastrointest Endosc* 1994, **40**:780–781. **[51].**
Ueno J, Davis SW, Tanakami A, Seo K, Yoshida S, Nishitani H, *et al.*: **Ectopic Gastric**
• **Mucosa in the Upper Esophagus: Detection and Radiographic Findings.** *Radiology* 1994, **191**:751–753. **[19].**
Warren WH, Smith C, Faber LP: **Clinical Experience with Montgomery Salivary**
• **Bypass Stents in the Esophagus.** *Ann Thorac Surg* 1994, **57**:1102–1106; Discussion 1106–1107. **[57].**
Wilcox CM: **Short Report: Time Course of Clinical Response with Fluconazole for**
• **Candida Oesophagitis in Patients with AIDS.** *Aliment Pharmacol Ther* 1994, **8**:347–350. **[33].**
Wilcox CM, Schwartz DA: **Comparison of Two Corticosteroid Regimens for the**
• **Treatment of HIV-associated Idiopathic Esophageal Ulcer.** *Am J Gastroenterol* 1994, **89**:2163–2167. **[32].**
Wilcox CM, Straub RF, Schwartz DA: **Prospective Characterization of**
•• **Cytomegalovirus Esophagitis in AIDS.** *Gastrointest Endosc* 1994, **40**:481–484. **[31].**
Wu WC, Katon RM, Saxon RR, Barton RE, Uchida BT, Keller FS, *et al.*: **Silicone-covered**
• **Self-expanding Metallic Stents for the Palliation of Malignant Esophageal Obstruction and Esophagorespiratory Fistulas: Experience in 32 Patients and a Review of the Literature.** *Gastrointest Endosc* 1994, **40**:22–33. **[61].**

## Endoscopy of the stomach

Adachi Y, Mori M, Maehara Y, Sugimachi K: **Dukes' Classification: a Valid Prognostic**
• **Indicator for Gastric Cancer.** *Gut* 1994, **35**:1368–1471. **[40].**
Adang RP, Vismans JFJFE, Talmon JL, Hasman A, Ambergen AW, Stockbrugger RW:
• **The Diagnostic Outcome of Upper Gastrointestinal Endoscopy: are Referral Sources and Patient Age Determining Factors?** *Eur J Gastroenterol Hepatol* 1994, **6**:329–335. **[1].**

Alassi MT, Genta RM, Karttunen TJ, Graham DY: **Clarithromycin Amoxycillin Therapy for Helicobacter Pylori Infection.** *Aliment Pharmacol Ther* 1994, **8**:453–456.

Alassi MT, Ramirez FC, Lew GM, Genta RM, Graham DY: **Clarithromycin, Tetracycline, and Bismuth: a New Non-metronidazole Therapy for Helicobacter Pylori Infection.** *Am J Gastroenterol* 1994, **89**:1203–1205.

Alcantara M, Rodriguez R, Potenciano JLM, Carrobles JL, Munoz C, Gomez R: **Endoscopic and Bioptic Findings in the Upper Gastrointestinal Tract in Patients with Crohn's Disease.** *Endoscopy* 1993, **25**:282–286.

Ali W, Sikora SS, Banerjee D, Kapoor VK, Saraswat VA, Saxena R, Kaushik SP: **Gastroduodenal Tuberculosis.** *Aust N Z J Surg* 1993, **63**:466–467.

Anon: **Is Upper Endoscopy Justified when the Stool Hemoccult is Positive But the Colonoscopy is Negative?** *Gastroenterology* 1993, **105**:297.

Ashorn M, Ruuska T, Karikoszki R, Miettinen A, Maki M: ***Helicobacter Pylori* Gastritis**
• **in Dyspeptic Children. A Long-term Follow-up after Treatment with Colloidal Bismuth Subcitrate and Tinidazole.** *Scand J Gastroenterol* 1994, **29**:203–208. **[32].**

Bayerdorffer E, Ritter MM, Hatz R, Brooks W, Ruckdeschel G, Stolte M: **Healing of**
• **Protein Losing Hypertrophic Gastropathy by Eradication of *Helicobacter Pylori*. Is *Helicobacter Pylori* a pathogenic Factor in Menetrier's Disease.** *Gut* 1994, **35**:701–704. **[39].**

Bell GD, Powell KU: **Eradication of Helicobacter-pylori and Its Effect in Peptic Ulcer Disease.** *Scand J Gastroenterol* 1993, **28** (suppl 196):7–11.

Block R, Jankowski J, Johnston D, Colvin JR, Wormsley KG: **The Administration of Supplementary Oxygen to Prevent Hypoxia During Upper Alimentary Endoscopy.** *Endoscopy* 1993, **25**:269–273.

Borody TJ, Andrews P, Mancuso H, McCauley D, Jankiewicz E, Ferch N, *et al.*:
•• ***Helicobacter Pylori* Reinfection Rate, in Patients with Cured Duodenal Ulcer.** *Am J Gastroenterol* 1994, **89**:529–532. **[12].**

Bowling TE, Hadjiminas CL, Polson RJ, Baron JH, Foale RA: **Effects of Supplemental Oxygen on Cardiac Rhythm During Upper Gastrointestinal Endoscopy: a Randomised Controlled Double Blind Trial.** *Gut* 1993, **34**:1492–1497.

Boyd HK, Zaterka S, Eisig JN, Chinzon D, Iriya K, Laudanna AA, Boyd EJS: **Helicobacter Pylori and Refractory Duodenal Ulcers: Cross-over Comparison of Continued Cimetidine with Cimetidine Plus Antimicrobials.** *Am J Gastroenterol* 1994, **89**:1505–1510.

Bytzer P, Moller Hansen J, Schaffalitzky De Muckadell OB: **Empirical $H_2$ Blocker**
• **Therapy or Prompt Endoscopy in Management of Dyspepsia.** *Lancet* 1994, **343**:811–816. **[2].**

Cappell MS, Sidhom O: **A Multicenter, Multiyear Study of the Safety and Clinical**
• **Utility of Esophago-gastroduodenoscopy in 20 Consecutive Pregnant Females with Follow-up of Fetal Outcome.** *Am J Gastroenterol* 1993, **88**:1900–1905. **[5].**

Chen YK, Gladden DR, Kestenbaum DJ, Collen MJ: **Is There a Role for**
• **Gastrointestinal Endoscopy in the Evaluation of Patients with Occult Blood-positive Stool and Negative Colonoscopy?** *Am J Gastroenterol* 1993, **88**:2026–2029. **[4].**

Chong J, Marshall BJ, Barkin JS, McCallum RW, Reiner DK, Hoffman SR, *et al.*:
• **Occupational Exposure To *Helicobacter Pylori* for the Endoscopy Professional: a Sera Epidemiological Study.** *Am J Gastroenterol* 1994, **88**:1987–1992. **[10].**

Cowan RE, Manning AP, Ayliffe GAJ, Axon ATR, Causton JS, Cripps JS, Hall R, Hanson PJV, Harrison J, Leicester RJ, Neumann C, Wicks J: **Aldehyde Disinfectants and Health in Endoscopy Units. The Report of a Working Party of the British Society of Gastroenterology Endoscopy Committee.** *Gut* 1993, **34**:1641–1645.

Craanen ME, Blok P, Dekker W, Tytgat GNJ: ***Helicobacter Pylori* and Early Gastric**
•• **Cancer.** *Gut* 1994, **35**:1372–1374. **[20].**

Cullen DJE, Collins BJ, Christiansen KJ, Epis J, Warren JR, Surveyor I, *et al.*: **When is**
• ***Helicobacter Pylori* Infection Acquired?** *Gut* 1993, **34**:1681–1682. **[11].**

De Boer WA, Driessen WMM, Potters VPJ, Tytgat GNJ: **Randomized Study Comparing**
• **1 with 2 Weeks of Quadruple Therapy for Eradicating *Helicobacter Pylori*.** *Am J Gastroenterol* 1994, **89**:1993–1997. **[57].**

Deboni M, Deboni M, Cielo R: **Helicobacter Pylori and Pre-neoplastic and Neoplastic Gastric Lesions.** *Ital J Gastroenterol* 1994, **26** (suppl 1):29–34.

Dellaratta RK, Corapi MJ, Horowitz BR, Calio AJ: **Risk of Postoperative Upper Gastrointestinal Tract Hemorrhage in Patients with Active Peptic Ulcer Disease Undergoing Nonulcer Surgery.** *Arch Intern Med* 1993, **153**:2141–2144.

DiSaario JA, Fennerty MB, Tietze CC, Hutson WR, Burt RW: **Endoscopic Balloon**
• **Dilation for Ulcer-induced Gastric Outlet Obstruction.** *Am J Gastroenterol* 1994, **89**:868–871. **[47].**

Duckworth PF Jr, Kirby DF, McHenry L, DeLegge MH, Foxx-Orenstein A: **Percutaneous**
• **Endoscopic Gastrojejunostomy Made Easy: a New Over-the-wire Technique.** *Gastrointest Endosc* 1994, **3**:350–353. **[46].**

Fertitta AM, Comin U, Terruzzi V, Minoli G, Zambelli A, Cannatelli G, Bodini P, Bertoli G, Negri R, Brunati S, Fiocca R, Turpini F, Prada A, Ceretti E, Gullotta R, Cornaggia M: **Clinical Significance of Gastric Dysplasia — a Multicenter Follow-Up Study.** *Endoscopy* 1993, **25**:265–268.

Fiocca R, Luinetti O, Villani L, Chiaravalli A, Cornaggia M, Stella G, *et al.*: **High**
•• **Incidence Of *Helicobacter Pylori* Colonization in Early Gastric Cancer and the Possible Relationship to Carcinogenesis.** *Eur J Gastroenterol Hepatol* 1993, **5** (suppl 2):S2–S8. **[19].**

Fishbein VA, Rosen AM, Lack EE, Montgomery EA, Fleischer D: **Diffuse Hemorrhagic**
• **Gastroenteropathy: Report of a New Entity.** *Gastroenterology* 1994, **106**:500–505. **[50].**

Frazzoni M, Lonardo A, Grisendi A, Dellacasa G, Pulvirenti M, Ferrari AM, Digregorio C, Melini L: **Are Routine Duodenal and Antral Biopsies Useful in the Management of Functional Dyspepsia? A Diagnostic and Therapeutic Study.** *J Clin Gastroenterol* 1993, **17**:101–108.

Goggin PM, Collins DA, Jazrawi RP, Jackson PA, Corbishley CM, Bourke BE, *et al.*:
• **Prevalence Of *Helicobacter Pylori* Infection and Its Effects on Symptoms and Non-steroidal Anti-inflammatory Drug Induced Gastrointestinal Damage in Patients with Rheumatoid Arthritis.** *Gut* 1993, **34**:1677–1680. **[24].**

Graham DY, Karttunen TJ, Genta RM: **The Evaluation of Treatment of *H. Pylori***
• **Infections: Strategies for the Design of Clinical Trials.** *Jpn J Endoscopy* 1994, **8**:991–1002. **[26].**

Hayashi N, Kawano S, Tsuji S, Tokai Y, Nagano K, Fusamoto H, *et al.*: **Identification**
• **and Diameter Assessment of Gastric Submucosal Vessels Using Infrared Electronic Endoscopy.** *Endoscopy* 1994, **26**:686–689. **[49].**

Henderson JM, Strodel WE, Gilinsky NH: **Limitations of Percutaneous Endoscopic Jejunostomy.** *JPEN J Parenter Enteral Nutr* 1993, **17**:546–550.

Heresbach D, Raoul JL, Bretagne JF, Minet J, Donnio PY, Ramee MP, *et al.*: ***Helicobacter Pylori*: Risk and Severity Factor of Non-steroidal Anti-inflammatory Drug Induced Gastropathy.** *Gut* 1992, **33**:1608–1611. **[25].**

Hussain ST, Allum WH: **Pernicious Anaemia and Multiple Gastric Polyps with Early Gastric Cancer.** *J R Soc Med* 1993, **86**:603.

Hussell T, Isaacson PG, Crabtree JE, Spencer J: **The Response of Cells from Low-**
• **grade B-cell Gastric Lymphomas of Mucosa-associated Lymphoid Tissue to *Helicobacter Pylori*.** *Lancet* 1993, **342**:571–574. **[23].**

Iber FL, Sutberry M, Gupta R, Kruss D: **Evaluation of Complications During and after Conscious Sedation for Endoscopy Using Pulse Oximetry.** *Gastrointest Endosc* 1993, **39**:620–625.

Isaacson PG: **Gastric Lymphoma and Helicobacter Pylori [Editorial].** *N Engl J Med* 1994, **330**:1310–1311.

Iwao T, Toyonaga A, Harada H, Harada K, Ban S, Ikegami M, Tanikawa K: **Arterial Oxygen Desaturation During Non-sedated Diagnostic Upper Gastrointestinal Endoscopy.** *Gastrointest Endosc* 1994, **40**:277–280.

Iwao T, Toyonaga A, Harada H, Harada K, Ban S, Minetoma T, Sumino M, Ikegami M, Tanikawa K: **Arterial Oxygen Desaturation During Non-sedated Diagnostic Upper Gastrointestinal Endoscopy in Patients with Cirrhosis.** *Gastrointest Endosc* 1994, **40**:281–284.

Karita M, Tada M: **Endoscopic and Histologic Diagnosis of Submucosal Tumors**
• **of the Gastrointestinal Tract Using Combined Strip Biopsy and Bite Biopsy.** *Gastrointest Endosc* 1994, **6**:749–753. **[42].**

Labenz J, Borsch G: **Evidence for the Essential Role of *Helicobacter Pylori* in**
• **Gastric Ulcer Disease.** *Gut* 1994, **35**:19–22. **[15].**

Labenz J, Borsch G: **Role Of *Helicobacter Pylori* Eradication in the Prevention of**
•• **Peptic Ulcer Bleeding Relapse.** *Digestion* 1994, **55**:19–23. **[16].**

Labenz J, Ruhl GH, Bertrams J, Borsch G: **Clinical Course of Duodenal Ulcer Disease**
• **One Year after Omeprazole Plus Amoxycillin or Triple Therapy Plus Ranitidine for Cure Of *Helicobacter Pylori* Infection.** *Eur J Gastroenterol Hepatol* 1994, **6**:293–297. **[29].**

Lazzaroni M, Porro GB: **The Relationship Between Duodenal Ulcer Disease and Helicobacter-Pylori Infection.** *Eur J Gastroenterol Hepatol* 1993, **5** (suppl 2):S70–S72.

Leitch DG, Wicks J, Elbeshir OA, Ali SAM, Chaudhury BK: **Topical Anesthesia with 50 Mg of Lidocaine Spray Facilitates Upper Gastrointestinal Endoscopy.** *Gastrointest Endosc* 1993, **39**:384–387.

Lin SK, Lambert JR, Schembri MA, Nicholson L, Korman MG: **Helicobacter Pylori Prevalence in Endoscopy and Medical Staff.** *J Gastroenterol Hepatol* 1994, **9**:319–324.

Lipscomb GR, *et al.*: **Blocked Gastrostomy Tubes [Letter].** *Lancet* 1994, **343**:801.

Loeb JM, Coble YD, Eisenbrey AB, Estes EH, Kennedy WR, Numann PJ, Scott WC, Skelton WD, Steinhilber RM, Strong JP, Toevs CC, Loeb JM, Rinaldi RC, Vatz JB: **The use of Pulse Oximetry During Conscious Sedation.** *JAMA* 1993, **270**:1463–1468.

Mansi C, Savarino V, Mela GS, Picciotto A, Mele MR, Celle G: **Are Clinical Patterns of Dyspepsia a Valid Guideline for Appropriate use of Endoscopy? A Report on 2253 Dyspeptic Patients.** *Am J Gastroenterol* 1993, **88**:1011–1015.

Marion MT, Zweng TN, Strodel WE: **One-stage Gastrostomy Button: an Assessment.**
• *Endoscopy* 1994, **26**:666–670. **[45].**

Marshall BJ: ***Helicobacter Pylori*.** *Am J Gastroenterol* 1994, **89** (suppl):S116–S128.

Matysiak-Budnik T, Gosciniak G, Brugmann D, Lubczynska-Kowalska W, Poniewierka E,
• Knapik Z, *et al.*: **Seroprevalence of *Helicobacter Pylori* Infection in Medical Staff in Poland.** *Eur J Gastroenterol Hepatol* 1994, **6**:309–311. **[9].**

Mendis RE, Gerdes H, Lightdale CJ, Botet JF: **Large Gastric Folds: a Diagnostic**
• **Approach Using Endoscopic Ultrasonography.** *Gastrointest Endosc* 1994, **4**:437–441. **[37].**

Menegatti M, Vaira D, Mule P, Miglioli M, Barbara L: **Comparison of Urease Tests for the Diagnosis of Helicobacter-Pylori Infection.** *Eur J Gastroenterol Hepatol* 1993, **5** (suppl 2):S38–S40.

Minocha A, Mokshagundam S, Gallo SH, Rahal PR: **Alterations in Upper**
• **Gastrointestinal Motility In *Helicobacter Pylori*-positive Nonulcer Dyspepsia.** *Am J Gastroenterol* 1994, **89**:1797–1800. **[36].**

Nagengast FM: **Sedation and Monitoring in Gastrointestinal Endoscopy.** *Scand J Gastroenterol* 1993, **28** (suppl 200):28–32.

NIH Consensus Development Panel: ***Helicobacter Pylori* in Peptic Ulcer Disease.**
•• *JAMA* 1994, **272**:65–69. **[17].**

Noach LA, Bertola MA, Schwartz MP, Rauws EA, Tytgat GNJ: **Treatment of Helicobacter Pylori Infection: an Evaluation of Various Therapeutic Trials.** *Eur J Gastroenterol Hepatol* 1994, **6**:585–592.

Nogueira AMMF, Ribeiro GM, Rodrigues MAG, Queiroz DMM, Mendes EN, Rocha GA, Barbosa AJA: **Prevalence of Helicobacter-Pylori in Brazilian Patients with Gastric Carcinoma.** *Am J Clin Pathol* 1993, **100**:236–239.

Nomura A, Stemmermann GN, Chyou PH, Perez-Perez GI, Blaser MJ: ***Helicobacter***
• ***Pylori* Infection and the Risk for Duodenal and Gastric Ulceration.** *Ann Intern Med* 1994, **120**:977–981. **[14].**

Paarsonnet J, Hansen S, Rodriguez L, Gelb AB, Warnke RA, Jellum E, *et al.*:
•• **Helicobacter Infection and Gastric Lymphoma.** *N Engl J Med* 1994, **18**:1267–1271. **[21].**

Panos MZ, Reilly H, Moran A, Wallis PJW, Wears R, Chesner IM: **Percutaneous**
• **Endoscopic Gastrostomy in a general Hospital: Prospective Evaluation of Indications, Outcome, and Randomized Comparison of Two Tube Designs.** *Gut* 1994, **35**:1551–1556. **[44].**

Parikh SS, Desai SB, Prabhu SR, Trivedi MH, Shankaran K, Bhukanwala FA, *et al.*:
• **Congestive Gastropathy: Factors Influencing Development, Endoscopic Features, *Helicobacter Pylori* Infection and Microvessel Disease.** *Am J Gastroenterol* 1994, **89**:1036–1042. **[48].**

Patel P, Mendall MA, Khulusi S, Molineaux N, Levy J, Maxwell JD, *et al.*: **Salivary**
• **Antibodies To *Helicobacter Pylori*: Screening Dyspeptic Patients Before Endoscopy.** *Lancet* 1994, **344**:511–512. **[13].**

Paterlini A, Rolfi F, Buffoli F, Cesari P, Graffeo M, Lanzani G, Pascarella A: **Endoscopy in the Diagnosis of *Helicobacter-Pylori* Infection.** *Eur J Gastroenterol Hepatol* 1993, **5** (suppl 2):S36–S37.

Penston JG: ***Helicobacter Pylori* Eradication — Understandable Caution But no Excuse for Inertia.** *Aliment Pharmacol Ther* 1994, **8**:369–389.

Peterson WL, Graham DY, Marshall B, Blaser MJ, Genta RM, Klein PD, Stratton CW, Drnec J, Prokocimer P, Siepman N: **Clarithromycin as Monotherapy for Eradication of *Helicobacter Pylori* — a Randomized, Double-Blind Trial.** *Am J Gastroenterol* 1993, **88**:1860–1864.

Pristautz H, Eherer A, Brezinschik R, Truschnig-Wilders M, Petritsch W, Schreiber
• F, *et al.*: **Prevalence of *Helicobacter Pylori* Antibodies in the Serum of Gastroenterologists in Austria.** *Endoscopy* 1994, **26**:690–696. **[8].**

Quine MA, Bell GD, McCloy RF, Dvelin HB, Hopkins A: **Appropriate use of Upper**
• **Gastrointestinal Endoscopy. A Prospective Audit. The Steering Group of the Upper Gastrointestinal Endoscopy Audit Committee.** *Gut* 1994, **35**:1209–1214. **[3].**

Qvist N, Rasmussen L, Axelsson CK: **Helicobacter Pylori-associated Gastritis**
• **and Dyspepsia. The Influence on Migrating Motor Complexes.** *Scand J Gastroenterol* 1994, **29**:133–137. **[34].**

Rao SSC, Murthy KVR: **Post-Bulbar and Coexisting Ulceration: Unique Features of Peptic Ulcer in Hyderabad.** *Gut* 1993, **34**:1327–1330.

Roosendaal R, Kuipers EJ, Van Den Brule AJC, Pena AS, Uyterlinde AM, Walboomers
• JMM, *et al.*: **Importance of the Fiberoptic Cleaning Procedure for Detection of *Helicobacter Pylori* in Gastric Biopsy Specimens for PCR.** *J Clin Microbiol* 1994, **4**:1123–1126. **[33].**

Sakaki N, Takemoto T: **The Relationship Between Endoscopic Findings of Gastric**
• **Ulcer Scar and Ulcer Relapse.** *J Clin Gastroenterol* 1993, **17** (suppl 1):S64–S69. **[18].**

Saunders BP, Trewby PN: **Open Access Endoscopy — is the Lost Outpatient Clinic of Value.** *Postgrad Med J* 1993, **69**:787–790.

Schrader JA, Peck HV, Notis WM, Shaw P, Venezia RA: **A Role for Culture in Diagnosis of Helicobacter Pylori-Related Gastric Disease.** *Am J Gastroenterol* 1993, **88**:1729–1733.

Sipponen P, Hyvarinen H: **Role of Helicobacter-pylori in the Pathogenesis of Gastritis, Peptic Ulcer and Gastric Cancer.** *Scand J Gastroenterol* 1993, **28** (suppl 196):3–6.

Smith MR, Bell GD: **Routine Oxygen During Endoscopy? An Editorial Review.** *Endoscopy* 1993, **25**:298–300.

Sobhani I: ***Helicobacter Pylori*, and Gastric Lymphoma and Adenocarcinoma.** *Gastroenterol Clin Biol* 1994, **18**:232–235.

Stanghellini V, MacCarini MR, Barbara G, Jadallah K, Cioffi G, Ferri A: **The Relationship Between Functional Dyspepsia and Helicobacter-Pylori Infection.** *Eur J Gastroenterol Hepatol* 1993, **5** (suppl 2):S64–S66.

Stolte M, Sticht T, Eidt S, Ebert D, Finkenzeller G: **Frequency, Location, and Age**
•• **and Sex Distribution of Various Types of Gastric Polyps.** *Endoscopy* 1994, **26**:659–665. **[41].**

Stucki G, Johannesson M, Liang MH: **Is Misoprostol Cost-effective in the Prevention of Nonsteroidal Anti-inflammatory Drug-induced Gastropathy in Patients with Chronic Arthritis? A Review of Conflicting Economic Evaluations.** *Arch Intern Med* 1994, **154**:2020–2025.

Suda K, Seki T, Kano Y, Sasagawa M: **Continuous 5-Fluorouracil Infusion Causing Acute Gastric Mucosal Lesions.** *Endoscopy* 1993, **25**:426–427.

Swarbrick ET, McCloy RF, Axon ATR, Morris AI, Hellier MD, Barnes RJ, Gear MLW: **Gastrointestinal Endoscopy in General Practice.** *Gut* 1994, **35**:1342.

Takeshita K, Ashikawa T, Watanuki S, Tani M, Saito N, Sunagawa M, Habu H, Endo M: **Endoscopic and Clinicopathological Features of Primary Gastric Lymphoma.** *Hepatogastroenterology* 1993, **40**:485–490.

Tatsuta M, Iishi H, Okuda S, Taniguchi H, Yokota Y: **The Association of Helicobacter-Pylori with Differentiated-Type Early Gastric Cancer.** *Cancer* 1993, **72**:1841–1845.

The EUROGAST Study Group: **Epidemiology Of, and Risk Factors For, *Helicobacter***
•• ***Pylori* Infection Among 3194 Asymptomatic Subjects in 17 Populations.** *Gut* 1993, **34**:1672–1676. **[6].**

Thijs JC, Van Zwet AA, Molenaar W, Oom JAJ, De Korte H, Runhaar EA: **Short Report:**
• **Clarithromycin, an Alternative to Metronidazole in the Triple Therapy of *Helicobacter Pylori* Infection.** *Aliment Pharmacol Ther* 1994, **8**:131–134. **[28].**

Thompson GB, Van Heerden JA, Sarr MG: **Adenocarcinoma of the Stomach: are we Making Progress?** *Lancet* 1993, **342**:713–717.

Trespi E, Broglia F, Villani L, Luinetti O, Fiocca R, Solcia E: **Distinct Profiles of**
• **Gastritis in Dyspepsia Subgroups. Their Different Clinical Responses to Gastritis Healing after *Helicobacter Pylori* Eradication.** *Scand J Gastroenterol* 1994, **29**:884–888. **[35].**

Tsuji S, Kawano S, Sato N, Hayashi N, Peng HB, Tsujii M, Nagano K, Takei Y, Chen SS, Kashiwagi T, Fusamoto H, Kamada T: **Comparison of Infrared Electronic Endoscopy Using Reflection and Transmission.** *Endoscopy* 1993, **25**:278–281.

Tytgat GNJ: **Treatments that Impact Favorably Upon the Eradication of**
• ***Helicobacter Pylori* and Ulcer Recurrence.** *Aliment Pharmacol Ther* 1994, **8**:359–368. **[30].**

Unge P, Ekstrom P: **Effects of Combination Therapy with Omeprazole and an Antibiotic on Helicobacter-pylori and Duodenal Ulcer Disease.** *Scand J Gastroenterol* 1993, **28** (suppl 196):17–18.

Uyub AM, Raj SM, Visvanathan R, Nazim M, Aiyar S, Anuar AK: ***Helicobacter Pylori***
• **Infection in North-eastern Peninsular Malaysia: Evidence for an Unusually Low Prevalence.** *Scand J Gastroenterol* 1994, **29**:209–213. **[7].**

Wang WM, Chen CY, Jan CM, Chen LT, Perng DS, Lin SR, *et al.*: **Long-term Follow-up**
• **and Serological Study after Triple Therapy of *Helicobacter Pylori*-associated Duodenal Ulcer.** *Am J Gastroenterol* 1994, **89**:1793–1796. **[31].**

Wotherspoon AC, Dogliono C, Diss TC, Pan L, Moschini A, De Boni M, *et al.*:
•• **Regression of Primary Low-grade B-cell Gastric Lymphoma of Mucosa-associated Lymphoid Tissue Type after Eradication of *Helicobacter Pylori*.** *Lancet* 1993, **342**:575–577. **[22].**

Yang R, Naaritoku W, Laine L: **Prospective Randomized Comparison of Disposable**
•• **and Reusable Biopsy Forceps in Gastrointestinal Endoscopy.** *Gastrointest Endosc* 1994, **40**:671–674. **[43].**

Yasunaga Y, Shinomura Y, Kanyama S, Yabu M, Nakanishi T, Miyazaki Y, *et al.*:
• **Improved Fold Width and Increased Acid Secretion after Eradication of the Organism In *Helicobacter Pylori*-associated Enlarged Fold Gastritis.** *Gut* 1994, **35**:1571–1574. **[38].**

Zerbib F, Vialette G, Cayla R, Rudelli A, Sauvet P, Bechade D, Seurat PL, Lamouliatte H: **Follicular Gastritis in Adults — Relation with Helicobacter Pylori, Histological and Endoscopic Features.** *Gastroenterol Clin Biol* 1993, **17**:529–534.


## Endoscopy of the small bowel


Albertiflor JJ, Hernandez ME, Ferrer JP: **Endoscopic Polypectomy of a Large Duodenal Carcinoid [Letter].** *Gastrointest Endosc* 1993, **39**:853–854.

Barkin JS, Chong J, Reiner DK: **First Generation Video Enteroscope-fourth**
•• **Generation Push-type Small Bowel Enteroscopy Utilizing Overtube.** *Gastrointest Endosc* 1994, **40**:743–747. **[1].**

Bertoni G, Sassatelli R, Tansimi P, Ricci E, Conigilano R, Bedogni G: **Jejunal Polyps in**
• **Familial Adenomatous Polyposis Assessed by Push Type Endoscopy.** *J Clin Gastroenterol* 1993, **17**:343–348. **[3].**

Bessell JR, Karatassas A, Allen PW: **Intestinal Ischaemia Associated with Carcinoid Tumour: a Case Report with Review of the Pathogenesis.** *J Gastroenterol Hepatol* 1994, **9**:304–307.

Cappell MS, Godil A: **A Multicenter Case Controlled Study of Percutaneous**
• **Endoscopic Gastrostomy in HIV Seropositive Patients.** *Am J Gastroenterol* 1993, **88**:2059–2066. **[8].**

Carneiro F, David L, Seruca R, Castedo S, Nesland JM, Sobrinhosimoes M: **Hyperplastic Polyposis and Diffuse Carcinoma of the Stomach — a Study of a Family.** *Cancer* 1993, **72**:323–329.

Chen YK, Gladden DR, Kestenbaum DKJ, Collen MJ: **Is There a Role for Upper Gastrointestinal Endoscopy in the Evaluation of Patients with Occult Blood-Positive Stool and Negative Colonoscopy?** *Am J Gastroenterol* 1993, **88**:2026–2029.

Chong J, Tagle M, Barkin JS, Reiner DK: **Small Bowel Push-type Fiberoptic**
•• **Enteroscopy for Patients with Occult Gastrointestinal Bleeding or Suspected Small Bowel Pathology.** *Am J Gastroenterol* 1994, **89**:2143–2146. **[2].**

Coben RM, Weintraub A, DiMarino AJ Jr, Cohen S: **Gastroesophageal Reflux During**
• **Gastrostomy Feeding.** *Gastroenterology* 1994, **106**:13–18. **[15].**

Cusso X, Mones J, Ocana J, Mendez C, Vilardell F: **Is Endoscopic Gastric Cytology Worthwhile? An Evaluation of 903 Cases of Carcinoma.** *J Clin Gastroenterol* 1993, **16**:336–339.

Dealmeida ACM, Dossantos NM, Aldeia FJ: **Long-Term Clinical and Endoscopic Assessment after Total Gastrectomy for Cancer.** *Surg Endosc* 1993, **7**:518–523.

Duckworth PF Jr, Kirby DF, McHenry L, DeLegge MH, Foxx-Orenstein A: **Percutaneous**
• **Endoscopic Gastrojejunostomy Made Easy: a New Over the Wire Technique.** *Gastrointest Endosc* 1994, **40**:350–353. **[11].**

Farinati F, Rugge M, Dimario F, Valiante F, Baffa R: **Early and Advanced Gastric Cancer in the Follow-Up of Moderate and Severe Gastric Dysplasia Patients — a Prospective Study.** *Endoscopy* 1993, **25**:261–264.

Fertitta AM, Comin U, Terruzzi V, Minoli G, Zambelli A, Cannatelli G, Bodini P, Bertoli G, Negri R, Brunati S, Fiocca R, Turpini F, Prada A, Ceretti E, Gullotta R, Cornaggia M: **Clinical Significance of Gastric Dysplasia — a Multicenter Follow-Up Study.** *Endoscopy* 1993, **25**:265–268.

Fregonese D, Difalco G: **Through the Nose Gastroscopy for the Placement of Feeding Tubes.** *Endoscopy* 1993, **25**:539–541.

Ghosh S, Palmer KR: **Double Percutaneous Endoscopic Gastrostomy Fixation — an Effective Treatment for Recurrent Gastric Volvulus.** *Am J Gastroenterol* 1993, **88**:1271–1272.

Ginsberg GG, Lipman TO, Fleischer DE: **Endoscopic Clip-assisted Placement of Enteral Feeding Tubes.** *Gastrointest Endosc* 1994, **40**:220–222.

Gorman RC, Morris JB, Metz CA, Mullen JL: **The Button Jejunostomy for Long-Term Jejunal Feeding — Results of a Prospective Randomized Trial.** *JPEN J Parenter Enteral Nutr* 1993, **17**:428–431.

Gottlieb K, Leya J, Kruss DM, Mobarhan S, Iber FL: **Intraluminal Fungal Colonization of Gastrostomy Tubes.** *Gastrointest Endosc* 1993, **39**:413–415.

Green JA, Barkin JS, Gregg PA, Kohen K: **Ulcerative Jejunitis in Refractory Celiac Disease — Enteroscopic Visualization.** *Gastrointest Endosc* 1993, **39**:584–585.

Harris A, Dabezies MA, Catalano MF, Krevsky B: **Early Experience with a Video Push Enteroscope.** *Gastrointest Endosc* 1994, **40**:62–64.

Inoue H, Noguchi O, Saito N, Takeshita K, Endo M: **Endoscopic Mucosectomy for Early Cancer Using a pre-looped Plastic Cap [Letter].** *Gastrointest Endosc* 1994, **40**:263–264.

Kadakia SC, Cassaday M, Shaffer RT: **Comparison of Fòley Catheter as a**
• **Replacement Gastrostomy Tube with Commercial Replacement Gastrostomy Tube: a Prospective Randomized Trial.** *Gastrointest Endosc* 1994, **40**:188–193. **[14].**

Kadakia SC, Parker A, Angueira C, Cassaday M: **Failure to Deflate the Balloon of Replacement Gastrostomy Tubes.** *Gastrointest Endosc* 1993, **39**:576–578.

Kaw M, Sekas G: **Long Term Follow Up of Consequences of Percutaneous**
•• **Endoscopic Gastrostomy Tubes in Nursing Home Patients.** *Dig Dis Sci* 1994, **39**:738–743. **[17].**

Keymling M, Wagner HJ, Vakil N, Knyrim K: **Relief of Malignant Duodenal Obstruction by Percutaneous Insertion of a Metal Stent.** *Gastrointest Endosc* 1993, **39**:439–441.

Kudo S: **Endoscopic Mucosal Resection of Flat and Depressed Types of Early Colorectal Cancer.** *Endoscopy* 1993, **25**:455–461.

Kuemmerle JF, Kirby DF: **Diagnostic Endoscopy Via Gastrostomy or PEG Stoma.** *Am*
• *J Gastroenterol* 1993, **88**:1445–1446. **[10].**

Kuo JY, Mo LR, Tsai CC, Yueh SK, Lin RC, Hwang MH: **Endoscopic Fragmentation of Gastric Phytobezoar by Electrohydraulic Lithotripsy.** *Gastrointest Endosc* 1993, **39**:706–708.

Leonbarua R, Gilman RH, Rodriguez C, Bonilla JJ, Yi A, Maurtua D, Sack RB: **Comparison of Three Methods to Obtain Upper Small Bowel Contents for Culture.** *Am J Gastroenterol* 1993, **88**:925–928.

Lim SG, Lipman MC, Squire S, Pillay D, Gillespie S, Sankey EA, Dhillon AP, Johnson MA, Lee CA, Pounder RE: **Audit of Endoscopic Surveillance Biopsy Specimens in HIV Positive Patients with Gastrointestinal Symptoms.** *Gut* 1993, **34**:1429–1432.

Lo AY, Shinya H: **Endoscopic Placement of Long Intestinal Tubes.** *Am Surg* 1993, **59**:626–627.

Logerfo P: **Feeding Gastrostomy.** *Surg Endosc* 1994, **8**:1049.

Luostarinen M, Isolauri J, Laitinen J, Koskinen M, Keyrilainen O, Markkula H, Lehtinen E, Uusitalo A: **Fate of Nissen Fundoplication after 20 Years — a Clinical, Endoscopical, and Functional Analysis.** *Gut* 1993, **34**:1015–1020.

Marin OE, Glassman MS, Schoen BT, Caplan DB: **Safety and Efficacy of Percutaneous**
• **Endoscopic Gastrostomy in Children.** *Am J Gastroenterol* 1994, **89**:357–361. **[9].**

Maurino E, Capizzano H, Niveloni S, Kogan Z, Valero J, Boerr L, *et al.*: **Value of**
• **Endoscopic Markers in Celiac Disease.** *Dig Dis Sci* 1993, **38**:2028–2033. **[4].**

Mellinger JD, Ponsky JL: **Percutaneous Endoscopic Gastrostomy.** *Endoscopy* 1994, **26**:55–59.

Moulis H, Vender RJ: **Percutaneous Endoscopic Gastrostomy for Treatment of Gas-Bloat Syndrome.** *Gastrointest Endosc* 1993, **39**:581–583.

Qureshi H, Zuberi SJ, Baqai R: **Giardia Lamblia in Patients Undergoing Upper GI Endoscopy [Letter].** *Am J Gastroenterol* 1994, **89**:459–460.

Rattan J, Arber N, Tiomny E, Moshkowitz M, Chapsky Y, Baratz M, Rozen P, Gilat T: **Gastric Polypoid Lesions — an 8-Year Study.** *Hepatogastroenterology* 1993, **40**:107–109.

Saeed ZA, Ramirez FC, Hepps KS, Dixon WB: **A Method for the Endoscopic Retrieval of Trichobezoars.** *Gastrointest Endosc* 1993, **39**:698–700.

Sali A, Wong PT, Read A, McQuillan T, Conboy D: **Percutaneous Endoscopic Gastrostomy — the Heidelberg Repatriation Hospital Experience.** *Aust N Z J Surg* 1993, **63**:545–550.

Schiano TD, Pfister D, Harrison L, Shike M: **Neoplastic Seeding as a Complication of**
• **Percutaneous Endoscopic Gastrostomy.** *Am J Gastroenterol* 1994, **89**:131–133. **[16].**

Seifert E, Schulte F, Weismuller J, Demas CR, Stolte M: **Endoscopic and Bioptic Diagnosis of Malignant Non-Hodgkins Lymphoma of the Stomach.** *Endoscopy* 1993, **25**:497–501.

Singh S, MacLeod G, Walker T, McKee G, Bailey ME: **Endoscopic Fine-needle Aspiration Cytology in the Diagnosis of Linitis Plastica.** *Br J Surg* 1994, **81**:1010.

Smedh K, Olaison G, Nystrom PO, Sjodahl R: **Intraoperative Enteroscopy in Crohn's**
•• **Disease.** *Br J Surg* 1993, **80**:897–900. **[6].**

Solt J, Papp Z: **Strecker Stent Implantation in Malignant Gastric Outlet Stenosis.** *Gastrointest Endosc* 1993, **39**:442–444.

Swaroop VS, Mohandas KM, Swaroop VD, Soman CS, Krishnamurthi S, Nagral A, Jagannath P, Desouza LJ: **Comparative Endoscopic Study of Primary Gastric Lymphoma Vs Gastric Carcinoma.** *J Surg Oncol* 1994, **56**:94–97.

Tada M, Murakami A, Karita M, Yanai H, Okita K: **Endoscopic Resection of Early Gastric Cancer.** *Endoscopy* 1993, **25**:445–450.

Takekoshi T, Baba Y, Ota H, Kato Y, Yanagisawa A, Takagi K, Noguchi Y: **Endoscopic Resection of Early Gastric Carcinoma — Results of a Retrospective Analysis of 308 Cases.** *Endoscopy* 1994, **26**:352–358.

Taranto D, Suozzo R, Romano M, Disapio M, Caporaso N, Blanco CD, Coltorti M: **Gastric Endoscopic Features in Patients with Liver Cirrhosis — Correlation with Esophageal Varices, Intravariceal Pressure, and Liver Dysfunction.** *Digestion* 1994, **55**:115–120.

Thakeb F, Salem SAM, Abdallah M, Elbatanouny M: **Endoscopic Diagnosis of Gastric Varices.** *Endoscopy* 1994, **26**:287–291.

Thompson GB, Van Heerden JA, Sarr MG: **Adenocarcinoma of the Stomach: are we Making Progress?** *Lancet* 1993, **342**:713–717.

Vargo JJ, Germain MM, Swenson JA, Harrison CR: **Ultrasound Assisted Percutaneous**
• **Endoscopic Gastrostomy in a patient with Advanced Ovarian Carcinoma and Recurrent Intestinal Obstruction.** *Am J Gastroenterol* 1993, **88**:1946–1948. **[13].**

Waye JD: **Endoscopy of the Small Bowel — Push, Sonde and Intra-Operative.** *Endoscopy* 1994, **26**:60–63.

Zwas FR, Bonheim NA, Berken CA, Gray S: **Ileoscopy as an Important Tool for the Diagnosis of Crohns Disease — a Report of Seven Cases.** *Gastrointest Endosc* 1994, **40**:89–91.

## Endoscopy of upper gastrointestinal bleeding

Acharya SK, Dasarathy S, Saksena S, Pande JN: **A Prospective Randomized Study to Evaluate Propranolol in Patients Undergoing Long-Term Endoscopic Sclerotherapy.** *J Hepatol* 1993, **19**:291–300.

Alemayehu G, Jarnerot G: **Same-Day Upper and Lower Endoscopy in Patients with Occult Bleeding, Melena, Hematochezia, and or Microcytic Anemia — a Retrospective Study of 224 Patients.** *Scand J Gastroenterol* 1993, **28**:667–672.

Anon: **Endoscopic Ligation Versus Sclerotherapy: is it Time to Jump on the Bandwagon?** *Gastroenterology* 1993, **105**:1915.

Anon: **Endoscopic Laser Therapy for Radiation-Induced Mucosal Hemorrhage: have we Seen the Light? [Summary].** *Gastroenterology* 1994, **106**:544–545.

Avgerinos A, Rekoumis G, Klonis C, Papadimitriou N, Gouma P, Pournaras S, Raptis S: **Propranolol in the Prevention of Recurrent Upper Gastrointestinal Bleeding in Patients with Cirrhosis Undergoing Endoscopic Sclerotherapy — a Randomized Controlled Trial.** *J Hepatol* 1993, **19**:301–311.

Baettig B, Haecki W, Lammer F, Jost R: **Dieulafoy's Disease: Endoscopic Treatment and Follow Up.** *Gut* 1993, **34**:1418–1421.

Barsoum MS, Boulos FI, Aly AMH, Saad M, Soliman MA, Doss WH, Zakaria S, Thakeb F: **Acute Variceal Hemorrhage — the Persistent Bleeder — a Plea for Management.** *World J Surg* 1994, **18**:273–278.

Bender JS, Bouwman DL, Weaver DW: **Bleeding Gastroduodenal Ulcers — Improved Outcome from a Unified Surgical Approach.** *Am Surg* 1994, **60**:313–315.

Berg PL, Barina W, Born P: **Endoscopic Injection of Fibrin Glue Versus Polidocanol in Peptic Ulcer Hemorrhage: a Pilot Study.** *Endoscopy* 1994, **26**:528–530.

Berner JS, Gaing AA, Sharma R, Almenoff PL, Muhlfelder T, Korsten MA: **Sequelae after Esophageal Variceal Ligation and Sclerotherapy: a Prospective Randomized Study.** *Am J Gastroenterol* 1994, **89**:852–858.

Bertoni G, Sassatelli R, Fornaciari G, Briglia R, Tansini P, Grisendi A, Pedretti G, Beltrami G, Conigliaro R, Pacchione D, Bedogni G: **Oral Isosorbide-5-Mononitrate Reduces the Rebleeding Rate During the Course of Injection Sclerotherapy for Esophageal Varices.** *Scand J Gastroenterol* 1994, **29**:363–370.

Binmoeller KF, Vadeyar HJ, Soehendra N: **Treatment of Esophageal Varices.**
•• *Endoscopy* 1994, **26**:42–47. **[29].**

Bornman PC, Krige JE, Terblanche J: **Management of Oesophageal Varices.** *Lancet*
•• 1994, **343**:1079–1084. **[30].**

Burroughs AK: **Octreotide in Variceal Bleeding.** *Gut* 1994, **35**:S23–S27. **[36].**

• Carter R, Anderson JR: **Randomized Trial of Adrenaline Injection and Laser Photocoagulation in the Control of Haemorrhage from Peptic Ulcer.** *Br J Surg* 1994, **81**:869–871.

Chan ACW, Chung SCS, Sung JY, Leung JWC, Li AKC: **A Double-blind Randomized**
• **Controlled Trial Comparing Sodium Tetradecyl Sulphate and Ethanolamine Oleate in the Sclerotherapy of Bleeding Oesophageal Varices.** *Endoscopy* 1993, **25**:513–517. **[28].**

Choudari CP, Elton RA, Palmer KR: **The Outcome of Peptic Ulcer Haemorrhage in Relation to Consumption of Nonsteroidal Anti-Inflammatory Drugs or Aspirin.** *Aliment Pharmacol Ther* 1994, **8**:457–460.

Choudari CP, Palmer KR: **Outcome of Endoscopic Injection Therapy for Bleeding Peptic Ulcer in Relation to the Timing of the Procedure.** *Eur J Gastroenterol Hepatol* 1993, **5**:951–953.

Choudari CP, Palmer KR: **Endoscopic Injection Therapy for Bleeding Peptic Ulcer; a**
• **Comparison of Adrenaline Alone with Adrenaline Plus Ethanolamine Oleate.** *Gut* 1994, **35**:608–610. **[12].**

Choudari CP, Rajgopal C, Palmer KR: **Acute Gastrointestinal Haemorrhage in Anticoagulated Patients: Diagnoses and Response to Endoscopic Treatment.** *Gut* 1994, **35**:464–466.

Chu KM, Lai ECS, Ng IOL: **Hereditary Hemorrhagic Telangiectasia Involving the Ampulla of Vater Presented with Recurrent Gastrointestinal Bleeding.** *Am J Gastroenterol* 1993, **88**:1116–1119.

Chung SCS, Leung JWC, Leong HT, Lo KK, Li AKC: **Adding a Sclerosant to Endoscopic Epinephrine Injection in Actively Bleeding Ulcers — a Randomized Trial.** *Gastrointest Endosc* 1993, **39**:611–615.

Colcher MD, Garjian PL, Gebhard RL, Goff JS, Kruss DM, Lance PM, *et al.*: **Sclerotherapy for Male Alcoholic Cirrhotic Patients Who have Bled from Esophageal Varices: Results of a randomized, Multicenter Clinical Trial.** *Hepatology* 1994, **20**:618–625.

Delpiano M, Montino F, Manfredda I, Occhipinti P: **Varices of the Entire Gastrointestinal Tract.** *Gastrointest Endosc* 1993, **39**:822–824.

Elomar MM, Jenkins AP, Hollowood K, Banerjee AK, Thompson RPH: **Gastric Telangiectasis — a Rare Cause of Severe Blood Loss in Crest Syndrome.** *Postgrad Med J* 1994, **70**:302–304.

Falk GL: **Bleeding Duodenal Ulceration — Reply.** *Aust N Z J Surg* 1993, **63**:653–654.

Foutch PG: **Angiodysplasia of the Gastrointestinal Tract [Review].** *Am J Gastroenterol* 1993, **88**:807–818.

Fox JG, Hunt PS: **Management of Acute Bleeding Gastric Malignancy.** *Aust N Z J Surg* 1993, **63**:462–465.

Freeman ML, Cass OW, Peine CJ, Onstad GR: **The Non-Bleeding Visible Vessel Versus the Sentinel Clot — Natural History and Risk of Rebleeding.** *Gastrointest Endosc* 1993, **39**:359–366.

Gatta A, Merkel C, Amodio P, Bellon S, Bellumat A, Bolognesi M, Borsato L, Butto M, Casson FT, Cavallarin G, Cielo R, Cristina P, Cucci E, Donada C, Donadon V, Enzo E, Marin R, Mazzaro C, Miori R, Noventa F, Torboli P, Ruol A: **Development and Validation of a Prognostic Index Predicting Death after Upper Gastrointestinal Bleeding in Patients with Liver Cirrhosis: a multicenter Study.** *Am J Gastroenterol* 1994, **89**:1528–1536.

Gertsch P, Fischer G, Kleber G, Wheatley AM, Geigenberger G, Sauerbruch T: **Manometry of Esophageal Varices: Comparison of an Endoscopic Balloon Technique with Needle Puncture.** *Gastroenterology* 1993, **105**:1159–1166.

Gimson AES, Ramage JK, Panos MZ, Hayllar K, Harrison PM, Williams R, Westaby D: **Randomised Trial of Variceal Banding Ligation Versus Injection Sclerotherapy for Bleeding Oesophageal Varices.** *Lancet* 1993, **342**:391–394.

Goenka MK, Mehta SK, Kochhar R, Nagi B, Sachdev A, Bhardwaj A, Gupta NM: **Primary Aortoduodenal Fistula in a 23 Year Old Man Without an Associated Aortic Aneurysm.** *Eur J Surg* 1993, **159**:371–372.

Goff JS: **Gastroesophageal Varices — Pathogenesis and Therapy of Acute Bleeding.** *Gastroenterol Clin North Am* 1993, **22**:779–800.

Goff JS: **Endoscopic Sclerotherapy for Esophageal and Gastric Varices — Safety and Efficacy.** *Endoscopy* 1994, **26**:483–485.

Gostout CJ, Viggiano TR, Balm RK: **Acute Gastrointestinal Bleeding from Portal Hypertensive Gastropathy — Prevalence and Clinical Features.** *Am J Gastroenterol* 1993, **88**:2030–2033.

Graham DY, Hepps KS, Ramirez FC, Lew GM, Saeed ZA: **Treatment of *Helicobacter***
• ***Pylori* Reduces the Rate of Rebleeding in Peptic Ulcer Disease.** *Scand J Gastroenterol* 1993, **28**:939–942. **[20].**

Greig JD, Garden OJ, Carter DC: **Prophylactic Treatment of Patients with**
• **Esophageal Varices — is it Ever Indicated?** *World J Surg* 1994, **18**:176–184. **[23].**

Grisendi A, Lonardo A, Dellacasa G, Frazzoni M, Pulvirenti M, Ferrari AM, Varoli M, Mezzanotte G, Melini L: **Combined Endoscopic and Surgical Management of Dieulafoy Vascular Malformation.** *J Am Coll Surg* 1994, **179**:182–186.

Gupta PK, Fleischer D: **Endoscopic Hemostasis in Nonvariceal Bleeding.** *Endoscopy* 1994, **26**:48–54.

Harris JM, Dipalma JA: **Clinical Significance of Mallory-Weiss Tears.** *Am J Gastroenterol* 1993, **88**:2056–2058.

Hawkey CJ: **Aspirin and Gastrointestinal Bleeding.** *Aliment Pharmacol Ther* 1994, **8**:141–146.

Heinrich D, Meier J, Wehrli H, Buhler H: **Upper Gastrointestinal Hemorrhage Preceding Development of Bouveret's Syndrome.** *Am J Gastroenterol* 1993, **88**:777–780.

Herold G, Preclik G, Stange F: **Gastroduodenal Ulcer Hemorrhage: Endoscopic Injection Therapy Using a Fibrin Sealant.** *Hepatogastroenterology* 1994, **41**:116–119.

Hill DB, Stokes BD, Gilinsky NH: **Arterial Oxygen Saturation During Emergency Esophagogastroduodenoscopy — the Effects of Nasal Oxygen.** *J Clin Gastroenterol* 1994, **18**:284–286.

Hintze RE, Binmoeller KF, Adler A, Veltzke W, Thonke F, Soehendra N: **Improved Endoscopic Management of Severe Upper Gastrointestinal Hemorrhage Using a New Wide-channel Endoscope.** *Endoscopy* 1994, **26**:613–616.

Hirata M, Ishihama S, Sanjo K, Idezuki Y: **Study of New Prognostic Factors of Esophageal Variceal Rupture by use of Image Processing with a Video Endoscope.** *Surgery* 1994, **116**:8–16.

Hsu PI, Lin XZ, Chan SH, Lin CY, Chang TT, Shin JS, *et al.*: **Bleeding Peptic Ulcer —**
• **Risk Factors for Rebleeding and Sequential Changes in Endoscopic Findings.** *Gut* 1994, **35**:746–749. **[10].**

Ishikawa M, Kikutsuji T, Miyauchi T, Sakakihara Y: **Limitations of Endoscopic Haemostasis by Ethanol Injection and Surgical Management for Bleeding Peptic Ulcer.** *J Gastroenterol Hepatol* 1994, **9**:64–68.

Iwase H, Morise K, Kawase T, Horiuchi Y: **Endoscopic Injection Sclerotherapy for Esophageal Varices During Pregnancy.** *J Clin Gastroenterol* 1994, **18**:80–83.

Jaramillo JL, Carmona C, Galvez C, De La Mata M, Mino G: **Efficacy of the Heater Probe in Peptic Ulcer with a Non-Bleeding Visible Vessel. A Controlled, Randomised Study.** *Gut* 1993, **34**:1502–1506.

Jensen DM, Cheng S, Kovacs T, Randall D, Jensen ME, Reedy T, *et al.*: •• **A Controlled Study of Ranitidine for the Prevention of Recurrent Hemorrhage from Duodenal Ulcer.** *N Engl J Med* 1994, **330**:382–386. **[19]**.

Kahn D, Krige JE, Terblanche J, Bornman PC, Robson SC: **A 15-Year Experience of Injection Sclerotherapy in Adult Patients with Extrahepatic Portal Venous Obstruction.** *Ann Surg* 1994, **219**:34–39.

Karrer FM, Holland RM, Allshouse MJ, Lilly JR: **Portal Vein Thrombosis: Treatment of Variceal Hemorrhage by Endoscopic Variceal Ligation.** *J Pediatr Surg* 1994, **29**:1149–1151.

Katschinski B, Logan R, Davies J, Faulkner G, Pearson J, Langman M: **Prognostic • Factors in Upper Gastrointestinal Bleeding.** *Dig Dis Sci* 1994, **39**:706–712. **[9]**.

Katz PO, Salas L: **Less Frequent Causes of Upper Gastrointestinal Bleeding.** *Gastroenterol Clin North Am* 1993, **22**:875–889.

Kitamura K, Ikebe M, Morita M, Matsuda H, Kuwano H, Sugimachi K: **The Evaluation of Submucosal Carcinoma of the Esophagus as a More Advanced Carcinoma.** *Hepatogastroenterology* 1993, **40**:236–239.

Kohler B, Rieman JF: **Does Doppler Ultrasound Improve the Prognosis of Acute Ulcer Bleeding.** *Hepatogastroenterology* 1994, **41**:51–53.

Kokawa H, Shijo H, Kubara K, Nakaoka K, Toriya H, Shirai Z, Okazaki M: **Long-Term Risk Factors for Bleeding after First Course of Endoscopic Injection Sclerotherapy — a Univariate and Multivariate Analysis.** *Am J Gastroenterol* 1993, **88**:1206–1211.

Labenz J, Borsch G: **Bleeding Watermelon Stomach Treated by Nd:YAG Laser Photocoagulation.** *Endoscopy* 1993, **25**:240–242.

Labenz J, Borsch G: **Role of Helicobacter Pylori Eradication in the Prevention of Peptic Ulcer Bleeding Relapse.** *Digestion* 1994, **55**:19–23.

Lai KH, Peng SN, Guo WS, Lee FY, Chang FY, Malik U, *et al.*: **Endoscopic Injection • for the Treatment of Bleeding Ulcers — Local Tamponade or Drug Effect.** *Endoscopy* 1994, **26**:338–341. **[13]**.

Laine L, Elnewihi HM, Migikovsky B, Sloane R, Garcia F: **Endoscopic Ligation Compared with Sclerotherapy for the Treatment of Bleeding Esophageal Varices.** *Ann Intern Med* 1993, **119**:1–7.

Laine L, Freeman M, Cohen H: **Lack of Uniformity in Evaluation of Endoscopic • Prognostic Features of Bleeding Ulcers.** *Gastrointest Endosc* 1994, **40**:411–417. **[6]**.

Laine L, Peterson WL: **Bleeding Peptic Ulcer.** *N Engl J Med* 1994, **331**:717–727. **[1]**.

Lam SK, Lai KC: **Endoscopic Haemostasis for Gastrointestinal Bleeding — the Dawning of a New Era [Editorial].** *J Gastroenterol Hepatol* 1994, **9**:69–74.

Lanza FL, Royer GL: **NSAID-Induced Gastric Ulceration is Dose Related by Weight — an Endoscopic Study with Flurbiprofen.** *Am J Gastroenterol* 1993, **88**:683–686.

Laws HL, McKernan JB: **Endoscopic Management of Peptic Ulcer Disease.** *Ann Surg* 1993, **217**:548–556.

Lin CY, Lin PW, Tsai HM, Lin XZ, Chang TT, Shin JS: **Influence of Paraesophageal Venous Collaterals on Efficacy of Endoscopic Sclerotherapy for Esophageal Varices.** *Hepatology* 1994, **19**:602–608.

Lin HJ, Perng CL, Lee SD: **Is Sclerosant Injection Mandatory after an Epinephrine Injection for Arrest of Peptic Ulcer Haemorrhage? A Prospective, Randomised, Comparative Study.** *Gut* 1993, **34**:1182–1185.

Lopes GM, Grace ND: **Gastroesophageal Varices — Prevention of Bleeding and Rebleeding.** *Gastroenterol Clin North Am* 1993, **22**:801–820.

Lubke HJ, Kauschitz D, Schumacher B: **Angiodysplasia of the Gastrointestinal Tract: Incidental Finding or Cause of Recurrent Gastrointestinal Bleeding.** *Z Gastroenterol* 1993, **31** (suppl 5):27–29.

Martin M, Zajko AB, Orons PD, Dodd G, Wright H, Colangelo J, Tartar R, Rikkers LF, Iwatsuki S, Wexler MJ, Pickleman J: **Transjugular Intrahepatic Portosystemic Shunt in the Management of Variceal Bleeding — Indications and Clinical Results.** *Surgery* 1993, **114**:719–727.

McKee RF, Garden OJ, Anderson JR, Carter DC: **A Trial of Elective Versus on Demand Sclerotherapy in Poor Risk Patients with Variceal Haemorrhage.** *Endoscopy* 1994, **26**:474–477.

Moreto M, Zaballa M, Ojembarrena E, Ibanez S, Suarez MJ, Steien F, *et al.*: **Combined • (short Term Plus Long Term) Sclerotherapy V Short Term Only Sclerotherapy: a Randomized Prospective Trial.** *Gut* 1994, **35**:687–691. **[26]**.

Mueller X, Rothenbuehler JM, Amery A, Harder F: **Bleeding Peptic Ulcer — an Audit of Conservative Management.** *J R Soc Med* 1994, **87**:132–134.

Mueller X, Rothenbuehler JM, Amery A, Meyer B, Harder F: **Outcome of Peptic Ulcer Hemorrhage Treated According to a Defined Approach.** *World J Surg* 1994, **18**:406–410.

Ohta M, Hashizume M, Kamakura T, Ueno K, Tomikawa M, Tanoue K, Kitano S, Sugimachi K: **Endoscopic Injection Sclerotherapy for Esophageal Varices in the Elderly.** *World J Surg* 1994, **18**:764–768.

Orr KB: **Bleeding Duodenal Ulceration.** *Aust N Z J Surg* 1993, **63**:653.

Paquet KJ, Lazar A, Bickhart J: **Massive and Recurrent Gastrointestinal Hemorrhage Due to Jejunal Varices in an Afferent Loop — Diagnosis and Management.** *Hepatogastroenterology* 1994, **41**:276–277.

Park KGM, Steele RJC, Masson J: **Endoscopic Injection of Adrenaline for Benign Oesophageal Ulcer Haemorrhage.** *Br J Surg* 1994, **81**:1317–1318.

Pimentel RR, Vanstolk RU: **Gastric Plasmacytoma — a Rare Cause of Massive Gastrointestinal Bleeding.** *Am J Gastroenterol* 1993, **88**:1963–1964.

Planas R, Quer JC, Boix J, Canet J, Armengol M, Cabre E, *et al.*: **A Prospective • Randomized Trial Comparing Somatostatin and Sclerotherapy in the Treatment of Acute Variceal Bleeding.** *Hepatology* 1994, **20**:370–375. **[35]**.

Pollack R, Lipsky H, Goldberg RI: **Duodenal Dieulafoys Lesion.** *Gastrointest Endosc* 1993, **39**:820–822.

Potiamiano S, Carter CR, Anderson JR: **Endoscopic Laser Treatment of Diffuse • Gastric Antral Vascular Ectasia.** *Gut* 1994, **35**:461–463. **[41]**.

Potzi R, Bauer P, Schofl R, Reichel W, Kerstan E, Renner F, Gangl A: **Prophylactic Endoscopic Sclerotherapy of Esophageal Varices in Liver Cirrhosis — Long-Term Follow-Up and Final Results of a Multicenter Prospective Controlled Randomized Trial in Vienna.** *Endoscopy* 1993, **25**:287–289.

Qvist P, Arnesen KE, Jacobsen CD, Rosseland AR: **Endoscopic Treatment and Restrictive Surgical Policy in the Management of Peptic Ulcer Bleeding — Five Years' Experience in a central Hospital.** *Scand J Gastroenterol* 1994, **29**:569–576.

Radosevich PM, Laberge JM, Gordon RL: **Current Status and Future Possibilities of Transjugular Intrahepatic Portosystemic Shunts in the Management of Portal Hypertension.** *World J Surg* 1994, **18**:785–789.

Richardson JD, Lordon RE: **Gastrointestinal Bleeding Caused by Angiodysplasia — a Difficult Problem in Patients with Chronic Renal Failure Receiving Hemodialysis Therapy.** *Am Surg* 1993, **59**:636–638.

Rolando N, Gimson A, Philpotthoward J, Sahathevan M, Casewell M, Fagan E, Westaby D, Williams R: **Infectious Sequelae after Endoscopic Sclerotherapy of Oesophageal Varices — Role of Antibiotic Prophylaxis.** *J Hepatol* 1993, **18**:290–294.

Rosandic-Pilas M, Kacic M, Salamon V, Pulanic R, Dujsin M, Radanovic B, Paar V: **Sclerotherapy of Bleeding Oesophageal Varices in Children with Prehepatic Portal Hypertension: a Prospective Evaluation Over 7 Years.** *Eur J Gastroenterol Hepatol* 1993, **5**:533–540.

Rossle M, Haag K, Ochs A, Sellinger M, Noldge G, Perarnau JM, *et al.*: **The Transjugular • Intrahepatic Portosystemic Stent-shunt Procedure for Variceal Bleeding.** *N Engl J Med* 1994, **330**:165–171. **[39]**.

Saeed ZA, Winchester CB, Michaletz PA, Woods KL, Graham DY: **A Scoring System to Predict Rebleeding after Endoscopic Therapy of Nonvariceal Upper Gastrointestinal Hemorrhage with a Comparison of Heat Probe and Ethanol Injection.** *Am J Gastroenterol* 1993, **88**:1842–1849.

Sakai P, Maluf F, Melo JM, Ishioka S: **Is Endoscopic Band Ligation of Esophageal Varices Contraindicated in Child-Pugh C Patients.** *Endoscopy* 1994, **26**:511–512.

Scottconne CEH, Subramony C: **Localization of Small Intestinal Bleeding — the Role of Intraoperative Endoscopy.** *Surg Endosc* 1994, **8**:915–917.

Siringo S, Bolondi L, Gaiani S, Sofia S, Difebo G, Zironi G, Rigamonti A, Miglioli M, Cavalli G, Barbara L: **The Relationship of Endoscopy, Portal Doppler Ultrasound Flowmetry, and Clinical and Biochemical Tests in Cirrhosis.** *J Hepatol* 1994, **20**:11–18.

Siringo S, Bolondi L, Gaiani S, Sofia S, Zironi G, Rigamonti A, Difebo G, Miglioli M, Cavalli G, Barbara L: **Timing of the First Variceal Hemorrhage in Cirrhotic Patients: Prospective Evaluation of Doppler Flowmetry, Endoscopy and Clinical Parameters.** *Hepatology* 1994, **20**:66–73.

Stanciu C, Cijevschi C, Stan M, Sandulescu E: **Endoscopic Intravascular Esophageal Pressure Measurements in Cirrhotic Patients — Response to Metoclopramide.** *Hepatogastroenterology* 1993, **40**:173–175.

Stringer MD, Howard ER: **Longterm Outcome after Injection Sclerotherapy for Oesophageal Varices in Children with Extrahepatic Portal Hypertension.** *Gut* 1994, **35**:257–259.

Strohm D, Rommele UE, Barton E, Paulmartin C: **Injection Treatment of Bleeding Peptic Ulcer with Fibrin or Polidocanol.** *Dtsch Med Wochenschr* 1994, **119**:249–256.

Taylor AJN, Hadjiminas D, Rosin RD, Hershman MJ, Tanner AG: **Pancreaticoduodenal Artery Aneurysm — Diagnostic and Management Difficulties.** *J R Soc Med* 1993, **86**:356–357.

Terblanche J, Stiegmann GV, Krige JEJ, Bornman PC: **Long-term Management of •• Variceal Bleeding: the Place of Varix Injection and Ligation.** *World J Surg* 1994, **18**:185–192. **[32]**.

Teres J, Bosch J, Bordas JM, Garcia-Pagan JC, Feu F, Cirera I, Rodes J: **Propranolol Versus Sclerotherapy in Preventing Variceal Rebleeding: a Randomized Controlled Trial.** *Gastroenterology* 1993, **105**:1508–1514.

Thakeb F, Salem SAM, Abdallah M, El Batanouny M: **Endoscopic Diagnosis of Gastric • Varices.** *Endoscopy* 1994, **26**:287–291. **[37]**.

The Veterans Affairs Cooperative Variceal Sclerotherapy Group: **Sclerotherapy for Male • Alcoholic Cirrhotic Patients Who have Bled from Esophageal Varices: Results of a randomized, Multicenter Clinical Trial.** *Hepatology* 1994, **20**:618–625. **[22]**.

Toh Y, Baba K, Ikebe M, Adachi Y, Kuwano H, Sugimachi K: **Endoscopic Ultrasonography in the Diagnosis of an Early Esophageal Carcinoma.** *Hepatogastroenterology* 1993, **40**:212–216.

Vanthiel DH, Dindzans VJ, Schade RR, Rabinovitz M, Gavaler JS: **Prophylactic Versus Emergency Sclerotherapy of Large Esophageal Varices Prior to Liver Transplantation.** *Dig Dis Sci* 1993, **38**:1505–1510.

Villanueva C, Balanzo J, Espinos JC, Fabrega E, Sainz S, Gonzalez D, Vilardell F: **Endoscopic Injection Therapy of Bleeding Ulcer — a Prospective and Randomized Comparison of Adrenaline Alone or with Polidocanol.** *J Clin Gastroenterol* 1993, **17**:195–200.

Villanueva C, Balanzo J, Torras X, Soriano G, Sainz S, Vilardell F: **Value of Second-look • Endoscopy after Injection Therapy for Bleeding Peptic Ulcer — a Prospective and Randomized Trial.** *Gastrointest Endosc* 1994, **40**:34–39. **[16]**.

Wachsberg RH, Simmons MZ: **Coronary Vein Diameter and Flow Direction in Patients with Portal Hypertension — Evaluation with Duplex Sonography and Correlation with Variceal Bleeding.** *AJR Am J Roentgenol* 1994, **162**:637–641.

Williams RA, Vartany A, Davis IP, Wilson SE: **Impact of Endoscopic Therapy on Outcome of Operation for Bleeding Peptic Ulcers.** *Am J Surg* 1993, **166**:712–715.

Williams SGI, Westaby D: **Fortnightly Review: Management of Variceal • Haemorrhage.** *BMJ* 1994, **308**:1213–1216. **[31]**.

Willson PD, Kunkler R, Blair SD, Reynolds KW: **Emergency Oesophageal Transection for Uncontrolled Variceal Haemorrhage.** *Br J Surg* 1994, **81**:992–995.

Wu CS, Tung SY: **Henoch-Schonlein Purpura Complicated by Upper Gastrointestinal Bleeding with an Unusual Endoscopic Picture.** *J Clin Gastroenterol* 1994, **19**:128–131.

Yoshida T, Hayashi N, Suzumi N, Miyazaki S, Terai S, Itoh T, Nishimura S, Noguchi T, Hino K, Yasunaga M, Tada M, Okita K: **Endoscopic Ligation of Gastric Varices Using a Detachable Snare.** *Endoscopy* 1994, **26**:502–505.

Zuccaro G: **Bleeding Peptic Ulcer — Pathogenesis and Endoscopic Therapy.** *Gastroenterol Clin North Am* 1993, **22**:737–750.

Zuckerman DA, Bocchini TP, Birnbaum EH: **Massive Hemorrhage in the Lower Gastrointestinal Tract in Adults — Diagnostic Imaging and Intervention.** *AJR Am J Roentgenol* 1993, **161**:703–711.

## Endosonography


Abe S, Lightdale CJ, Brennan MF: **The Japanese Experience with Endoscopic Ultrasonography in the Staging of Gastric Cancer [Review].** *Gastrointest Endosc* 1993, **39**:586–591.

Adams LS, Peltekian KM, Mitchell MJ: **Detection of Crohns Ileitis by Endovaginal Ultrasonography.** *Abdom Imaging* 1994, **19**:400–402.

•• Amouyal P, Amouyal G, Levy P, Tuzet S, Palazzo L, Vilgrain V, *et al.*: **Diagnosis of Choledocholithiasis by Endoscopic Ultrasonography.** *Gastroenterology* 1994, **106**:1062–1067. **[28].**

Avunduk C, Hampf F, Coughlin B: **Endoscopic Sonography of the Stomach: Findings in Benign and Malignant Lesions.** *AJR Am J Roentgenol* 1994, **163**:591–595.

Baillie J: **Complications of Endoscopy.** *Endoscopy* 1994, **26**:185–203.

Barthet M, Debonne JM, Klotz F, Sahel J: **Endoscopic Ultrasound Diagnosis of Anomalous Pancreaticobiliary Union Associated with Gallbladder Carcinoma [Letter].** *Gastroenterol Clin Biol* 1993, **17**:766–768.

Benamouzig R, Marteau P, Lavergne A, Palazzo L, Dahan H, Rambaud JC: **Gastroduodenal Linitis Plastica Infiltration Due to Metastatic Involvement from Bladder Cancer: Endosonographic Findings Correlated with Histology.** *Eur J Gastroenterol Hepatol* 1994, **6**:179–182.

Bhattacharya I: **Endoscopic Ultrasonography: Towards a More Perfect Union.** *Lancet* 1994, **344**:349.

• Boustiere C, Dumas O, Jouffre C, Letard JC, Patouillard B, Etaix JP, *et al.*: **Endoscopic Ultrasonography-classification of Gastric Varices in Patients with Cirrhosis. Comparison with Endoscopic Findings.** *J Hepatol* 1993, **19**:268–272. **[46].**

Burtin P: **Does Endoscopic Ultrasonography of the Gastrointestinal Tract have a Place in the Evaluation of Portal Hypertension in Cirrhosis.** *Gastroenterol Clin Biol* 1994, **18**:339–341.

•• Caletti G, Odegaard S, Rosch T, Sivak MV, Tio TL, Yasuda K: **Endoscopic Ultrasonography (EUS): a Summary of the Conclusions of the Working Party for the Tenth World Congress of Gastroenterology Los Angeles, California October, 1994.** *Am J Gastroenterol* 1994, **89** (suppl). **[9].**

Catalano MF, Sivak MV, Vanstolk R, Zuccaro G, Rice TW: **Initial Evaluation of a New-generation Endoscopic Ultrasound System.** *Gastrointest Endosc* 1994, **40**:356–359.

•• Catalano MF, Sivak MVJ, Rice T, Gragg LA, Van Dam J: **Endosonographic Features Predictive of Lymph Node Metastasis.** *Gastrointest Endosc* 1994, **40**:442–446. **[18].**

Cataldo PA, Senagore A, Luchtefeld MA: **Intrarectal Ultrasound in the Evaluation of Perirectal Abscesses.** *Dis Colon Rectum* 1993, **36**:554–558.

Chang KJ, Albers CG, Erickson RA, Butler JA, Wuerker RB, Lin F: **Endoscopic Ultrasound-Guided Fine Needle Aspiration of Pancreatic Carcinoma.** *Am J Gastroenterol* 1994, **89**:263–266.

•• Chang KJ, Katz KD, Durbin TE, Erickson RA, Butler JA, Lin F, *et al.*: **Endoscopic Ultrasound-guided Fine-needle Aspiration.** *Gastrointest Endosc* 1994, **40**:694–699. **[2].**

Cheong DMO, Nogueras JJ, Wexner SD, Jagelman DG: **Anal Endosonography for Recurrent Anal Fistulas: Image Enhancement with Hydrogen Peroxide.** *Dis Colon Rectum* 1993, **36**:1158–1160.

Cho ES, Nakajima M, Yasuda K, Ashihara T, Kawai K: **Endoscopic Ultrasonography in the Diagnosis of Colorectal Cancer Invasion.** *Gastrointest Endosc* 1993, **39**:521–527.

Constantinescu MA, Hunter DC, Allenmersh TG: **Abdominal Ultrasouind can be Helpful in Diagnosis of Obscure Small Bowel Haemorrhage.** *Eur J Surg Oncol* 1993, **19**:475–478.

Cuesta MA, Meijer S, Borgstein PJ, Mulder LS, Sikkenk AC: **Laparoscopic Ultrasonography for Hepatobiliary and Pancreatic Malignancy.** *Br J Surg* 1993, **80**:1571–1574.

Cushing GL, Fitzgerald PJ, Bommer WJ, Andrews MW, Cronan MS, Martineztorres GG, Jang YT, Belef WM, Prindiville TP: **Intraluminal Ultrasonography During ERCP with High-Frequency Ultrasound Catheters.** *Gastrointest Endosc* 1993, **39**:432–435.

Deen KI, Williams JG, Kumar D, Keighley MRB: **Anal Sphincter Surgery for Faecal Incontinence: the Role of Endosonography.** *Coloproctology* 1993, **15**:352–355.

Dhiman RK, Choudhuri G, Saraswat VA, Mukhopadhyay DK, Khan EM, Pandey R, Naik SR: **Endoscopic Ultrasonographic Evaluation of the Rectum in Cirrhotic Portal Hypertension.** *Gastrointest Endosc* 1993, **39**:635–640.

Donahue PE, Anan K, Doyle M, Nadimpalli V, Schlesinger P, Nyhus LM: **Endoscopic Ultrasonography Verifies Effect on Endoscopic Treatment of Reflux in Dogs and Man.** *Surg Endosc* 1993, **7**:524–528.

Eckardt VF, Jung B, Fischer B, Lierse W: **Anal Endosonography in Healthy Subjects and Patients with Idiopathic Fecal Incontinence.** *Dis Colon Rectum* 1994, **37**:235–242.

• Emblem R, Dhaenens G, Stien R, Morkric L, Aasen AO, Bergan A: **The Importance of Anal Endosonography in the Evaluation of Idiopathic Fecal Incontinence.** *Dis Colon Rectum* 1994, **37**:42–48. **[52].**

•• Engel AF, Kamm MA, Sultan AH, Bartram CI, Nicholls RJ: **Anterior Anal Sphincter Repair in Patients with Obstetric Trauma.** *Br J Surg* 1994, **81**:1231–1234. **[53].**

• Falk GW, Catalano MF, Sivak MV, Rice TW, Van Dam J: **Endosonography in the Evaluation of Patients with Barrett's Esophagus and High Grade Dysplasia.** *Gastrointest Endosc* 1994, **40**:207–212. **[13].**

Falk PM, Blatchford GJ, Cali RL, Christensen MA, Thorson AG: **Transanal Ultrasound and Manometry in the Evaluation of Fecal Incontinence.** *Dis Colon Rectum* 1994, **37**:468–472.

Feltbersma RJF, Cuesta MA: **Anorectal Endosonography in Benign Anorectal Disorders.** *Scand J Gastroenterol* 1993, **28** (suppl 200):70–73.

Fockens P, Vandullemen HM, Tytgat GNJ: **Endosonography of Stenotic Esophageal Carcinomas: Preliminary Experience with an Ultra-thin, Balloon-fitted Ultrasound Probe in Four Patients.** *Gastrointest Endosc* 1994, **40**:226–228.

Frank N, Grieshammer B, Zimmermann W: **A New Miniature Ultrasonic Probe for Gastrointestinal Scanning: Feasibility and Preliminary Results.** *Endoscopy* 1994, **26**:603–608.

Furukawa T, Tsukamoto Y, Naitoh Y, Hirooka Y, Katoh T: **Evaluation of Intraductal Ultrasonography in the Diagnosis of Pancreatic Cancer.** *Endoscopy* 1993, **25**:577–581.

• Furukawa T, Tsukamoto Y, Naitoh Y, Mitake M, Hirooka Y, Hayakawa T: **Differential Diagnosis of Pancreatic Diseases with an Intraductal Ultrasound System.** *Gastrointest Endosc* 1994, **40**:213–219. **[67].**

•• Giovannini M, Seitz JF: **Endoscopic Ultrasonography with a Linear-type Echoendoscope in the Evaluation Of 94 Patients with Pancreatobiliary Disease.** *Endoscopy* 1994, **26**:579–585. **[26].**

Giovannini M, Seitz JF, Rabbia I, Perrier H, Colonna MA, Houvenaeghel G, Delpero JR: **Linear Intrarectal Ultrasonography and Rectal Carcinoma — Results in 45 Patients.** *Gastroenterol Clin Biol* 1994, **18**:323–327.

Grech P: **Mirror-Image Artifact with Endoscopic Ultrasonography and Reappraisal of the Fluid-Air Interface.** *Gastrointest Endosc* 1993, **39**:700–703.

Greig JD, John TG, Mahadaven M, Garden OJ: **Laparoscopic Ultrasonography in the Evaluation of the Biliary Tree During Laparoscopic Cholecystectomy.** *Br J Surg* 1994, **81**:1202–1206.

Grimm H, Binmoeller KF, Hamper K, Koch J, Hennebruns D, Soehendra N: **Endosonography for Preoperative Locoregional Staging of Esophageal and Gastric Cancer.** *Endoscopy* 1993, **25**:224–230.

Hata J, Harumà K, Yamanaka H, Fujimura J, Yoshihara M, Shimamoto T, Sumii K, Kajiyama G, Yokoyama T: **Ultrasonographic Evaluation of the Bowel Wall in Inflammatory Bowel Disease — Comparison of Invivo and Invitro Studies.** *Abdom Imaging* 1994, **19**:395–399.

Hawes RH: **New Staging Techniques — Endoscopic Ultrasound.** *Cancer* 1993, **71** (suppl):4207–4213.

Heintz A, Mildenberger P, Georg M, Braunstein S, Junginger T: **Endoscopic Ultrasonography in the Diagnosis of Regional Lymph Nodes in Esophageal and Gastric Cancer — Results of Studies Invitro.** *Endoscopy* 1993, **25**:231–235.

Hirata N, Kawamoto K, Ueyama T, Iwashita I, Masuda K: **Endoscopic Ultrasonography in the Assessment of Colonic Wall Invasion by Adjacent Diseases.** *Abdom Imaging* 1994, **19**:21–26.

Hizawa K, Iida M, Suekane H, Mibu R, Mochizuki Y, Yao T, Fujishima M: **Mucosal Prolapse Syndrome: Diagnosis with Endoscopic US.** *Radiology* 1994, **191**:527–530.

Holscher AH, Dittler HJ, Siewert JR: **Staging of Squamous Esophageal Cancer: Accuracy and Value.** *World J Surg* 1994, **18**:312–320.

• Hordijk ML, Kok TC, Wilson JHP, Mulder AH: **Assessment of Response of Esophageal Carcinoma to Induction Chemotherapy.** *Endoscopy* 1993, **25**:592–596. **[16].**

• Hulsmans FJH, Tio TL, Fockens P, Bosma A, Tytgat GNJ: **Assessment of Tumor Infiltration Depth in Rectal Cancer with Transrectal Sonography: Caution is Necessary.** *Radiology* 1994, **190**:715–720. **[33].**

Jaspersen D: **Proctoscopic Doppler Ultrasound in Diagnostics and Treatment of Bleeding Hemorrhoids — Reply.** *Dis Colon Rectum* 1993, **36**:945.

Jaspersen D, Koerner T, Schorr W, Hammar CH: **Proctoscopic Doppler Ultrasound in Diagnostics and Treatment of Bleeding Hemorrhoids.** *Dis Colon Rectum* 1993, **36**:942–945.

Kalantzis N, Laoudi F, Kallimanis G, Gabriel P, Farmakis N: **The Role of Endoscopic Ultrasonography in Diagnosis of Benign Lesions of the Upper G1 Tract.** *Eur J Surg Oncol* 1993, **19**:449–454.

•• Kamm MA: **Obstetric Damage and Faecal Incontinence.** *Lancet* 1994, **344**:730–733. **[50].**

• Kawamoto K, Ueyama T, Iwashita I, Utsunomiya T, Honda H, Onitsuka H, *et al.*: **Colonic Submucosal Tumors: Comparison of Endoscopic US and Target Air-enema CT with Barium Enema Study and Colonoscopy.** *Radiology* 1994, **192**:697–702. **[43].**

Kochman ML, Scheiman J: **Endosonography — is it Sound for the Masses?** *J Clin Gastroenterol* 1994, **19**:2–5.

Kohler B, Riemann JF: **Endoscopic Injection Therapy of Forrest-II and Forrest-III Gastroduodenal Ulcers Guided by Endoscopic Doppler Ultrasound.** *Endoscopy* 1993, **25**:219–223.

Lee SH: **Transrectal Ultrasound in the Diagnosis of Ano-Rectal Varices.** *Clin Radiol* 1994, **49**:69–70.

Leung FW, Wong DNW, Lau J, Bondoc EM, Hsu R, Leung JWC: **Endoscopic Assessment of Blood Flow in Duodenal Ulcers.** *Gastrointest Endosc* 1994, **40**:334–341.

Limberg B, Osswald B: **Diagnosis and Differential Diagnosis of Ulcerative Colitis and Crohn's Disease by Hydrocolonic Sonography.** *Am J Gastroenterol* 1994, **89**:1051–1057.

Machi J, Sigel B, Zaren HA, Kurohiji T, Yamashita Y: **Operative Ultrasonography During Hepatobiliary and Pancreatic Surgery.** *World J Surg* 1993, **17**:640–646.

Madsen EL, Zagzebski JA, Medina IR, Frank GR: **Performance Testing of Transrectal US Scanners.** *Radiology* 1994, **190**:77–80.

Malde H, Nagral A, Shah P, Joshi MS, Bhatia SJ, Abraham P: **Detection of Rectal and Pararectal Varices in Patients with Portal Hypertension — Efficacy of Transvaginal Sonography.** *AJR Am J Roentgenol* 1993, **161**:335–337.

•• Mendis RE, Gerdes H, Lightdale CJ, Botet JF: **Large Gastric Folds: a Diagnostic Approach Using Endoscopic Ultrasonography.** *Gastrointest Endosc* 1994, **40**:437–441. **[22].**

Miller LS, Liu J-B, Klenn PJ, Holahan MP, Varga J, Feld RI, Troshinsky M, Jimenez SA, Castell DO, Goldberg BB: **Endoluminal Ultrasonography of the Distal Esophagus in Systemic Sclerosis.** *Gastroenterology* 1993, **105**:31–39.

• Milsom JW, Czyrko C, Hull TL, Strong SA, Fazio VW: **Preoperative Biopsy of Pararectal Lymph Nodes in Rectal Cancer Using Endoluminal Ultrasonography.** *Dis Colon Rectum* 1994, **37**:364–368. **[1].**

Miro JRA, Benjamin S, Binmoeller Ķ, Boyce HW, Caletti GC, Classen M, Cotton PB, Geenen JE, Hawes R, Kawai K, Lambert R, Lehman G, Lightdale C, Rey JF, Riemann JF, Rosch T, Sivak MV, Soehendra N, Tio TL, Yamao K, Yasuda K, Zuccaro G: **Clinical Applications of Endoscopic Ultrasonography in Gastroenterology — State of the Art 1993 — Results of a Consensus Conference, Orlando, Florida, 19 January 1993.** *Endoscopy* 1993, **25**:358–366.

Mortensen MB, Pedersen SA, Hovendal CP: **Preoperative Assessment of Resectability in Gastroesophageal Carcinoma by Linear Array Endoscopic Ultrasonography.** *Scand J Gastroenterol* 1994, **29**:341–345.

• Motoo Y, Okai T, Ohta H, Satomura Y, Watanabe H, Yamakawa O, *et al.*: **Endoscopic Ultrasonography in the Diagnosis of Extraluminal Compressions Mimicking Gastric Submucosal Tumors.** *Endoscopy* 1994, **26**:239–242. **[41].**

•• Muller MF, Meyenberger C, Bertschinger P, Schaer R, Marincek B: **Pancreatic Tumors: Evaluation with Endoscopic US, CT, and MR Imaging.** *Radiology* 1994, **190**:745–751. **[30].**

Nagita A, Amemoto K, Yoden A, Yamazaki T, Mino M, Miyoshi H: **Ultrasonographic Diagnosis of Juvenile Colonic Polyps.** *J Pediatr* 1994, **124**:535–540.

• Nattermann C, Dancygier H: **Endosonography in the Diagnosis and Staging of Malignant Gastric Tumors. A Prospective Comparative Study Between Endoscopic Sonography, Computed Tomography and Conventional Ultrasound.** *Z Gastroenterol* 1993, **31**:719–726. **[20].**

• Nattermann C, Goldschmidt AJW, Dancygier H: **Endosonography in Chronic Pancreatitis — a Comparison Between Endoscopic Retrograde Pancreatography and Endoscopic Ultrasonography.** *Endoscopy* 1993, **25**:565–570. **[32].**

• Nielsen MB, Dammegaard L, Pedersen JF: **Endosonographic Assessment of the Anal Sphincter after Surgical Reconstruction.** *Dis Colon Rectum* 1994, **37**:434–438. **[59].**

Nielsen MB, Rasmussen OO, Pedersen JF, Christiansen J: **Risk of Sphincter Damage and Anal Incontinence after Anal Dilatation for Fissure-in-Ano — an Endosonographic Study.** *Dis Colon Rectum* 1993, **36**:677–680.

Okai T, Mouri I, Yamaguchi Y, Ohta H, Motoo Y, Sawabu N: **Acute Gastric Anisakiasis — Observations with Endoscopic Ultrasonography.** *Gastrointest Endosc* 1993, **39**:450–452.

•• Palazzo L, Roseau G, Ruskone Fourmestraux A, Rougier P, Chaussade S, Rambaud J, *et al.*: **Endoscopic Ultrasonography in the Local Staging of Primary Gastric Lymphoma.** *Endoscopy* 1993, **25**:502–508. **[24].**

Papachrysostomou M, Pye SD, Wild SR, Smith AN: **Anal Endosonography in Asymptomatic Subjects.** *Scand J Gastroenterol* 1993, **28**:551–556.

• Peters JH, Hoeft SF, Heimbucher J, Bremner RM, De Meester TR, Bremner CG, *et al.*: **Selection of Patients for Curative or Palliative Resection of Esophageal Cancer Based on Preoperative Endoscopic Ultrasonography.** *Arch Surg* 1994, **129**:534–539. **[10].**

• Ramirez JM, Mortensen NJM, Takeuchi N, Humphreys MMS: **Endoluminal Ultrasonography in the Follow-up of Patients with Rectal Cancer.** *Br J Surg* 1994, **81**:692–694. **[35].**

Rosch T: **Endoscopic Ultrasonography — More Questions Than Answers [Editorial].** *Endoscopy* 1993, **25**:600–602.

Rosch T: **Endoscopic Ultrasonography.** *Endoscopy* 1994, **26**:148–168.

• Roseau G, Palazzo L, Colardelle P, Chaussade S, Couturier D, Paolaggi JA: **Endoscopic Ultrasonography in the Staging and Follow-up of Epidermoid Carcinoma of the Anal Canal.** *Gastrointest Endosc* 1994, **40**:447–450. **[36].**

Rothlin MA, Schlumpf R, Largiader F: **Laparoscopic Sonography — an Alternative to Routine Intraoperative Cholangiography?** *Arch Surg* 1994, **129**:694–700.

Roubein LD, Dubrow R, David C, Lynch P, Fornage B, Ajani J, Roth J, Levin B: **Endoscopic Ultrasonography in the Quantitative Assessment of Response to Chemotherapy in Patients with Adenocarcinoma of the Esophagus and Esophagogastric Junction.** *Endoscopy* 1993, **25**:587–591.

Rosch T: **Endoscopic Ultrasonography.** *Endoscopy* 1994, **26**:148–168. **[7].**

• Schafer A, Enck P, Furst G, Kahn T, Frieling T, Lubke HJ: **Anatomy of the Anal Sphincters: Comparison of Anal Endosonography to Magnetic Resonance Imaging.** *Dis Colon Rectum* 1994, **37**:777–781. **[49].**

Schafer A, Enck P, Heyer T, Gantke B, Frieling T, Lubke HJ: **Endosonography of the Anal Sphincters — Incontinent and Continent Patients and Healthy Controls.** *Z Gastroenterol* 1994, **32**:328–331.

• Schratter-Sehn AU, Lochs H, Vogelsang H, Schurawitzki H, Herold C, Schratter M: **Endoscopic Ultrasonography Versus Computed Tomography in the Differential Diagnosis of Perianorectal Complications in Crohn's Disease.** *Endoscopy* 1993, **25**:582–586. **[60].**

• Schuder G, Hildebrandt U, Kreissler Haag D, Seitz G, Feifel G: **Role of Endosonography in the Surgical Management of Non-Hodgkin's Lymphoma of the Stomach.** *Endoscopy* 1993, **25**:509–512. **[25].**

Sentovich SM, Blatchford GJ, Falk PM, Thorson AG, Christensen MA: **Transrectal Ultrasound of Rectal Tumors.** *Am J Surg* 1993, **166**:638–642.

• Smith JW, Brennan MF, Botet JF, Gerdes H, Lightdale CJ: **Preoperative Endoscopic Ultrasound can Predict the Risk of Recurrence after Operation for Gastric Carcinoma.** *J Clin Oncol* 1993, **11**:2380–2385. **[21].**

•• Snady H, Bruckner H, Siegel J, Cooperman A, Neff R, Kiefer L: **Endoscopic Ultrasonographic Criteria of Vascular Invasion by Potentially Resectable Pancreatic Tumors.** *Gastrointest Endosc* 1994, **40**:326–333. **[29].**

•• Solomon M, McLeod RS, Cohen EK, Simons ME, Wilson S: **Reliability and Validity Studies of Endoluminal Ultrasonography for Anorectal Disorders.** *Dis Colon Rectum* 1994, **37**:546–551. **[34].**

Souquet JC, Napoleon B, Pujol B, Ponchon T, Keriven O, Lambert R: **Echoendoscopy Prior to Endoscopic Tumor Therapy — More Safety.** *Endoscopy* 1993, **25**:475–478.

• Squillace SJ, Johnson DA, Sanowski RA: **The Endosonographic Appearance of a Dieulafoy's Lesion.** *Am J Gastroenterol* 1994, **89**:276–277. **[47].**

•• Sultan AH, Kamm MA, Hudson CN, Bartram CI: **Third Degree Obstetric and Sphincter Tears: Risk Factors and Outcome of Primary Repair.** *BMJ* 1994, **308**:887–891. **[57].**

•• Sultan AH, Kamm MA, Talbot IC, Nicholls RJ, Bartram CI: **Anal Endosonography for Identifying External Sphincter Defects Confirmed Histologically.** *Br J Surg* 1994, **81**:463–465. **[56].**

Tacke W, Kruis W, Zehnter E, Ziegenhagen D, Velasco S, Diehl V: **Endoscopic Ultrasound of the Upper Gastrointestinal Tract in the Staging of Malignant Lymphomas.** *Z Gastroenterol* 1994, **32**:431–435.

• Tio TL, Blank LECM, Wijers OB, Hartog Jager FCAD, Van Dijk JDP, Tytgat GNJ: **Staging and Prognosis Using Endosonography in Patients with Inoperable Esophageal Carcinoma Treated with Combined Intraluminal and External Irradiation.** *Gastrointest Endosc* 1994, **40**:304–310. **[17].**

Tjandra JJ, Milsom JW, Schroeder T, Fazio VW: **Endoluminal Ultrasound is Preferable to Electromyography in Mapping Anal Sphincteric Defects.** *Dis Colon Rectum* 1993, **36**:689–692.

Vandam J, Rice TW, Catalano MF, Kirby T, Sivak MV: **High-Grade Malignant Stricture is Predictive of Esophageal Tumor Stage — Risks of Endosonographic Evaluation.** *Cancer* 1993, **71**:2910–2917.

• Vilmann P, Hancke S, Henriksen FW, Jacobsen GK: **Endosonographically-guided Fine Needle Aspiration Biopsy of Malignant Lesions in the Upper Gastrointestinal Tract.** *Endoscopy* 1993, **25**:523–527. **[6].**

• Wegener M, Adamek RJ, Wedmann B, Pfaffenbach B: **Endosonographically Guided Fine-needle Aspiration Puncture of Paraesophagogastric Mass Lesions: Preliminary Results.** *Endoscopy* 1994, **26**:586–591. **[4].**

Wiersema MJ, Hassig WM, Hawes RH, Wonn MJ: **Mediastinal Lymph Node Detection with Endosonography.** *Gastrointest Endosc* 1993, **39**:788–793.

•• Wiersema MJ, Kochman ML, Cramer HM, Tao LC, Wiersema LM: **Endosonography-guided Real-time Fine-needle Aspiration Biopsy.** *Gastrointest Endosc* 1994, **40**:700–707. **[3].**

Wiersema MJ, Wiersema LM, Khusro Q, Cramer HM, Tao LC: **Combined Endosonography and Fine-needle Aspiration Cytology in the Evaluation of Gastrointestinal Lesions.** *Gastrointest Endosc* 1994, **40**:199–206.

•• Wiersema MJ, Wiersema LM, Khusro Q, Cramer HM, Tao LC: **Combined Endosonography and Fine-needle Aspiration Cytology in the Evaluation of Gastrointestinal Lesions.** *Gastrointest Endosc* 1994, **40**:199–206. **[5].**

Yang YK, Wexner SD, Nogueras JJ, Jagelman DG: **The Role of Anal Ultrasound in the Assessment of Benign Anorectal Diseases.** *Coloproctology* 1993, **15**:260–265.

Yoshikane H, Tsukamoto Y, Niwa Y, Goto H, Hase S, Mizutani K, Nakamura T: **Carcinoid Tumors of the Gastrointestinal Tract — Evaluation with Endoscopic Ultrasonography.** *Gastrointest Endosc* 1993, **39**:375–383.

• Yoshikane H, Tsukamoto Y, Niwa Y, Goto H, Hase S, Shimodaira M, Maruta S, *et al.*: **Superficial Esophageal Carcinoma: Evaluation by Endoscopic Ultrasonography.** *Am J Gastroenterol* 1994, **89**:702–707. **[12].**

Zerbi A, Balzano G, Bottura R, Dicarlo V: **Reliability of Pancreatic Cancer Staging Classifications.** *Int J Pancreatol* 1994, **15**:13–18.

## Endoscopy and the pancreas

Alkarawi MA, Mohamed ARE, Alshahri MG, Yasawy MI: **Endoscopic Sphincterotomy in Acute Gallstone Pancreatitis and Cholangitis — a Saudi Hospital Experience.** *Hepatogastroenterology* 1993, **40**:396–401.

Alvarez C, Hunt K, Ashley SW, Reber HA: **Emphysematous Cholecystitis after ERCP.** *Dig Dis Sci* 1994, **39**:1719–1723.

Alvarez C, Robert M, Sherman S, Reber HA: **Histologic Changes after Stenting of the Pancreatic Duct.** *Arch Surg* 1994, **129**:765–768.

•• Ammann R, Muellhaupt B, Meyenberger C, Heitz P: **Alcoholic Nonprogressive Chronic Pancreatitis: Prospective Long-term Study of a Large Cohort with Alcoholic Acute Pancreatitis (1976–1992).** *Pancreas* 1994, **9**:365–373. **[4].**

Angelini G, Sgarbi D, Castagnini A, Cavallini G, Bovo P: **Common Bile Duct Involvement in Chronic Pancreatitis.** *Ital J Gastroenterol* 1994, **26**:79–82.

Balaji LN, Tandon RK, Tandon BN, Banks PA: **Prevalence and Clinical Features of Chronic Pancreatitis in Southern India.** *Int J Pancreatol* 1994, **15**:29–34.

Banks PA: **Acute Pancreatitis: Medical and Surgical Management.** *Am J Gastroenterol* 1994, **89** (suppl):S78–S85.

Bardaxoglou E, Campion JP, Maddern G, Siriser F, Launois B: **A Simple Method to Control Intractable Bleeding after Endoscopic Sphincterotomy.** *Am J Surg* 1994, **167**:277–278.

Bedford RA, Howerton DH, Geenen JE: **The Current Role of ERCP in the Management of Benign Pancreatic Disease.** *Endoscopy* 1994, **26**:113–119.

Bejanin H: **Endoscopic Drainage of Pancreatic Pseudocysts — a Report of 26 Cases (Vol 17, Pg 804, 1993).** *Gastroenterol Clin Biol* 1994, **18**:401.

Blackstone MG: **Balloon Sphincteroplasty Vs Endoscopic Papillotomy for Bileduct Stones.** *Lancet* 1993, **342**:1314.

Blind PJ, Mellbring G, Hjertkvist M, Sandzen B: **Diagnosis of Traumatic Pancreatic Duct Rupture by On-Table Endoscopic Retrograde Pancreatography.** *Pancreas* 1994, **9**:387–389.

Boender J, Nix GAJJ, Deridder MAJ, Van Blankenstein M, Schutte HE, Dees J, Wilson JHP: **Endoscopic Papillotomy for Common Bile Duct Stones — Factors Influencing the Complication Rate.** *Endoscopy* 1994, **26**:209–216.

Born P, Barina W, Terfloth R, Fiebig A, Paul F: **Pancreatic Duct Stenosis Mimicking a Tumor Due to an Aberrant Vessel.** *Endoscopy* 1994, **26**:260–261.

Botoman VA, Kozarek RA, Novell LA, Patterson DJ, Ball TJ, Wechter DG, Neal LA: **Long-term Outcome after Endoscopic Sphincterotomy in Patients with Biliary Colic and Suspected Sphincter of Oddi Dysfunction.** *Gastrointest Endosc* 1994, **40**:165–170.

Boujaoude J, Pelletier G, Fritsch J, Choury A, Lefebvre JF, Roche A, Frouge C, Liguory C, Etienne JP: **Management of Clinically Relevant Bleeding Following Endoscopic Sphincterotomy.** *Endoscopy* 1994, **26**:217–221.

• Bozkurt T, Braun U, Leferink S, Gilly G, Lux G: **Comparison of Pancreatic Morphology and Exocrine Functional Impairment in Patients with Chronic Pancreatitis.** *Gut* 1994, **35**:1132–1136. **[1].**

• Bradley EL: **A Clinically Based Classification System for Acute Pancreatitis.** *Arch Surg* 1993, **128**:586–590. **[8].**

Burdick JS, Schmalz MJ, Geenen JE: **Guidewire Fracture During Endoscopic Sphincterotomy.** *Endoscopy* 1993, **25**:251–252.

• Chen YK, Foliente RL, Santoro MJ, Walter MH, Collen MJ: **Endoscopic Sphincterotomy-induced Pancreatitis: Increased Risk Associated with Nondilated Bile Ducts and Sphincter of Oddi Dysfunction.** *Am J Gastroenterol* 1994, **89**:327–333. **[37].**

Chen YK, McCarter TL, Santoro MJ, Hanson BL, Collen MJ: **Utility of Endoscopic Retrograde Cholangiopancreatography in the Evaluation of Idiopathic Abdominal Pain.** *Am J Gastroenterol* 1993, **88**:1355–1358.

Cho KC: **Focal Parenchymal Opacification of the Liver by Overinjection of Contrast Material During ERCP.** *AJR Am J Roentgenol* 1994, **162**:1123–1124.

Choudhry U, Ruffolo T, Jamidar P, Hawes R, Lehman G: **Sphincter of Oddi Dysfunction in Patients with Intact Gallbladder — Therapeutic Response to Endoscopic Sphincterotomy.** *Gastrointest Endosc* 1993, **39**:492–495.

Cohen SA, Kasmin FE, Siegel JH: **Alterations of Pancreatic Stents [Letter].** *Gastrointest Endosc* 1994, **40**:256–257.

• Coleman SD, Eisen GM, Troughton AB, Cotton PB: **Endoscopic Treatment in Pancreas Divisum.** *Am J Gastroenterol* 1994, **89**:1152–1155. **[24].**

• Costamagna G, Gabbrielli A, Mutignani M, Perri V, Crucitti F: **Treatment of 'obstructive' Pain by Endoscopic Drainage in Patients with Pancreatic Head Carcinoma.** *Gastrointest Endosc* 1993, **39**:774–777. **[42].**

Cotton PB: **Towards Safer Endoscopic Retrograde Cholangiopancreatography (ERCP) [Letter].** *Gut* 1994, **35**:284.

Cuer JC, Dapoigny M, Bommelaer G: **The Effect of Midazolam on Motility of the Sphincter of Oddi in Human Subjects.** *Endoscopy* 1993, **25**:384–386.

Funnell IC, Bornman PC, Krige JEJ, Beningfield SJ, Terblanche J: **Endoscopic Drainage of Traumatic Pancreatic Pseudocyst.** *Br J Surg* 1994, **81**:879–881.

Gazelle GS, Mueller PR, Raafat N, Halpern EF, Cardenosa G, Warshaw AL: **Cystic Neoplasms of the Pancreas: Evaluation with Endoscopic Retrograde Pancreatography.** *Radiology* 1993, **188**:633–636.

Grace PA, Williamson RCN: **Modern Management of Pancreatic Pseudocysts [Review].** *Br J Surg* 1993, **80**:573–581.

Gronlund B, Svendsen LB: **Management of Endoscopic Impaction During Routine ERCP Using the Gastric Grip.** *Endoscopy* 1993, **25**:375–376.

• Guelrud M, Mujica C, Jaen D, Plaz J, Arias J: **The Role of ERCP in the Diagnosis and Treatment of Idiopathic Recurrent Pancreatitis in Children and Adolescents.** *Gastrointest Endosc* 1994, **40**:428–436. **[34].**

Hartle RJ, McGarrity TJ, Conter RL: **Treatment of a Giant Biloma and Bile Leak by ERCP Stent Placement.** *Am J Gastroenterol* 1993, **88**:2117–2118.

Heinerman M, Mann R, Boeckl O: **An Unusual Complication in Attempted Non-Surgical Treatment of Pancreatic Bile Duct Stones.** *Endoscopy* 1993, **25**:248–250.

Heinerman PM, Graf AH, Boeckl O: **Does Endoscopic Sphincterotomy Destroy the Function of Oddi's Sphincter?** *Arch Surg* 1994, **129**:876–880.

Heyman MB, Zwass M, Applebaum M, Rudolph CD, Gordon R, Ring EJ: **Chronic Recurrent Esophageal Strictures Treated with Balloon Dilation in Children with Autosomal Recessive Epidermolysis Bullosa Dystrophica.** *Am J Gastroenterol* 1993, **88**:953–957.

Howell DA, Holbrook RF, Bosco JJ, Muggia RA, Biber BP: **Endoscopic Needle Localization of Pancreatic Pseudocysts Before Transmural Drainage.** *Gastrointest Endosc* 1993, **39**:693–698.

• Huibregtse K, Smits ME: **Endoscopic Management of Diseases of the Pancreas.** *Am J Gastroenterol* 1994, **89**:S66–S77. **[44].**

• Ikenberry SO, Sherman S, Hawes RH, Smith M, Lehman GA: **The Occlusion Rate of Pancreatic Stents.** *Gastrointest Endosc* 1994, **40**:611–613. **[26].**

Jowell PS, Baillie J: **Towards Safer Endoscopic Retrograde Cholangiopancreatography (ERCP) [Letter].** *Gut* 1994, **35**:284.

Jung W, Neubrand M, Luderitz B: **Application of High Frequency Current in Patients with Cardiac Pacemakers During Endoscopy Procedures.** *Z Gastroenterol* 1994, **32**:479–482.

• Karanjia ND, Widdison AL, Leung F, Alvarez C, Lutrin FJ, Reber HA: **Compartment Syndrome in Experimental Chronic Obstructive Pancreatitis: Effect of Decompressing the Main Pancreatic Duct.** *Br J Surg* 1994, **81**:259–264. **[17].**

Kiil J, Ronning H: **Pancreatic Fistula Cured by an Endoprosthesis in the Pancreatic Duct.** *Br J Surg* 1993, **80**:1316–1317.

Kimdeobald J, Kozarek RA, Ball TJ, Patterson DJ, Brandabur JJ, Raltz S: **Prospective Evaluation of Costs of Disposable Accessories in Diagnostic and Therapeutic ERCP.** *Gastrointest Endosc* 1993, **39**:763–765.

Klinkenbijl JHG, Jeekel J, Schmitz PIM, Rombout PAR, Nix GAJJ, Bruining HA, Van Blankenstein M: **Carcinoma of the Pancreas and Periampullary Region — Palliation Versus Cure.** *Br J Surg* 1993, **80**:1575–1578.

• Kozarek RA, Ball TJ. Patterson DJ, Brandabur JJ, Traverso LW, Raltz S: **Endoscopic Pancreatic Duct Sphincterotomy: Indications, Technique, and Analysis of Results.** *Gastrointest Endosc* 1994, **40**:592–598. **[27].**

Kozarek RA, Jiranek GC, Traverso L: **Endoscopic Treatment of Pancreatic Ascites.** *Am J Surg* 1994, **168**:223–226.

Kuo YC, Wu CS: **Role of Endoscopic Retrograde Pancreatography in Pancreatic Ascites.** *Dig Dis Sci* 1994, **39**:1143–1146.

Ladas SD, Tassios PS, Katsogridakis J, Giorgiotis K, Tastemiroglou T, Raptis SA: **The Clinical Need for Sphincter of Oddi Manometry in Gastrointestinal Endoscopy Units.** *Endoscopy* 1993, **25**:387–391.

Lai ECS, Lo CM: **Acute Pancreatitis — the Role of ERCP in 1994.** *Endoscopy* 1994, **26**:488–492.

Lang IM, Martin DF: **Gallbladder Function after Endoscopic Sphincterotomy — a Dynamic Ultrasound Assessment.** *Br J Radiol* 1993, **66**:585–587.

• Laugier R: **Dynamic Endoscopic Manometry in Response to Secretin in Patients with Chronic Pancreatitis.** *Endoscopy* 1994, **26**:222–227. **[21].**

• Layer P, Yamamoto H, Kalthoff L, Clain JE, Bakken LJ, DiMagno EP: **The Different Courses of Early- and Late-onset Idiopathic and Alcoholic Chronic Pancreatitis.** *Gastroenterology* 1994, **107**:1481–1487. **[6].**

Little TE, Kozarek RA: **Pancreatic Stones as a Cause of Bile Duct and Ampullary Obstruction — Endoscopic Treatment Approaches.** *Gastrointest Endosc* 1993, **39**:709–712.

Lo SK, Patel A: **Treatment of Endoscopic Sphincterotomy-Induced Hemorrhage — Injection of Bleeding Site with ERCP Contrast Solution Using a Minor Papilla Diagnostic Catheter.** *Gastrointest Endosc* 1993, **39**:436–439.

•• Lowenfels AB, Maisonneuve P, Cavallini G, Ammann RW, Lankisch PG, Andersen JR, *et al.*: **Prognosis of Chronic Pancreatitis: an International Multicenter Study.** *Am J Gastroenterol* 1994, **89**:1467–1471. **[5].**

MacMathuna P, *et al.*: **Balloon Sphincteroplasty Vs Endoscopic Papillotomy for Bileduct Stones [Letter].** *Lancet* 1994, **343**:486.

MacMathuna P, White P, Clarke E, Lennon J, Crowe J: **Endoscopic Sphincteroplasty — a Novel and Safe Alternative to Papillotomy in the Management of Bile Duct Stones.** *Gut* 1994, **35**:127–129.

Manoukian AV, Schmalz MJ, Geenen JE, Hogan WJ, Venu RP, Johnson GK: **The Incidence of Post-Sphincterotomy Stenosis in Group II Patients with Sphincter of Oddi Dysfunction.** *Gastrointest Endosc* 1993, **39**:496–498.

Marshall JB: **Acute Pancreatitis — a Review with an Emphasis on New Developments [Review].** *Arch Intern Med* 1993, **153**:1185–1198.

Matory YL, Gaynor J, Brennan M: **Carcinoma of the Ampulla of Vater.** *Surg Gynecol Obstet* 1993, **177**:366–370.

Mollison LC, Desmond PV, Stockman KA, Andrew JH, Watson K, Shaw G, Breen K: **A Prospective Study of Septic Complications of Endoscopic Retrograde Cholangiopancreatography.** *J Gastroenterol Hepatol* 1994, **9**:55–59.

Nakamura R, Machado R, Amikura K, Ruebner B, Frey CF: **Role of Fine Needle Aspiration Cytology and Endoscopic Biopsy in the Preoperative Assessment of Pancreatic and Peripancreatic Malignancies.** *Int J Pancreatol* 1994, **16**:17–21.

Neoptolemos JP: **Endoscopic Sphincterotomy in Acute Gallstone Pancreatitis.** *Br J Surg* 1993, **80**:547–549.

• Neoptolemos JP, Stonelake P, Radley S: **Endoscopic Sphincterotomy for Acute Pancreatitis.** *Hepatogastroenterology* 1993, **40**:550–555. **[10].**

Newton J, Hawes R, Jamidar P, Harig J, Lehman G: **Survey of Informed Consent for Endoscopic Retrograde Cholangiopancreatography.** *Dig Dis Sci* 1994, **39**:1714–1718.

Ng WT, Kong CK, Book KS, Auyeung MC: **Isolated Ventral Chronic Calcific Pancreatitis in Pancreas Divisum: an Explanation [Letter].** *Gastrointest Endosc* 1994, **40**:264.

Nishihara K, Fukuda T, Tsuneyoshi M, Kominami T, Maeda S, Saku M: **Intraductal Papillary Neoplasm of the Pancreas.** *Cancer* 1993, **72**:689–696.

Nitsche R, Folsch UR: **Early Treatment of Acute Biliary Pancreatitis by Endoscopic Papillotomy.** *Z Gastroenterol* 1994, **32**:182–183.

Obara T, Maguchi H, Saitoh Y, Sohma M, Tsuji K, Koike Y, Takemura K, Ura H, Namiki M: **Intraductal Papillary Neoplasms of the Pancreas — Diagnosis by Endoscopic Pancreatic Biopsy.** *Endoscopy* 1993, **25**:290–293.

Ott DJ, Young GP, Mitchell RG, Chen MYM, Gelfand DW: **Therapeutic ERCP — Spectrum of Procedures Performed in 60 Consecutive Patients.** *Abdom Imaging* 1994, **19**:30–33.

Portis M, Meyers P, McDonald JC, Gholson CF: **Traumatic Pancreatitis in a Patient with Pancreas Divisum — Clinical and Radiographic Features.** *Abdom Imaging* 1994, **19**:162–164.

Rao R, Fedorak I, Prinz RA, Keith RG, Vitale G, Grosfeld JL, Fried GM, Baker RJ: **Effect of Failed Computed Tomography-Guided and Endoscopic Drainage on Pancreatic Pseudocyst Management.** *Surgery* 1993, **114**:843–849.

Riemann JF, Kohler B: **Endoscopy of the Pancreatic Duct — Value of Different Endoscope Types.** *Gastrointest Endosc* 1993, **39**:367–370.

Rolny P, Arleback A: **Effect of Midazolam on Sphincter of Oddi Motility.** *Endoscopy* 1993, **25**:381–383.

Rolny P, Geenen JE, Hogan WJ: **Post-Cholecystectomy Patients with Objective Signs of Partial Bile Outflow Obstruction — Clinical Characteristics, Sphincter of Oddi Manometry Findings, and Results of Therapy.** *Gastrointest Endosc* 1993, **39**:778–781.

Saeed ZA, Ramirez FC, Hepps KS: **Endoscopic Stent Placement for Internal and External Pancreatic Fistulas.** *Gastroenterology* 1993, **105**:1213–1217.

Sand J, Nordback I: **Prospective Randomized Trial of the Effect of Nifedipine on Pancreatic Irritation after Endoscopic Retrograde Cholangiopancreatography.** *Digestion* 1993, **54**:105–111.

Scioscia PJ, Dillon PW, Cilley RE, Hoover WC, Krummel TM: **Endoscopic Sphincterotomy in the Management of Posttraumatic Biliary Fistula.** *J Pediatr Surg* 1994, **29**:3–6.

Shaw MJ, Dorsher PJ, Vennes JA: **Cystic Duct Anatomy — an Endoscopic Perspective.** *Am J Gastroenterol* 1993, **88**:2102–2106.

Sherman S: **ERCP and Endoscopic Sphincterotomy-Induced Pancreatitis.** *Am J Gastroenterol* 1994, **89**:303–305.

Sherman S, Alvarez C, Robert M, Ashley SW, Reber HA, Lehman GA: **Polyethylene Pancreatic Duct Stent-Induced Changes in the Normal Dog Pancreas.** *Gastrointest Endosc* 1993, **39**:658–664.

•• Sherman S, Hawes RH, Rathgaber SW, Uzer MF, Smith MT, Khusro QE, *et al.*: **Post-ERCP Pancreatitis: Randomized, Prospective Study Comparing a Low- and High osmolality Contrast Agent.** *Gastrointest Endosc* 1994, **40**:422–427. **[35].**

Shim KS, Suh JM, Yang YS, Choi JY, Park YH: **3-Dimensional Demonstration and Endoscopic Treatment of Pancreatic-Peritoneal Fistula.** *Am J Gastroenterol* 1993, **88**:1775–1779.

Shimizu S, Tada M, Kawai K: **Diagnostic ERCP.** *Endoscopy* 1994, **26**:88–92.

Siegel JH, Cohen SA, Kasmin FE, Veerappan A: **Stent-guided Sphincterotomy.** *Gastrointest Endosc* 1994, **40**:567–572.

Siegel JH, Veerappan A, Cohen SA, Kasmin FE: **Endoscopic Sphincterotomy for Biliary Pancreatitis: an Alternative to Cholecystectomy in High-risk Patients.** *Gastrointest Endosc* 1994, **40**:573–575.

Sisken RB, Fearnot NE, Smith HJ: **Electrosurgical Safety of Guide Wires During Endoscopic Sphincterotomy.** *Gastrointest Endosc* 1993, **39**:770–773.

• Smithline A, Silverman W, Rogers D, Nisi R, Wiersema M, Jamidar P, *et al.*: **Effect of Prophylactic Main Pancreatic Duct Stenting on the Incidence of Biliary Endoscopic Sphincterotomy-induced Pancreatitis in High-risk Patients.** *Gastrointest Endosc* 1993, **39**:652–657. **[38].**

Studley JGN, Sami AR, Williamson RCN: **Dissemination of Pancreatic Carcinoma Following Endoscopic Sphincterotomy.** *Endoscopy* 1993, **25**:301–302.

Tajiri H, Kobayashi M, Niwa H, Furui S: **Clinical Application of an Ultra-Thin Pancreatoscope Using a Sequential Video Converter.** *Gastrointest Endosc* 1993, **39**:371–374.

•• Takehara Y, Ichijo K, Tooyama N, Kodaira N, Yamamoto H, Tatami M, *et al.*: **Breath-hold MR Cholangiopancreatography with a Long-echo-train Fast Spin-echo Sequence and a Surface Coil in Chronic Pancreatitis.** *Radiology* 1994, **192**:73–78. **[3].**

Tham TCK, Kennedy R, O'Connor FA: **Early Complications and Mean 8-Year Follow-Up after Endoscopic Sphincterotomy in Young Fit Patients.** *Eur J Gastroenterol Hepatol* 1994, **6**:621–624.

Uomo G, Rabitti PG, Laccetti M, Visconti M: **Pancreatico-Choledochal Junction and Pancreatic Duct System Morphology in Acute Biliary Pancreatitis — a Prospective Study with Early ERCP.** *Int J Pancreatol* 1993, **13**:187–191.

Vahlensieck M, Vogel J, Kreft B, Reiser M: **Mucinous Cystadenoma of the Pancreatic Tail with Ductal Communication.** *J Comput Assist Tomogr* 1993, **17**:502–503.

• Van Der Hul R, Plaisier P, Jeekel J, Terpstra O, Den Toom R, Bruining H: **Extracorporeal Shock-wave Lithotripsy of Pancreatic Duct Stones: Immediate and Long-term Results.** *Endoscopy* 1994, **26**:573–578. **[28].**

Vellacott KD, Ogunbiyi OA: **Results of Endoscopic Retrograd Cholangio-Pancreatography Using a Mobile Image Intensifier.** *J R Coll Surg Edinb* 1993, **38**:216–219.

• Vestergaard H, Kruse A, Rokkjaer M, Frobert O, Thommesen P, Funch-Jensen P: **Endoscopic Manometry of the Sphincter of Oddi and the Pancreatic and Biliary Ducts in Patients with Chronic Pancreatitis.** *Scand J Gastroenterol* 1994, **29**:188–192. **[20].**

Weitemeyer R: **The Treatment of Ampullary Stenosis by Endoscopic Sphincterotomy (EST).** *Am J Surg* 1994, **167**:493–496.

•• Wiersema MJ, Hawes RH, Lehman GA, Kochman ML, Sherman S, Kopecky KK: **Prospective Evaluation of Endoscopic Ultrasonography and Endoscopic Retrograde Cholangiopancreatography in Patients with Chronic Abdominal Pain of Suspected Pancreatic Origin.** *Endoscopy* 1993, **25**:555–564. **[2].**

Yamaguchi K, Nagai E, Ueki T, Nishihara K, Tamaka M: **Carcinoma of the Ampulla of Vater.** *Aust N Z J Surg* 1993, **63**:256–262.

## Endoscopy and gallstones

Adam A, Roddie ME, Benjamin IS: **Mirizzi Syndrome — Treatment with Metallic Endoprosthesis.** *Clin Radiol* 1993, **48**:198–201.

Amouyal P, Amouyal G, Levy P, Tuzet S, Palazzo L, Vilgrain V, *et al.*: **Diagnosis of**
•• **Choledocholithiasis by Endoscopic Ultrasonography.** *Gastroenterology* 1994, **106**:1062–1067. **[36].**

Axelrad AM, Fleischer DE, Strack LL, Benjamin SB, Alkawas FH: **Performance of ERCP**
• **for Symptomatic Choledocholithiasis During Pregnancy — Techniques to Increase Safety and Improve Patient Management.** *Am J Gastroenterol* 1994, **89**:109–112. **[65].**

Barkun AN, Barkun JS, Fried GM, Ghitulescu G, Steinmetz O, Pham C *et al.*, and the
•• McGill Gallstone Treatment Group: **Useful Predictors of Bile Duct Stones in Patients Undergoing Laparoscopic Cholecystectomy.** *Ann Surg* 1994, **220**:32–39. **[10].**

Benattar JM, Carolibosc FX, Harris AG, Dumas R, Delmont J: **Endoscopic Sphincterotomy for Common Bile Duct Calculi in Patients Without Stones in the Gallbladder.** *Dig Dis Sci* 1993, **38**:2225–2227.

Binmoeller KF, Bruckner M, Thonke F, Soehendra N: **Treatment of Difficult Bile Duct Stones Using Mechanical, Electrohydraulic and Extracorporeal Shock Wave Lithotripsy.** *Endoscopy* 1993, **25**:201–206.

Binmoeller KF, Soehendra N, Liguory C: **The Common Bile Duct Stone: Time to**
• **Leave it to the Laparoscopic Surgeon?** *Endoscopy* 1994, **26**:315–319. **[17].**

Binmoeller KF, Thonke F, Soehendra N: **Endoscopic Treatment of Mirizzi's Syndrome.** *Gastrointest Endosc* 1993, **39**:532–536.

Boender J, Nix GA, De Ridder MA, Van Blankestein M, Schutte HE, Dees J, *et al.*:
• **Endoscopic Papillotomy for Common Bile Duct Stones: Factors Influencing the Complication Rate.** *Endoscopy* 1994, **26**:209–216. **[51].**

Bohorfoush AG, Ballinger PJ, Hogan WJ: **A New Method for Exchange of Endoprostheses in the Biliary and Pancreatic Ducts.** *Gastrointest Endosc* 1993, **39**:799–802.

Bose SM, Lobo DN, Singh G, Wig JD: **Bile Duct Cysts — Presentation in Adults.** *Aust N Z J Surg* 1993, **63**:853–857.

Boujouade J, Pelletier G, Fritsch J, Choury A, Lefebvre JF, Roche A, *et al.*: **Management**
• **of Clinically Relevant Bleeding Following Endoscopic Sphincterotomy.** *Endoscopy* 1994, **26**:217–221. **[54].**

Brooks DC, Connors PJ, Apstein MD, Carrlocke DL: **Failure of Piezoelectric Lithotripsy of a Gallstone Impacted in the Gallbladder Neck.** *Am J Gastroenterol* 1993, **88**:768–770.

Brugge WR: **Expanding the Diagnostic Capabilities of Endoscopy: Common Bile Duct Stones.** *Hepatology* 1994, **20**:1095–1096.

Carroll BJ, Fallas MH, Phillips EH: **Laparoscopic Transcystic Choledochoscopy.** *Surg*
• *Endosc* 1994, **8**:310–314. **[23].**

Chen K, Foliente RL, Santoro MJ, Walter MH, Collen MJ: **Endoscopic Sphincterotomy-**
• **induced Pancreatitis: Increased Risk Associated with Non Dilated Bile Ducts and Sphincter of Oddi Dysfunction.** *Am J Gastroenterol* 1994, **89**:327–333. **[52].**

Chijiiwa K, Ichimiya H, Kuroki S, Koga A, Nakayama F: **Late Development of Cholangiocarcinoma after the Treatment of Hepatolithiasis.** *Surg Gynecol Obstet* 1993, **177**:279–282.

Cisek PL, Greaney GC: **The Role of Endoscopic Retrograde Cholangiopancreatography with Laparoscopic Cholecystectomy in the Management of Choledocholithiasis.** *Am Surg* 1994, **60**:772–776.

Clair DG, Carrlocke DL, Becker JM, Brooks DC, Orlando R, Thayer BA, Maini BS, Baute PB, Rattner DW: **Routine Cholangiography is not Warranted During Laparoscopic Cholecystectomy.** *Arch Surg* 1993, **128**:551–555.

Costamagna G, Mutignani M, Perri V, Gabrielli A, Locicero P, Crucitti F: **Diagnostic and**
• **Therapeutic ERCP in Patients with Billroth II Gastrectomy.** *Acta Gastroenterol Belg* 1994, **57**:155–162. **[55].**

Cotton PB, Chung SC, Davis WZ, Gibson RM, Ransohoff DF, Strasberg SM: **Issues in**
•• **Cholecystectomy and Management of Duct Stones.** *Am J Gastroenterol* 1994, **89** (suppl):S169–S176. **[53].**

Ell C, Hochberger J, May A, Fleig WE, Bauer R, Mendez L, Hahn EG: **Laser Lithotripsy of Difficult Bile Duct Stones by Means of a Rhodamine-6G Laser and an Integrated Automatic Stone-Tissue Detection System.** *Gastrointest Endosc* 1993, **39**:755–762.

Feretis C, Apostolidis N, Mallas E, Manouras A, Papadimitriou J: **Endoscopic Drainage of Acute Obstructive Cholecystitis in Patients with Increased Operative Risk.** *Endoscopy* 1993, **25**:392–395.

Fireman Z, Kyzer S, Michalevicz D, Shapiro G, Lurie B, Chiamoff C: **Esophageal Perforation after Endoscopic Sphincterotomy During Stone Extraction from the Common Bile Duct.** *J Clin Gastroenterol* 1994, **19**:173–175.

Fletcher DR: **Changes in the Practice of Biliary Surgery and ERCP During the Introduction of Laparoscopic Cholecystectomy to Australia — Their Possible Significance.** *Aust N Z J Surg* 1994, **64**:75–80.

Foutch PG, Harlan JR, Hoefer M: **Endoscopic Therapy for Patients with a Post-Operative Biliary Leak.** *Gastrointest Endosc* 1993, **39**:416–421.

Franceschi D, Brandt C, Margolin D, Szopa B, Ponsky J, Priebe P, Stellato T, Eckhauser ML, Hawasli A, Pickleman J: **The Management of Common Bile Duct Stones in Patients Undergoing Laproscopic Cholecystectomy.** *Am Surg* 1993, **59**:525–532.

Frazee RC, Roberts J, Symmonds R, Hendricks JC, Snyder S, Smith R, Custer MD, Stoltenberg P, Avots A: **Combined Laparoscopic and Endoscopic Management of Cholelithiasis and Choledocholithiasis.** *Am J Surg* 1993, **166**:702–706.

Goldberg HI: **Helical Cholangiography: Complementary or Substitute Study for Endoscopic Retrograde Cholangiography?** *Radiology* 1994, **192**:615–616.

Goldschmiedt M, Wolf L, Shires T: **Treatment of Symptomatic Choledocholithiasis During Pregnancy.** *Gastrointest Endosc* 1993, **39**:812–814.

Graham SM, Flowers JL, Scott TR, Bailey RW, Scovill WA, Zucker KA, Imbembo AL: **Laparoscopic Cholecystectomy and Common Bile Duct Stones — the Utility of Planned Perioperative Endoscopic Retrograde Cholangiography and Sphincterotomy — Experience with 63 Patients.** *Ann Surg* 1993, **218**:61–67.

Guibaud L, Bret PM, Reinhold C, Atri M, Barkun AN: **Diagnosis of Choledocholithia-**
• **sis: Value of MR Cholangiography.** *AJR Am J Roentgenol* 1994, **163**:847–850. **[45].**

Hainsworth PJ, Rhodes M, Gompertz RH, Armstrong CP, Lennard TW: **Imaging of the**
•• **Common Bile Duct in Patients Undergoing Laparoscopic Cholecystectomy.** *Gut* 1994, **35**:991–995. **[3].**

Harshfield DL, Teplick SK, Brandon JC: **Pain Control During Interventional Biliary Procedures — Epidural Anesthesia Vs IV Sedation.** *AJR Am J Roentgenol* 1993, **161**:1057–1059.

Hawasli A, Lloyd L, Pozios V, Veneri R: **The Role of Endoscopic Retrograde Cholangiopancreatogram in Laparoscopic Cholecystectomy.** *Am Surg* 1993, **59**:285–289.

Ji ZL, Chen HR, Wang EH, Yang DT, Gao NR, Yang JZ, Liu BY: **Percutaneous Endoscopic Polypectomy of Gallbladder Polyps.** *Endoscopy* 1994, **26**:609–612.

Johlin FC, Neil GA: **Drainage of the Gallbladder in Patients with Acute Acalculous Cholecystitis by Transpapillary Endoscopic Cholecystotomy.** *Gastrointest Endosc* 1993, **39**:645–651.

Johnson GK, Geenen JE, Venu RP, Schmalz MJ, Hogan WJ: **Treatment of Non-Extractable Common Bile Duct Stones with Combination Ursodeoxycholic Acid Plus Endoprostheses.** *Gastrointest Endosc* 1993, **39**:528–531.

Kalloo AN, Thuluvath PJ, Pasricha PJ: **Treatment of High-risk Patients with**
• **Symptomatic Cholelithiasis by Endoscopic Gallbladder Stenting.** *Gastrointest Endosc* 1994, **40**:608–610. **[58].**

Kent AL, Cox MR, Wilson TG, Padbury RTA, Toouli J: **Endoscopic Retrograde Cholangiopancreatography Following Laparoscopic Cholecystectomy.** *Aust N Z J Surg* 1994, **64**:407–412.

Khuroo MS, Dar MY, Yattoo GN, Khan BA, Boda MI, Zargar SA, Javid G, Allai MS: **Serial Cholangiographic Appearances in Recurrent Pyogenic Cholangitis.** *Gastrointest Endosc* 1993, **39**:674–679.

Kozarek RA, Ball TJ, Patterson DJ, Brandabur JJ, Raltz S, Traverso LW: **Endoscopic**
• **Treatment of Biliary Injury in the Era of Laparoscopic Cholecystectomy.** *Gastrointest Endosc* 1994, **40**:10–16. **[32].**

Lancaster JF, Strong RW, McIntyre A, Kerlin P: **Gallstone Ileus Complicating Endoscopic Sphincterotomy.** *Aust N Z J Surg* 1993, **63**:416–417.

Lauri A, Horton RC, Davidson BR, Burroughs AK, Dooley JS: **Endoscopic Extraction of Bile Duct Stones — Management Related to Stone Size.** *Gut* 1993, **34**:1718–1721.

Leitman IM, Fisher ML, McKinley MJ, Rothman R, Ward RJ, Reiner DS, Tortolani AJ: **The Evaluation and Management of Known or Suspected Stones of the Common Bile Duct in the Era of Minimal Access Surgery.** *Surg Gynecol Obstet* 1993, **176**:527–533.

Leung JWC, Ling TKW, Chan RCY, Cheung SW, Lai CW, Sung JJY *et al.*: **Antibiotics,**
• **Biliary Sepsis, and Bile Duct Stones.** *Gastrointest Endosc* 1994, **40**:716–721. **[5].**

Linder S, Vonrosen A, Wiechel KL: **Bile Duct Pressure, Hormonal Influence and Recurrent Bile Duct Stones.** *Hepatogastroenterology* 1993, **40**:370–374.

Lingam K, Carter R, Drury JK: **Retained Gallstones Following Laparoscopic Cholecystectomy.** *J R Coll Surg Edinb* 1993, **38**:353.

MacMathuna P, White P, Clarke E, Lennon J, Crowe J: **Endoscopic Sphincteroplasty:**
•• **a Novel and Safe Alternative to Papillotomy in the Management of Bile Duct Stones.** *Gut* 1994, **35**:127–129. **[47].**

Maetani I, Hoshi H, Ohashi S, Yoshioka H, Sakai Y: **Cholangioscopic Extraction of Intrahepatic Stones Associated with Biliary Strictures Using a Rendezvous Technique.** *Endoscopy* 1993, **25**:303–306.

May GR, Cotton PB, Edmunds SEJ, Chong W: **Removal of Stones from the Bile Duct at ERCP Without Sphincterotomy.** *Gastrointest Endosc* 1993, **39**:749–754.

Mitchell SA, Jacyna MR, Chadwick S: **Common Bile Duct Stones — a Controversy Revisited — for Debate.** *Br J Surg* 1993, **80**:759–760.

Neuhaus H: **Cholangioscopy.** *Endoscopy* 1994, **26**:120–125. **[56].**

Neuhaus H, Hoffman W, Gottlieb K, Classen M: **Endoscopic Lithotripsy of Bile Duct**
• **Stones Using a New Laser with Automatic Recognition System.** *Gastrointest Endosc* 1994, **39**:755–762. **[50].**

Niederau C, Pohlmann U, Lubke H, Thomas L: **Prophylactic Antibiotic Treatment**
•• **in Therapeutic or Complicated Diagnostic ERCP: Results of a Randomized Controlled Clinical Study.** *Gastrointest Endosc* 1994, **40**:533–537. **[6].**

Orourke NA, Askew AR, Cowen AE, Roberts R, Fielding GA: **The Role of ERCP and Endoscopic Sphincterotomy in the Era of Laparoscopic Cholecystectomy.** *Aust N Z J Surg* 1993, **63**:3–7.

Pencev D, Brady PG, Pinkas H, Boulay J: **The Role of ERCP in Patients after Laparoscopic Cholecystectomy.** *Am J Gastroenterol* 1994, **89**:1523–1527.

Perissat J, Huibregtse K, Keane FBV, Russell RCG, Neoptolemos JP: **Management**
•• **of Bile Duct Stones in the Era of Laparoscopic Cholecystectomy.** *Br J Surg* 1994, **81**:799–810. **[15].**

Petelin JB: **Clinical Results of Common Bile Duct Exploration.** *Endosc Surg All*
• *Technol* 1993, **3**:125–129. **[25].**

Phillips EH: **Controversies in the Management of Common Duct Calculi.** *Surg Clin*
• *North Am* 1994, **74**:931–948. **[18].**

Pitt HA, Venbrux AC, Coleman J, Prescott CA, Johnson MS, Osterman FA Jr, *et al.*:
• **Intrahepatic Stones. The Transhepatic Team Approach.** *Ann Surg* 1994, **219**:527–535. **[57].**

Plaisier PW, Vanbuuren HR, Nix GAJJ, Vanderhul RL, Bruining HA: **Extracorporeal Shock Wave Lithotripsy as a Troubleshooter for a Dormia Basket Impacted in the Common Bile Duct [Letter].** *Gastrointest Endosc* 1994, **40**:259–260.

Plaisier PW, Vanderhul RL, Terpstra OT, Bruining HA: **Current Treatment Modalities for Symptomatic Gallstones [Review].** *Am J Gastroenterol* 1993, **88**:633–639.

Prat F, Fritsch J, Choury AD, Frouge C, Marteau V, Etienne JP: **Laser Lithotripsy of Difficult Biliary Stones.** *Gastrointest Endosc* 1994, **40**:290–295.

Rothlin MA, Schlumpf R, Largiader F: **Laparoscopic Sonography. an Alternative to**
• **Routine Intraoperative Cholangiography?** *Arch Surg* 1994, **129**:694–700. **[42].**

Schlumpf R, Klotz HP, Wehrli H, Herzog U: **A Nation's Experience in Laparoscopic**
• **Cholecystectomy. Prospective Multicenter Analysis of 3722 Cases.** *Surg Endosc* 1994, **8**:35–41. **[22].**

Schneider HT, Weisshaar E, Anderegg A, Delmont JP, Benattar JM, Coendoz S, Ell C: **Piezoelectric Shockwave Lithotripters — Differences in Fragmentation Efficiency Invitro.** *Scand J Gastroenterol* 1993, **28**:460–464.

Schoonjans R, Deman M, Aerts P, Vanderspek P, Vansteenberge R, Lepoutre L: **Combined Percutaneous Balloon Dilation and Extracorporeal Shock Wave Lithotripsy for Treatment of Biliary Stricture and Common Bile Duct Stones.** *Am J Gastroenterol* 1994, **89**:1573–1576.

Schulman A: **Intrahepatic Biliary Stones — Imaging Features and a Possible Relationship with Ascaris Lumbricoides.** *Clin Radiol* 1993, **47**:325–332.

Shaw MJ, Mackie RD, Moore JP, Dorsher PJ, Freeman ML, Meier PB, Potter T, Hutton SW, Vennes JA: **Results of a Multicenter Trial Using a Mechanical Lithotripter for the Treatment of Large Bile Duct Stones.** *Am J Gastroenterol* 1993, **88**:730–733.

Sheenchen SM, Chou FF: **Postoperative Choledochoscopy — is Routine Antibiotic Prophylaxis Necessary — a Prospective Randomized Study.** *Surgery* 1994, **115**:170–175.

Sheridan J, Williams TM, Yeung E, Ho CS, Thurston W: **Percutaneous Transhepatic Management of an Impacted Endoscopic Basket.** *Gastrointest Endosc* 1993, **39**:444–446.

Sherman S, Hawes RH, Uzer MF, Smith MT, Lehman GA: **Endoscopic Stent Exchange Using a Guide Wire and Mini-Snare.** *Gastrointest Endosc* 1993, **39**:794–799.

Shian WJ, Wang YJ, Chi CS: **Choledochal Cysts — a 9-Year Review.** *Acta Paediatr* 1993, **82**:383–386.

Siddiqui MN, Hamid S, Khan H, Ahmed M: **Per-operative Endoscopic Retrograde Cholangio-pancreatography for Common Bile Duct Stones.** *Gastrointest Endosc* 1994, **40**:348–350.

Siegel JH: **Re: Endoscopic Stent Treatment of the Sump Syndrome [Letter].** *Am J Gastroenterol* 1994, **89**:139.

Siegel JH, Rodriguez R, Cohen SA, Kasmin FE, Cooperman AM: **Endoscopic Management of Cholangitis: Critical Review of an Alternative Technique and Report of a Large Series.** *Am J Gastroenterol* 1994, **89**:1142–1146.

•• Steiner CA, Bass EB, Talamini MA, Pitt HA, Steinberg EP: **Surgical Rates and Operative Mortality for Open and Laparoscopic Cholecystectomy in Maryland.** *N Engl J Med* 1994, **330**:403–408. **[7].**

• Stockberger SM, Wass JL, Sherman S, Lehman GA, Kopecky KK: **Intravenous Cholangiography with Helical CT: Comparison with Endoscopic Retrograde Cholangiography.** *Radiology* 1994, **192**:675–680. **[44].**

Sugiyama M, Atomi Y, Kuroda A, Muto T: **Treatment of Choledocholithiasis in Patients with Liver Cirrhosis — Surgical Treatment or Endoscopic Sphincterotomy.** *Ann Surg* 1993, **218**:68–73.

Surick B, Washington M, Ghazi A: **Endoscopic Retrograde Cholangiopancreatography in Conjunction with Laparoscopic Cholecystectomy.** *Surg Endosc* 1993, **7**:388–392.

Testoni PA, Lella F, Masci E, Bagnolo F, Colombo E, Tittobello A: **Combined Endoscopic and Extracorporeal Shock-Wave Treatment in Difficult Bile Duct Stones — Early and Long-Term Results.** *Ital J Gastroenterol* 1994, **26**:294–298.

Van Der Hul RL, Plaisier PW, Hamming JF, Bruining HA, Van Blankenstein M: **Detection and Management of Common Bile Duct Stones in the Era of Laparoscopic Cholecystectomy.** *Scand J Gastroenterol* 1993, **28**:929–933.

Vandullemen H, Stuifbergen WNHM, Juttmann JR, Vanderwerken C: **Simple Release of an Impacted Dormia Basket During Endoscopic Bile Duct Stone Extraction.** *Endoscopy* 1993, **25**:374.

Vergunst H, Terpstra OT, Brakel K, Nijs HGT, Lameris JS, Tenkate FJW, Schroder FH: **Biliary Extracorporeal Shockwave Lithotripsy — Short-Term and Long-Term Observations in an Animal Model.** *Hepatogastroenterology* 1993, **40**:388–395.

• Voyles CR, Sanders DL, Hogan R: **Common Bile Duct Evaluation in the Era of Laparoscopic Cholecystectomy. 1050 Cases Later.** *Ann Surg* 1994, **219**:744–750. **[9].**

•• Wetter LA, Hamadeh RM, Griffiss JM, Oesterle A, Aagaard B Way LW: **Differences in Outer Membrane Characteristics Between Gallstone-associated Bacteria and Normal Bacterial Flora.** *Lancet* 1994, **343**:444–448. **[2].**

• Widdison AL, Longstaff AJ, Armstrong CP: **Combined Laparoscopic and Endoscopic Treatment of Gallstones and Bile Duct Stones: a Prospective Study.** *Br J Surg* 1994, **81**:595–597. **[12].**

Wilson TG, Jeans PL, Anthony A, Cox MR, Toouli J: **Laparoscopic Cholecystectomy and Management of Choledocholithiasis.** *Aust N Z J Surg* 1993, **63**:443–450.

• Windsor JA, Vokes DE: **Early Experience with Minimally Invasive Surgery: a New Zealand Audit.** *Aust N Z J Surg* 1994, **64**:81–87. **[8].**

Wu WC, Katon RM, McAfee JH: **Endoscopic Management of Common Bile Duct Stones Resulting from Metallic Surgical Clips (Cats Eye Calculi).** *Gastrointest Endosc* 1993, **39**:712–715.


## Endoscopy and non-calculus biliary obstruction


Anderson ID, Manson JM, Martin DF, Tweedle DEF: **Palliation of Biliary Obstruction in Patients with Advanced Breast Cancer Using Endoscopic Stents [Letter].** *Br J Surg* 1994, **81**:148.

Asbun HJ, Rossi RL, Lowell JA, Munson JL: **Bile Duct Injury During Laparoscopic Cholecystectomy — Mechanism of Injury, Prevention, and Management.** *World J Surg* 1993, **17**:547–552.

•• Ballinger AB, McHugh M, Catnach SM, Alstead EM, Clark ML: **Symptom Relief in Quality of Life after Stenting for Malignant Bile Duct Obstruction.** *Gut* 1994, **35**:467–470. **[9].**

• Baron TH, Lee JG, Wax TD, Schmitt CM, Cotton PB, Leung JWC: **An in Vitro, Randomized, Prospective Study to Maximize Cellular Yield During Bile Duct Brush Cytology.** *Gastrointest Endosc* 1994, **40**:146–149. **[4].**

Benhamou Y, Caumes E, Gerosa Y, Cadranel JF, Dohin E, Katlama C, Amouyal P, Canard JM, Azar N, Hoang C, Lecharpentier Y, Gentilini M, Opolon P, Valla D: **AIDS-Related Cholangiopathy — Critical Analysis of a Prospective Series of 26 Patients.** *Dig Dis Sci* 1993, **38**:1113–1118.

• Botoman VA, Kozarek RA, Novell LA, Patterson DJ, Ball TJ, Wechter DG, *et al.*: **Long-term Outcome after Endoscopic Sphincterotomy in Patients with Biliary Colic and Suspected Sphincter of Oddi Dysfunction.** *Gastrointest Endosc* 1994, **40**:165–170. **[26].**

Branum G, Schmitt C, Baillie J, Suhocki P, Baker M, Davidoff A, Branch S, Chari R, Cucchiaro G, Murray E, Pappas T, Cotton P, Meyers WC: **Management of Major Biliary Complications after Laparoscopic Cholecystectomy.** *Ann Surg* 1993, **217**:532–541.

Buffet C, Couderc T, Fritsch J, Choury A, Lefebvre JF, Marteau V, Ink O, Bonnel D, Liguory C, Etienne JP: **Palliative Endoscopic Drainage of Malignant Strictures of the Extrahepatic Biliary Tree.** *Gastroenterol Clin Biol* 1993, **17**:629–635.

Cainzos M: **Biliary Drainage in Obstructive Jaundice: Experimental and Clinical Aspects [Letter].** *Br J Surg* 1994, **81**:625–626.

Callea F, Sergi C, Fabbretti G, Brisigotti M, Cozzutto C, Medicina D: **Precancerous Lesions of the Biliary Tree.** *J Surg Oncol* 1993, (suppl 3):131–133.

Cates JA, Tompkins RK, Zinner MJ, Busuttil RW, Kallman C, Roslyn JJ: **Biliary Complications of Laparoscopic Cholecystectomy.** *Am Surg* 1993, **59**:243–247.

Chen MF, Jan YY, Jeng LB, Hwang TL, Wang CS, Chen SC: **Obstructive Jaundice Secondary to Ruptured Hepatocellular Carcinoma into the Common Bile Duct — Surgical Experiences of 20 Cases.** *Cancer* 1994, **73**:1335–1340.

Cherqui D: **Treatment of Jaundice Due to Malignant Obstruction of the Distal Common Bile Duct.** *Gastroenterol Clin Biol* 1993, **17**:626–628.

Cherqui D, Palazzo L, Piedbois P, Charlotte F, Duvoux C, Duron JJ, Fagniez PL, Valla D: **Common Bile Duct Stricture as a Late Complication of Upper Abdominal Radiotherapy.** *J Hepatol* 1994, **20**:693–697.

Costamagna G, Gabbrielli A, Mutignani M, Perri V, Crucitti F: **Treatment of Obstructive Pain by Endoscopic Drainage in Patients with Pancreatic Head Carcinoma.** *Gastrointest Endosc* 1993, **39**:774–777.

Cucchiara G, Gandini G, Simonetti G, Bracci F, Daffina A: **Palliative Treatment of Extrahepatic Bile Ducts Tumors.** *J Surg Oncol* 1993, (suppl 3):154–157.

Dasilva F, Boudghene F, Lecomte I, Delage Y, Grange JD, Bigot JM: **Sonography in AIDS-Related Cholangitis — Prevalence and Cause of an Echogenic Nodule in the Distal End of the Common Bile Duct.** *AJR Am J Roentgenol* 1993, **160**:1205–1207.

Davids PHP, Ringers J, Rauws EAJ, De Wit LT, Huibregtse K, VanDer Heyde MN, Tytgat GNJ: **Bile Duct Injury after Laparoscopic Cholecystectomy: the Value of Endoscopic Retrograde Cholangiopancreatography.** *Gut* 1993, **34**:1250–1254.

Deviere J, Cremer M, Baize M, Love J, Sugai B, Vandermeeren A: **Management of Common Bile Duct Stricture Caused by Chronic Pancreatitis with Metal Mesh Self Expandable Stents.** *Gut* 1994, **35**:122–126.

Dolan R, Pinkas H, Brady PG: **Acute Cholecystitis after Palliative Stenting for Malignant Obstruction of the Biliary Tree.** *Gastrointest Endosc* 1993, **39**:447–449.

Donovan J: **Nonsurgical Management of Biliary Tract Disease after Liver Transplantation.** *Gastroenterol Clin North Am* 1993, **22**:317–336.

•• Elta GH, Barnett JL: **Meperidine Need not be Proscribed During Sphincter of Oddi Manometry.** *Gastrointest Endosc* 1994, **40**:7–9. **[23].**

Escourrou J, Berthelemy P: **Biliary Complications Following Laparoscopic Cholecystectomy. Role of ERCP in Diagnosis and Treatment [Review].** *Eur J Gastroenterol Hepatol* 1993, **5**:667–676.

Farman J, Brunetti J, Baer JW, Freiman H, Comer GM, Scholz FJ, Koehler RE, Laffey K, Green P, Clemett AR: **AIDS-Related Cholangiopancreatographic Changes.** *Abdom Imaging* 1994, **19**:417–422.

• Ferrari AP Jr, Lichtenstein DR, Slivka A, Chang C, Carr-Locke DL: **Brush Cytology During ERCP for the Diagnosis of Biliary and Pancreatic Malignancies.** *Gastrointest Endosc* 1994, **40**:140–145. **[3].**

Foutch PG: **Diagnosis of Cancer by Cytologic Methods Performed During ERCP.** *Gastrointest Endosc* 1994, **40**:249–252.

Funnell IC, Bornman PC, Krige JEJ, Beningfield SJ, Terblanche J: **Complete Common Bile Duct Division at Laparoscopic Cholecystectomy — Management by Percutaneous Drainage and Endoscopic Stenting — Case Report.** *Br J Surg* 1993, **80**:1053–1054.

Gaing AA, Geders JM, Cohen SA, Siegel JH: **Endoscopic Management of Primary Sclerosing Cholangitis — Review, and Report of an Open Series [Review].** *Am J Gastroenterol* 1993, **88**:2000–2008.

• Gillams A, Gardener J, Richards R, Tan AC, Linney A, Lees WR: **Three Dimensional Computed Tomography Cholangiography: a New Technique for Biliary Tract Imaging.** *Br J Radiol* 1994, **67**:445–448. **[8].**

• Goldin E, Beyar M, Safra T, Globerman O, Verstandig A, Wengrower D, *et al.*: **A New Self-expandable and Removable Metal Stent for Biliary Obstruction — a Preliminary Report.** *Endoscopy* 1993, **25**:597–599. **[13].**

Goldin RD, Hunt J: **Biliary Tract Pathology in Patients with AIDS.** *J Clin Pathol* 1993, **46**:691–693.

Guthrie CM, Haddock G, Debeaux AC, Garden OJ, Carter DC: **Changing Trends in the Management of Extrahepatic Cholangiocarcinoma.** *Br J Surg* 1993, **80**:1434–1439.

Hamour AA, Bonnington A, Hawthorne B, Wilkins EGL: **Successful Treatment of AIDS-Related Cryptosporidial Sclerosing Cholangitis — Short Communication.** *AIDS* 1993, **7**:1449–1451.

Hanafy M, McDonald P: **Villous Adenoma of the Common Bile Duct.** *J R Soc Med* 1993, **86**:603–604.

• Helling TS: **Carcinoma of the Proximal Bile Duct.** *J Am Coll Surg* 1994, **178**:97–106. **[16].**

Hoepffner N, Foerster EC, Hogemann B, Domschke W: **Long-term Experience in Wallstent Therapy for Malignant Choledochal Stenosis.** *Endoscopy* 1994, **26**:597–602.

• Hoffman BJ, Cunningham JT, Marsh WH, O'Brien JJ, Watson J: **An *in Vitro* Comparison of Biofilm Formation on Various Biliary Stent Materials.** *Gastrointest Endosc* 1994, **50**:581–583. **[11].**

Howe CD, Hill DB, Gubbins G: **Polycystic Liver Disease Mimicking Sclerosing Cholangitis During Endoscopic Retrograde Cholangiopancreatography.** *Am J Gastroenterol* 1994, **89**:128–129.

Huibregtse K: **Plastic or Expandable Biliary Endoprostheses.** *Scand J Gastroenterol* 1993, **28** (suppl 200):3–7.

Ikenberry SO, Sherman S, Hawes RH, Smith M, Lehman GA: **The Occlusion Rate of Pancreatic Stents.** *Gastrointest Endosc* 1994, **40**:611–613.

Jablonowski H, Szelenyi H, Becker K, Lubke H, Borchard F, Strohmeyer G, Hengels KJ: **Sclerosing Cholangitis with Papillary Stenosis in a HIV-Infected Patient with Cryptosporidiosis.** *Z Gastroenterol* 1994, **32**:441–443.

Karsten TM, Davids PHP, Vangulik TM, Bosma A, Tytgat GNJ, Klopper PJ, Vanderheyde MN: **Effects of Biliary Endoprostheses on the Extrahepatic Bile Ducts in Relation to Subsequent Operation of the Biliary Tract.** *J Am Coll Surg* 1994, **178**:343–352.

Knyrim K, Wagner HJ, Pausch J, Vakil N: **A Prospective, Randomized, Controlled Trial of Metal Stents for Malignant Obstruction of the Common Bile Duct.** *Endoscopy* 1993, **25**:207–212.

• Kozarek RA, Ball TJ, Patterson DJ, Brandebur JJ, Raltz S, Traverso LW: **Endoscopic Treatment of Biliary Injury in the Era of Laparoscopic Cholecystectomy.** *Gastrointest Endosc* 1994, **40**:10–16. **[19].**

Kubota Y, Takaoka M, Tani K, Ogura M, Kin H, Fujimura K, *et al.*: **Endoscopic Transpapillary Biopsy for Diagnosis of Patients with Pancreaticobiliary Strictures.** *Am J Gastroenterol* 1993, **88**:1700–1704. **[6].**
•• 
Kuo PC, Lewis WD, Stokes K, Pleskow D, Simpson MA, Jenkins RL: **A Comparison of Operation, Endoscopic Retrograde Cholangiopancreatography, and Percutaneous Transhepatic Cholangiography in Biliary Complications after Hepatic Transplantation.** *J Am Coll Surg* 1994, **179**:177–181. **[21].**
• 
Kurzawinski T, Deery A, Dooley J, Dick R, Hobbs KEF, Davidson BR: **A Prospective Study of Biliary Cytology in 100 Patients with Bile Duct Strictures.** *Hepatology* 1993, **18**:1399–1403. **[2].**
• 
Lai ECS, Mok FPT, Fan ST, Lo CM, Chu KM, Leio CL, *et al.*: **Preoperative Endoscopic Training for Malignant Obstructive Jaundice.** *Br J Surg* 1994, **81**:1195–1198. **[18].**
•• 
Lallier M, Stvil D, Luks FI, Laberge JM, Bensoussan AL, Guttman FM, Blanchard H: **Biliary Tract Complications in Pediatric Orthotopic Liver Transplantation.** *J Pediatr Surg* 1993, **28**:1102–1105.

Lemmer ER, Bornman PC, Krige JEJ, Wright JP, Beningfield S, Jaskiewicz K, Kirsch RE, Kahn D, Terblanche JT, Robson SC: **Primary Sclerosing Cholangitis — Requiem for Biliary Drainage Operations?** *Arch Surg* 1994, **129**:723–728.

Lipsky H, Barkin JS, Grauer L: **Bile Duct Drainage with Lavage by Nasobiliary Tube in a Patient with Mucin-Producing Cystic Pancreatic Tumor.** *Gastrointest Endosc* 1993, **39**:574–576.

Low RN, Sigeti JS, Francis IR, Weinman D, Bower B, Shimakawa A, *et al.*: **Evaluation of Malignant Biliary Obstruction: Efficacy of Fast Multi-planar Spoiled Gradient-recalled MR Imaging Vs. Spin-echo MR Imaging, CT and Cholangiography.** *AJR Am J Roentgenol* 1994, **162**:315–323. **[7].**
• 
Maetani I, Hoshi H, Ohashi S, Yoshioka H, Sakai Y: **Cholangioscopic Extraction of Intrahepatic Stones Associated with Biliary Strictures Using a Rendezvous Technique.** *Endoscopy* 1993, **25**:303–306.

Magistrelli P, Masetti R, Coppola R, Coco C, Antinori A, Nuzzo G, Picciocchi A: **Changing Attitudes in the Palliation of Proximal Malignant Biliary Obstruction.** *J Surg Oncol* 1993, (suppl 3):151–153.

Mairiang E, Haswellelkins MR, Mairiang P, Sithithaworn P, Elkins DB: **Reversal of Biliary Tract Abnormalities Associated with Opisthorchis-Viverrini Infection Following Praziquantel Treatment.** *Trans R Soc Trop Med Hyg* 1993, **87**:194–197.

Manoukian AV: **Endoscopic Treatment of Problems Encountered after Cholecystectomy (Vol 39, Pg 9, 1993).** *Gastrointest Endosc* 1993, **39**:615.

Martin DF: **Combined Percutaneous and Endoscopic Procedures for Bile Duct Obstruction.** *Gut* 1994, **35**:1011–1012. **[14].**
• 
Maxwell P, Davis RI, Sloan JM: **Carcinoembryonic Antigen (CEA) in Benign and Malignant Epithelium of the Gall Bladder, Extrahepatic Bile Ducts, and Ampulla of Vater.** *J Pathol* 1993, **170**:73–76.

McAllister EW, Carey LC, Brady PG, Heller R, Kovacs SG: **The Role of Polymeric Surface Smoothness of Biliary Stents in Bacterial Adherence, Biofilm Deposition, and Stent Occlusion.** *Gastrointest Endosc* 1993, **39**:422–425.

Mitchell PLR, Harvey VJ, Lane MR, Evans BD, Thompson PI, Hamilton I: **Palliation of Biliary Obstruction in Patients with Advanced Breast Cancer Using Endoscopic Stents.** *Br J Surg* 1993, **80**:1188–1189.

Mohandas KM, Swaroop VS, Gullar SU, Dave UR, Jagannath P, DeSouza LJ: **Diagnosis of Malignant Obstructive Jaundice by Bile Cytology: Results Improved by Dilating the Bile Duct Strictures.** *Gastrointest Endosc* 1994, **40**:150–155. **[1].**
• 
Morenogonzalez E, Gomez R, Loinaz C, Garcia I, Gonzalezpinto I, Maffettone V, Delacalle A, Palomo JC, Palma F: **Surgical Resection of Biliary Tract Malignancies after Interventional Radiology Treatment.** *J Surg Oncol* 1993, (suppl 3):200–202.

Neuhaus H, Gottlieb K, Classen M: **The Stent Through Wire Mesh Technique for Complicated Biliary Strictures.** *Gastrointest Endosc* 1993, **39**:553–556.

Oda K, Itoh J, Hachisuka K, Yamaguchi A, Isogai M, Utsunomiya H, Osamura RY, Watanabe K: **Value of Computer Image Analysis in Improving ERCP Images in Metastatic Tumor of the Pancreas — Case Report.** *AJR Am J Roentgenol* 1993, **161**:885–886.

Ohtomo K, Baron RL, Dodd GD III, Federle MP, Miller WJ, Campbell WL, Confer SR, Weber KM: **Confluent Hepatic Fibrosis in Advanced Cirrhosis: Appearance at CT.** *Radiology* 1993, **188**:31–36.

Osorio RW, Freise CE, Stock PG, Lake JR, Laberge JM, Gordon RL, Ring EJ, Ascher NL, Roberts JP: **Nonoperative Management of Biliary Leaks after Orthotopic Liver Transplantation.** *Transplantation* 1993, **55**:1074–1077.

Rantis PC, Greenlee HB, Pickleman J, Prinz RA, Stellato, Hawasli A, Lloyd: **Laparoscopic Cholecystectomy Bile Duct Injuries — More Than Meets the Eye.** *Am Surg* 1993, **59**:533–540.

Raute M, Podlech P, Jaschke W, Manegold BC, Trede M, Chir B: **Management of Bile Duct Injuries and Strictures Following Cholecystectomy.** *World J Surg* 1993, **17**:553–562.

Reeders JWAJ, Bartelsman JFWM, Huibregtse K: **AIDS-Related Manifestations of the Bile Duct System — a Common Finding — Editorial Commentary.** *Abdom Imaging* 1994, **19**:423–424.

Rolny P, Geenen JE, Hogan WJ: **Post-cholecystectomy in Patients with 'objective Signs' of Partial Bile Outflow Obstruction: Clinical Characteristics, Sphincter of Oddi Findings, and Results of Therapy.** *Gastrointest Endosc* 1993, **39**:778–781. **[27].**
• 
Schoenthaler R, Phillips TL, Castro J, Efird JT, Better A, Way LW: **Carcinoma of the Extrahepatic Bile Ducts — the University of California at San Francisco Experience.** *Ann Surg* 1994, **219**:267–274.

Schofl R, Brownstone E, Reichel W, Fortunat W, Doblhofer F, Samec HJ, Brandstatter G, Stupnicki T, Pamperl H, Schreiber P, Gangl A: **Malignant Bile-duct Obstruction: Experience with Self-expanding Metal Endoprostheses (Wallstents) in Austria.** *Endoscopy* 1994, **26**:592–596.

Seitz U, Vadeyar H, Soehendra H: **Prolonged Patency with a New-designed Teflon Biliary Prosthesis.** *Endoscopy* 1994, **26**:478–482. **[10].**
• 
Sheng R, Zajko AB, Campbell WL, Abuelmagd K: **Biliary Strictures in Hepatic Transplants — Prevalence and Types in Patients with Primary Sclerosing Cholangitis Vs those with Other Liver Diseases.** *AJR Am J Roentgenol* 1993, **161**:297–300.

Sherman S, Lehman GA: **Opioids and the Sphincter of Oddi.** *Gastrointest Endosc* 1994, **49**:105–106. **[24].**
•• 
Sherman S, Rahaman S, Gottlieb K, Male R, Uzer M, Smith M, *et al.*: **Effect of Meperidine on Sphincter of Oddi Motility [Abstract].** *Gastrointest Endosc* 1994, **40**:P127. **[25].**
• 
Sherman S, Shaked A, Cryer HM, Goldstein LI, Busuttil RW: **Endoscopic Management of Biliary Fistulas Complicating Liver Transplantation and Other Hepatobiliary Operations.** *Ann Surg* 1993, **218**:167–175.

Silvis SE, Sievert CE, Vennes JA, Abeyta BK, Brennecke LH: **Comparison of Covered Versus Uncovered Wire Mesh Stents in the Canine Biliary Tract.** *Gastrointest Endosc* 1994, **140**:17–21. **[12].**
• 
Smith AC, Dowsett JF, Russell RCG, Hatfield ARW, Cotton PB: **Randomized Trial of Endoscopic Stenting Versus Surgical Bypass in Malignant Low Bile Duct Obstruction.** *Lancet* 1994, **344**:1655–1660. **[17].**
•• 
Smith MD, Robbins PD, Cullingford GL, Levitt MD: **Cholangiocarcinoma and Familial Adenomatous Polyposis.** *Aust N Z J Surg* 1993, **63**:324–327.

Soper NJ, Flye MW, Brunt LM, Stockmann PT, Sicard GA, Picus D, Edmundowicz SA, Aliperti G: **Diagnosis and Management of Biliary Complications of Laparoscopic Cholecystectomy.** *Am J Surg* 1993, **165**:663–669.

Springer DJ, Gaing AA, Siegel JH: **Radiologic Regression of Primary Sclerosing Cholangitis Following Combination Therapy with an Endoprosthesis and Ursodeoxycholic Acid.** *Am J Gastroenterol* 1993, **88**:1957–1959.

Sung JJY, Chung SCS, Tsui CP, Co AL, Li AKC: **Omitting Side-holes in Biliary Stents Does not Improve Drainage of the Obstructed Biliary System: a Prospective Randomized Trial.** *Gastrointest Endosc* 1994, **40**:321–325.

Tait NP: **Biliary Peritonitis Following Wallstent Insertion.** *Clin Radiol* 1993, **48**:210–212.

Tanaka K, Nishimura A, Yamada K, Ishibe R, Ishizaki N, Yoshimine M, Hamada N, Taira A: **Cancer of the Gallbladder Associated with Anomalous Junction of the Pancreatobiliary Duct System Without Bile Duct Dilatation.** *Br J Surg* 1993, **80**:622–624.

Theilmann L, Kuppers B, Kadmon M, Roeren T, Notheisen H, Stiehl A, *et al.*: **Biliary Tract Strictures after Orthoptic Liver Transplantation: Diagnosis and Management.** *Endoscopy* 1994, **26**:517–522. **[22].**
• 
Thervet L, Faulques B, Pissas A, Bremondy A, Monges B, Salducci J, Grimaud JC: **Endoscopic Management of Obstructive Jaundice Due to Portal Cavernoma.** *Endoscopy* 1993, **25**:423–425.

Thompson JF, Mathur MN, Coates AS: **Common Bile Duct Obstruction Due to Intraluminal Metastatic Melanoma.** *Aust N Z J Surg* 1993, **63**:502–504.

Tokunaga Y, Mukaihara S, Kubo S, Yang SM, Yo M, Nakayama H, Fujita T, Yokoyama T, Okamura R, Tanaka M, Noguchi M, Hayakawa K, Majima M: **Metallic Expanding Biliary Stents in Malignant Obstruction — Cases with Stent in Stent.** *J Clin Gastroenterol* 1993, **17**:153–157.

Traverso LW, Kozarek RA, Ball TJ, Brandabur JJ, Hunter JA, Jolly PC, Patterson DJ, Ryan JA, Thirlby RC, Wechter DG: **Endoscopic Retrograde Cholangiopancreatography after Laparoscopic Cholecystectomy.** *Am J Surg* 1993, **165**:581–586.

Van Der Hul RL, Plaisier PW, Lameris JS, Veeze-Kuijpers B, Van Blankenstein M, Terpstra OT: **Proximal Cholangiocarcinoma: a Multi-disciplinary Approach.** *Eur J Surg* 1994, **160**:213–218. **[15].**
• 
Vandenbosch RP, Van Der Schelling GP, Klinkenbijl JHG, Mulder PGH, Van Blankenstein M, Jeekel J: **Guidelines for the Application of Surgery and Endoprostheses in the Palliation of Obstructive Jaundice in Advanced Cancer of the Pancreas.** *Ann Surg* 1994, **219**:18–24.

Vansonnenberg E, Dagostino HB, Easter DW, Sanchez RB, Christensen RA, Kerlan RK, Moossa AR: **Complications of Laparoscopic Cholecystectomy — Coordinated Radiologic and Surgical Management in 21 Patients.** *Radiology* 1993, **188**:399–404.

Vanthiel DH, Fagiuoli S, Wright HI, Rodriguezrilo H, Silverman W: **Biliary Complications of Liver Transplantation [Review].** *Gastrointest Endosc* 1993, **39**:455–460.

Verstandig AG, Goldin E, Sasson T, Weinberger G, Wengrower D, Fich A, Lax E: **Combined Transhepatic and Endoscopic Procedures in the Biliary System.** *Postgrad Med J* 1993, **69**:384–388.

Vitale GC, Stephens G, Wienman TJ, Larson GM: **Use of Endoscopic Retrograde Cholangiopancreatography in the Management of Biliary Complications after Laparoscopic Cholecystectomy.** *Surgery* 1993, **114**:806-814. **[20].**
• 
Wagner HJ, Knyrim K, Vakil N, Klose KJ: **Plastic Endoprostheses Versus Metal Stents in the Palliative Treatment of Malignant Hilar Biliary Obstruction — a Prospective and Randomized Trial.** *Endoscopy* 1993, **25**:213–218.

Wagner HJ, Vakil N, Knyrim K: **Improved Biliary Stenting Using a Balloon Catheter and the Combined Technique for Difficult Stenoses.** *Gastrointest Endosc* 1993, **39**:688–693.

Wagner HJ, Werhand J, Schwerk WB, Rothmund M, Arnold R, Klose KJ: **Palliative Treatment of Complex Hilar Biliary Obstruction with Self-Expandable Metal Stents.** *Dtsch Med Wochenschr* 1993, **118**:1871–1877.

Wootton FT, Hoffman BJ, Cunningham JT: **A New Approach to Stenting a Tight, Angulated Post-Operative Biliary Stricture.** *Gastrointest Endosc* 1993, **39**:551–552.

Wu CS, Wu SS, Chen PC, Chiu CT, Lin SM, Jan YY, Hung CF: **Cholangiography of Icteric Type Hepatoma.** *Am J Gastroenterol* 1994, **89**:774–777.

Yau MP, Tsai CC, Mo LR, Lin RC, Kuo JY, Lin YW, Hwang MH: **Diagnostic and Therapeutic Interventions in Post-Laparoscopic Cholecystectomy Biliary Complications.** *Hepatogastroenterology* 1993, **40**:139–144.

Yeaton P, Kiss R, Deviere J, Salmon I, Bourgeois N, Pasteels JL, Cremer M: **Use of Cell Image Analysis in the Detection of Cancer from Specimens Obtained During Endoscopic Retrograde Cholangiopancreatography.** *Am J Clin Pathol* 1993, **100**:497–501.

## Laparoscopy

Apelgren KN, Scheeres DE: **Aortic Injury. A Catastrophic Complication of Laparoscopic Cholecystectomy.** *Surg Endosc* 1994, **8**:689–691. **[41].**
• 
Arnot RS: **Laparoscopy and Acalculous Cholecystitis.** *Aust N Z J Surg* 1994, **64**:405–406.

Babineau TJ, Lewis WD, Jenkins RL, Bleday R, Steele GD Jr, Forse RA: **Role of Staging Laparoscopy in the Treatment of Hepatic Malignancy.** *Am J Surg* 1994, **167**:151–155. **[6].**
•

Baigrie RJ, Krahenbuhl L, Dowling BL: **Laparoscopic Cholangiography Through the Gallbladder.** *J Am Coll Surg* 1994, **178**:175–176.

• Banwell PE, Hill ADK, Menzies-Gow N, Darzi A: **Laparoscopic Cholecystectomy: Safe and Feasible in Emphysematous Cholecystitis.** *Surg Laparosc Endosc* 1994, **4**:189–191. **[14].**

Barkun AN, Barkun JS, Fried GM, Ghitulescu G, Steinmetz O, Pham C, Meakins JL, Goresky CA: **Useful Predictors of Bile Duct Stones in Patients Undergoing Laparoscopic Cholecystectomy.** *Ann Surg* 1994, **220**:32–39.

Barkun JS, Fried GM, Barkun AN, Sigman HH, Hinchey EJ, Garzon J, Wexler MJ, Meakins JL: **Cholecystectomy Without Operative Cholangiography — Implications for Common Bile Duct Injury and Retained Common Bile Duct Stones.** *Ann Surg* 1993, **218**:371–379.

Battaglia SA, Pizzi WF, Khaneja SC, Bulauitan M: **Hepatic Duct Transection During Laparoscopic Cholecystectomy.** *Am Surg* 1993, **59**:664–665.

Berci G, Morgenstern L: **Laparoscopic Management of Common Bile Duct Stones — a Multi-Institutional SAGES Study.** *Surg Endosc* 1994, **8**:1168–1175.

Berry AR: **Bile Duct Injury after Laparoscopic Cholocystectomy [Letter].** *Gut* 1994, **35**:288.

• Berry SM, Ose KJ, Bell RH, Fink AS: **Thermal Injury of the Posterior Duodenum During Laparoscopic Cholecystectomy.** *Surg Endosc* 1994, **8**:197–200. **[38].**

Birkett DH: **3-D Imaging in Gastrointestinal Laparoscopy.** *Surg Endosc* 1993, **7**:556–557.

•• Bittner HB, Meyers WC, Brazer SR, Pappas TN: **Laparoscopic Nissen Fundoplication: Operative Results and Short-term Follow-up.** *Am J Surg* 1994, **167**:193–200. **[20].**

• Bloch P, Modiano P, Foster D, Bouhot F, Gompel H: **Recurrent Hemobilia after Laparoscopic Cholecystectomy.** *Surg Laparosc Endosc* 1994, **4**:375–377. **[39].**

Brandt CP, Priebe PP, Jacobs DG: **Value of Laparoscopy in Trauma ICU Patients with Suspected Acute Acalculous Cholecystitis.** *Surg Endosc* 1994, **8**:361–365.

Buckley RC, Hall TJ, Muakkassa FF, Anglin B, Rhodes RS, Scottconner CEH: **Laparoscopic Appendectomy: is it Worth It.** *Am Surg* 1994, **60**:30–34.

Byrne P, Nduka CC, Darzi A, Cameron A: **Teaching Laparoscopic Surgery [Letter].** *BMJ* 1994, **308**:1435.

• Callery MP, Aliperti G, Soper NJ: **Laparoscopic Duodenal Diverticulectomy Following Hemorrhage.** *Surg Laparosc Endosc* 1994, **4**:134–138. **[28].**

• Cappuccino H, Campanile F, Knecht J: **Laparoscopy-guided Drainage of Hepatic Abscess.** *Surg Laparosc Endosc* 1994, **4**:234–237. **[25].**

• Cappuccino H, Cargill N, Nguyen T: **Laparoscopic Cholecystectomy: 563 Cases at a Community Teaching Hospital and a Review of 12,201 Cases in the Literature.** *Surg Laparosc Endosc* 1994, **4**:213–221. **[12].**

• Cervantes J, Rojas GA, Ponte R: **Intrahepatic Subcapsular Biloma. A Rare Complication of Laparoscopic Cholecystectomy.** *Surg Endosc* 1994, **8**:208–210. **[37].**

Chan ACW, Shung SCS, Lau JWY, Brockwell J, Li MKW, Tate JJT, Au KT, Li AKC: **Laparoscopic Cholecystectomy: Results of First 300 Cases in Hong Kong.** *J R Coll Surg Edinb* 1994, **39**:26–30.

• Chardavoyne R, Wise L: **Exploratory Laparoscopy for Perforation Following Colonoscopy.** *Surg Laparosc Endosc* 1994, **4**:241–243. **[31].**

• Chu CM, Lin SM, Peng SM, Wu CS, Liaw YF: **The Role of Laparoscopy in the Evaluation of Ascites of Unknown Origin.** *Gastrointest Endosc* 1994, **40**:285–289. **[8].**

Cocks J, Johnson W, Cade R, Collopy B, Ewing H, Rogerson J, Rosengarten D, Thompson G, Turner P, Wale R, Davies E: **Bile Duct Injury During Laparoscopic Cholecystectomy — a Report of the Standards Sub-Committee of the Victorian State Committee of the Royal-Australasian-College-of-Surgeons.** *Aust N Z J Surg* 1993, **63**:682–683.

Cohen SA, Kasmin FE, Siegel JH, Cohen D: **ERCP after Laparoscopic Cholecystectomy [Letter].** *Gastrointest Endosc* 1994, **40**:255–256.

Collard JM, Degheldere CA, Dekock M, Otte JB, Kestens PJ: **Laparoscopic Antireflux Surgery — what is Real Progress?** *Ann Surg* 1994, **220**:146–154.

•• Corbitt Jr JD, Yusem SO: **Laparoscopic Cholecystectomy with Operative Cholangiogram.** *Surg Endosc* 1994, **8**:292–295. **[16].**

Corr P, Tate JJT, Lau WY, Dawson JW, Li AKC: **Preoperative Ultrasound to Predict Technical Difficulties and Complications of Laparoscopic Cholecystectomy.** *Am J Surg* 1994, **168**:54–56.

Cox MR, McCall JL, Wilson TG, Padbury RTA, Jeans PL, Toouli J: **Laparoscopic Appendicectomy: a Prospective Analysis.** *Aust N Z J Surg* 1993, **63**:840–847.

Cox MR, Wilson TG, Luck AJ, Jeans PL, Padbury RTA, Toouli J: **Laparoscopic Cholecystectomy for Acute Inflammation of the Gallbladder.** *Ann Surg* 1993, **218**:630–634.

•• Crantock LR, Dillon FJ, Hayes PC: **Diagnostic Laparoscopy in Liver Disease: Experience of 200 Cases.** *Aust N Z J Med* 1994, **24**:258–262. **[2].**

• Crockett HC, De Virgilio C, Shimaoka E, Bongard FS, Klein SR: **Acute Fatty Liver of Pregnancy: Laparoscopy-assisted Diagnosis.** *Surg Laparosc Endosc* 1994, **4**:230–233. **[11].**

Cuesta MA, Borgstein PJ, Meijer S: **Laparoscopy in the Diagnosis and Treatment of Acute Abdominal Conditions [Clinical Review].** *Eur J Surg* 1993, **159**:455–456.

Cuschieri A, Shimi S, Banting S, Nathanson LK, Pietrabissa A: **Intraoperative Cholangiography During Laparoscopic Cholecystectomy — Routine Vs Selective Policy.** *Surg Endosc* 1994, **8**:302–305.

Darzi A, Super P, Guillou PJ, Monson JRT: **Laparoscopic Sigmoid Colectomy: Total Laparoscopic Approach.** *Dis Colon Rectum* 1994, **37**:268–271.

Dunn D, Nair R, Fowler S, McCloy R: **Laparoscopic Cholecystectomy in England and Wales — Results of an Audit by the Royal College of Surgeons of England.** *Ann R Coll Surg Engl* 1994, **76**:269–275.

• Edelman DS: **Bile Leak from the Liver Bed Following Laparoscopic Cholecystectomy.** *Surg Endosc* 1994, **8**:205–207. **[36].**

• Eisenhauer DM, Saunders CJ, Ho HS, Wolfe BM: **Hemodynamic Effects of Argon Pneumoperitioneum.** *Surg Endosc* 1994, **8**:315–321. **[5].**

Elerding SC: **Laparoscopic Cholecystectomy in Pregnancy.** *Am J Surg* 1993, **165**:625–627.

• Felix EL, Michas CA, McKnight RL: **Laparoscopic Herniorrhaphy: Trans-abdominal Preperitoneal Floor Repair.** *Surg Endosc* 1994, **8**:100–104. **[18].**

• Felix EL, Michas CA, McKnight RL: **Laparoscopic Repair of Recurrent Groin Hernias.** *Surg Laparosc Endosc* 1994, **4**:200–204. **[19].**

Ferzli GS, Massaad A, Dysarz FA, Kopatsis A: **A Study of 101 Patients Treated with Extraperitoneal Endoscopic Laparoscopic Herniorrhaphy.** *Am Surg* 1993, **59**:707–708.

Ferzli GS, Massaad A, Kiel T, Worth MH: **The Utility of Laparoscopic Common Bile Duct Exploration in the Treatment of Choledocholithiasis.** *Surg Endosc* 1994, **8**:296–298.

Fielding GA, Orourke NA: **Laparoscopic Common Bile Duct Exploration.** *Aust N Z J Surg* 1993, **63**:113–115.

Fletcher DR: **Common Bile Duct Calculi at Laparoscopic Cholecystectomy — a Technique for Management.** *Aust N Z J Surg* 1993, **63**:710–714.

• Franklin Jr ME, Pharand D, Rosenthal D: **Laparoscopic Common Bile Duct Exploration.** *Surg Laparosc Endosc* 1994, **4**:119–124. **[17].**

Fried GM, Barkun JS, Sigman HH, Joseph L, Clas D, Garzon J, Hinchey EJ, Meakins JL: **Factors Determining Conversion to Laparotomy in Patients Undergoing Laparoscopic Cholecystectomy.** *Am J Surg* 1994, **167**:35–41.

•• Geagea T: **Laparoscopic Nissen–Rossetti Fundoplication.** *Surg Endosc* 1994, **8**:1080–1084. **[22].**

Geller AJ, Kolts BE, Achem SR, Wears R: **The High Frequency of Upper Gastrointestinal Pathology in Patients with Fecal Occult Blood and Colon Polyps.** *Am J Gastroenterol* 1993, **88**:1184–1187.

•• Genyk YS, Keller FS, Halpern NB: **Hepatic Artery Pseudoaneurysm and Hemobilia Following Laser Laparoscopic Cholecystectomy.** *Surg Endosc* 1994, **8**:201–204. **[40].**

• Goh PMY, Kum CK, Chia YW, Ti TK: **Laparoscopic Repair of Perforation of the Colon During Laparoscopy.** *Gastrointest Endosc* 1994, **40**:496–497. **[32].**

Halevy A, Golddeutch R, Negri M, Lin G, Shlamkovich N, Evans S, Cotariu D, Scapa E, Bahar M, Sackier JM: **Are Elevated Liver Enzymes and Bilirubin Levels Significant after Laparoscopic Cholecystectomy in the Absence of Bile Duct Injury.** *Ann Surg* 1994, **219**:362–364.

• Heinzelmann M, Schob O,Schlumpf R, Decurtins M, Himmelmann A, Largiader F: **Preoperative Diagnosis of Meckel's Diverticulum by Pertechnetate Scan and Laparoscopic Resection.** *Surg Laparosc Endosc* 1994, **4**:378–381. **[29].**

Horvath KD: **Strategies for the Prevention of Laparoscopic Common Bile Duct Injuries [Review].** *Surg Endosc* 1993, **7**:439–444.

Huang SM, Wu CW, Hong HT, Liu M, King KL, Lui WY: **Bile Duct Injury and Bile Leakage in Laparoscopic Cholecystectomy.** *Br J Surg* 1993, **80**:1590–1592.

Hutchinson CH, Traverso LW, Lee FT: **Laparoscopic Cholecystectomy — do Preoperative Factors Predict the Need to Convert to Open.** *Surg Endosc* 1994, **8**:875–878.

• Isaac J, Tekant Y, Kong KC, Ngoi SS, Goh P: **Laparoscopic Repair of Perforated Duodenal Ulcer.** *Gastrointest Endosc* 1994, **40**:68–69. **[30].**

• Jahns F, Reddy V, Sherman KE: **Ascites Secondary to Renal-cell Carcinoma Diagnosed at Laparoscopy.** *J Clin Gastroenterol* 1994, **18**:259–260. **[7].**

Jamieson GG, Watson DI, Brittenjones R, Mitchell PC, Anvari M: **Laparoscopic Nissen Fundoplication.** *Ann Surg* 1994, **220**:137–145.

• Jeffers LJ, Alzate I, Aguilar H, Reddy KR, Idrovo V, Cheinquer H, *et al.*: **Laparoscopic and Histologic Findings in Patients with the Human Immunodeficiency Virus.** *Gastrointest Endosc* 1994, **40**:160–164. **[10].**

John TG, Garden OJ: **Laparoscopic Ultrasonography — Extending the Scope of Diagnostic Laparoscopy.** *Br J Surg* 1994, **81**:5–6.

•• John TG, Greig JD, Crosbie JL: **Superior Staging of Liver Tumors with Laparoscopy and Laparoscopic Ultrasound.** *Ann Surg* 1994, **220**:711–719. **[9].**

Jorgensen JO, Hunt DR: **Laparoscopic Management of Pneumatic Dilatation Resistant Achalasia.** *Aust N Z J Surg* 1993, **63**:386–388.

• Khoury G, Geagea T, Hajj A, Jabbour-Khoury S, Baraka A, Nabbout G: **Laparoscopic Treatment of Hydatid Cysts of the Liver.** *Surg Endosc* 1994, **8**:1103–1104. **[26].**

• Kraemer SJM, Aye R, Kozarek RA, Hill LD: **Laparoscopic Hill Repair.** *Gastrointest Endosc* 1994, **40**:155-159. **[21].**

• Kum CK, Goh PMY: **Laparoscopic Cholecystectomy: the Singapore Experience.** *Surg Laparosc Endosc* 1994, **4**:22–24. **[13].**

• Libutti SK, Starker PM: **Laparoscopic Resection of a Nonparasitic Liver Cyst.** *Surg Endosc* 1994, **8**:1105–1107. **[27].**

MacIntyre IMC, Wilson RG: **Laparoscopic Cholecystectomy [Review].** *Br J Surg* 1993, **80**:552–559.

McAnena OJ, Willson PD: **Diathermy in Laparoscopic Surgery.** *Br J Surg* 1993, **80**:1094–1096.

McMahon AJ, Baxter JN, Odwyer PJ: **Preventing Complications of Laparoscopy.** *Br J Surg* 1993, **80**:1593–1594.

Modesto VL, Harkins B, Calton WC, Martindale RG: **Laparoscopic Gastrostomy Using Four-Point Fixation.** *Am J Surg* 1994, **167**:273–276.

Moran J, Delgrosso E, Wills JS, Hagy JA, Baker R: **Laparoscopic Cholecystectomy — Imaging of Complications and Normal Postoperative CT Appearance.** *Abdom Imaging* 1994, **19**:143–146.

Morgenstern L, Berci G, Pasternak EH: **Bile Leakage after Biliary Tract Surgery — a Laparoscopic Perspective [Review].** *Surg Endosc* 1993, **7**:432–438.

Murison MSC, Gartell PC, McGinn FP: **Does Selective Peroperative Cholangiography Result in Missed Common Bile Duct Stones?** *J R Coll Surg Edinb* 1993, **38**:220–224.

•• Musser DJ, Boorse RC, Madera F, Reed III JF: **Laparoscopic Colectomy: at what Cost?** *Surg Laparosc Endosc* 1994, **4**:1–5. **[23].**

Newman L, Newman C, Baird DR, Eubanks S, Mason E, Duncan T, Lucas GW: **An Institutional Review of the Management of Choledocholithiasis in 1616 Patients Undergoing Laparoscopic Cholecystectomy.** *Am Surg* 1994, **60**:273–277.

Orlando R, Russell JC, Lynch J, Mattie A, Rattner, Brooks DC, Braasch JW, Quinlan RM, Dunlop GR: **Laparoscopic Cholecystectomy — a Statewide Experience.** *Arch Surg* 1993, **128**:494–499.

Patel JC, McInnes GC, Bagley JS, Needham G, Krukowski ZH: **The Role of Intravenous Cholangiography in Pre-Operative Assessment for Laparoscopic Cholecystectomy.** *Br J Radiol* 1993, **66**:1125–1127.

Patterson M, Walters D, Browder W: **Postoperative Bowel Obstruction Following Laparoscopic Surgery.** *Am Surg* 1993, **59**:656–657.

Peters JH, Miller J, Nichols KE, Ollila D, Avrodopolous D: **Laparoscopic Cholecystectomy in Patients Admitted with Acute Biliary Symptoms.** *Am J Surg* 1993, **166**:300–303.

• Peters JH, Ollila D, Nichols KE, Gibbons GD, Dvanzo MA, Miller J, *et al.*: **Diagnosis and Management of Bile Leaks Following Laparoscopic Cholecystectomy.** *Surg Laparosc Endosc* 1994, **4**:163–170. **[35].**

Phillips E, Pleatman MA, Saxe A: **A 2-Person, 2-Handed Technique for Laparoscopic Cholecystectomy.** *Am Surg* 1993, **59**:639–641.

Phillips EH, Carroll BJ, Fallas MJ: **Laparoscopically Guided Cholecystectomy — a Detailed Report of the First 453 Cases Performed by One Surgical Team.** *Am Surg* 1993, **59**:235–242.

Qureshi MA, Brindley NM, Osborne DH, Bouchierhayes DJ, Burke PE, Leahy AL, Broe PJ, Grace PA: **Post-Cholecystectomy Symptoms after Laparoscopic Cholecystectomy.** *Ann R Coll Surg Engl* 1993, **75**:349–353.

• Rademaker BM, Odom JA, DeWitt LTH: **Hemodynamic Effects of Pneumoperitoneum for Laparoscopic Surgery: a comparison of CO2 with N2O Insufflation.** *Eur J Anesth* 1984, **11**:301–305. **[3].**

Ress AM, Sarr MG, Nagorney DM, Farnell MB, Donohue JH, McIlrath DC: **Spectrum and Management of Major Complications of Laparoscopic Cholecystectomy.** *Am J Surg* 1993, **165**:655–662.

Richardson AJ, Brancatisano R, Avramovic J, Roney W, Little JM: **Injuries to the Bile Duct Resulting from Laparoscopic Cholecystectomy.** *Aust N Z J Surg* 1993, **63**:684–689.

Roberts RH, Pettigrew RA, Vanrij AM: **Bile Leakage after Laparoscopic Cholecystectomy — Biliary Anatomy Revisited.** *Aust N Z J Surg* 1994, **64**:254–257.

Ronning H, Raundahl U, Kiil J: **Temporary use of a Biliary Endoprosthesis for Unsuspected Bile Duct Stones Found at Laparoscopic Cholecystectomy.** *Br J Surg* 1993, **80**:1443–1444.

Salky B, Bauer J: **Intravenous Cholangiography, ERCP, and Selective Operative Cholangiography in the Performance of Laparoscopic Cholecystectomy.** *Surg Endosc* 1994, **8**:289–291.

Salky BA: **Laparoscopic Management of Common Bile Duct Stones.** *Surg Endosc* 1994, **8**:1161–1162.

• Sardi A, McKinnon WMP: **Laparoscopic Adrenalectomy in Patients with Primary Aldosteronism.** *Surg Laparosc Endosc* 1994, **4**:86–91. **[24].**

•• Schier F, Waldschmidt J: **Laparoscopic in Children with Ill-defined Abdominal Pain.** *Surg Endosc* 1994, **8**:97–99. **[33].**

•• Schrenk P, Woisetschdlger R, Wayand WU: **Diagnostic Laparoscopy: Survey of 92 Patients.** *Am J Surg* 1994, **168**:348–351. **[1].**

See WA, Cooper CS, Fisher RJ: **Predictors of Laparoscopic Complications after Formal Training in Laparoscopic Surgery.** *JAMA* 1993, **270**:2689–2692.

Smith RS, Fry WR, Tsoi EKM, Henderson VJ, Hirvela ER, Koehler RH, Brams DM, Morabito DJ, Peskin GW: **Gasless Laparoscopy and Conventional Instruments — the Next Phase of Minimally Invasive Surgery.** *Arch Surg* 1993, **128**:1102–1107.

Soper NJ, Brunt LM, Callery MP, Edmundowicz SA, Aliperti G: **Role of Laparoscopic Cholecystectomy in the Management of Acute Gallstone Pancreatitis.** *Am J Surg* 1994, **167**:42–51.

Sosa JL, Sleeman D, Puente I, McKenney MG, Hartmann R: **Laparoscopic-Assisted Colostomy Closure after Hartmanns Procedure.** *Dis Colon Rectum* 1994, **37**:149–152.

Standsby G, Davidson B, Hobbs KEF: **Delayed Diagnosis of Biliary Leak Due to Bile Duct Division During Cholecystectomy.** *J R Coll Surg Edinb* 1994, **39**:49–50.

•• Steiner CA, Bass EB, Talamini MA, Pitt HA, Steinberg EP: **Surgical Rates and Operative Mortality for Open and Laparoscopic Cholecystectomy in Maryland.** *N Engl J Med* 1994, **330**:403–408. **[15].**

Sugrue M: **Prospective Comparison of Laparoscopic and Conventional Anterior Resection [Letter].** *Br J Surg* 1994, **81**:625.

Taylor TV, Bhandarkar DS: **Laparoscopic Vagotomy — an Operation for the 1990s.** *Ann R Coll Surg Engl* 1993, **75**:385–386.

Trondsen E, Reiertsen O, Andersen OK, Kjaersgaard P: **Laparoscopic and Open Cholecystectomy — a Prospective, Randomized Study.** *Eur J Surg* 1993, **159**:217–221.

Vallina VL, Velasco JM, McCulloch CS: **Laparoscopic Versus Conventional Appendectomy.** *Ann Surg* 1993, **218**:685–692.

Vanbeers BE, Lacrosse M, Trigaux JP, Decanniere L, Deronde T, Pringot J: **Noninvasive Imaging of the Biliary Tree Before or after Laparoscopic Cholecystectomy: use of Three-dimensional Spiral CT Cholangiography.** *AJR Am J Roentgenol* 1994, **162**:1331–1335.

Vancampenhout I, Prosmanne O, Gagner M, Pomp A, Deslandres E, Levesque HP: **Routine Operative Cholangiography During Laparoscopic Cholecystectomy — Feasibility and Value in 107 Patients.** *AJR Am J Roentgenol* 1993, **160**:1209–1211.

Velanovich V, Kaufmann C: **Two Pitfalls of Laparoscopic Balloon Cholangiography — Recognition and Correction.** *Am Surg* 1993, **59**:290–292.

Voyles CR, Sanders DL, Hogan R: **Common Bile Duct Evaluation in the Era of Laparoscopic Cholecystectomy — 1050 Cases Later.** *Ann Surg* 1994, **219**:744–752.

Wachsberg RH, Cho KC, Raina S: **Liver Infarction Following Unrecognized Right Hepatic Artery Ligation at Laparoscopic Cholecystectomy.** *Abdom Imaging* 1994, **19**:53–54.

Watson DI, Reed MWR, Johnson AG, Stoddard CJ: **Laparoscopic Fundoplication for Gastro-Oesophageal Reflux.** *Ann R Coll Surg Engl* 1994, **76**:264–268.

Wayand WU, Gitter T, Woisetschlager R: **Laparoscopic Cholecystectomy: the Austrian Experience.** *J R Coll Surg Edinb* 1993, **38**:152–153.

• Whitley MS, Laws SAM, Wise MH: **Use of a hand-held Doppler to Avoid Abdominal Wall Vessels in Laparoscopic Surgery.** *Ann R Coll Surg Engl* 1994, **76**:348–350. **[4].**

Windsor JA, Vokes DE: **Early Laparoscopic Biliary Injury: Experience in New Zealand.** *Br J Surg* 1994, **81**:1208–1211.

•• Woods MS, Traverso LW, Kozarek RA, Tsao J, Rossi RL, Gough D, *et al.*: **Characteristics of Biliary Tract Complications During Laparoscopic Cholecystectomy: a multi-institutional Study.** *Am J Surg* 1994, **167**:27–34. **[34].**

Woods SDS, Polglase AL: **Laparoscopically Assisted Anterior Resection for Villous Adenoma of the Rectum.** *Aust N Z J Surg* 1993, **63**:146–148.


## Paediatric endoscopy


Albanese CT, Towbin RB, Ulman I, Lewis J, Smith SD: **Percutaneous Gastrojejunostomy Versus Nissen Fundoplication for Enteral Feeding of the Neurologically Impaired Child with Gastroesophageal Reflux.** *J Pediatr* 1993, **123**:371–375.

Ashorn M, Ruuska T, Karikoski R, Valipakka J, Maki M: **Gastric Mucosal Cell Densities in Helicobacter Pylori-Positive and -Negative Dyspeptic Children and Healthy Controls.** *J Pediatr Gastroenterol Nutr* 1994, **18**:146–151.

Bahalomara N, Nahata MC, Murray RD, Linscheid TR, Williams T, Heitlinger LA, Li BUK, McClung HJ, Lininger B: **Efficacy of Diazepam and Meperidine in Ambulatory Pediatric Patients Undergoing Endoscopy — a Randomized, Double-Blind Trial.** *J Pediatr Gastroenterol Nutr* 1993, **16**:387–392.

Benninga MA, Wijers OB, Vanderhoeven CWP, Taminiau JAJM, Klopper PJ, Tytgat GNJ, Akkermans LMA: **Manometry, Profilometry, and Endosonography — Normal Physiology and Anatomy of the Anal Canal in Healthy Children.** *J Pediatr Gastroenterol Nutr* 1994, **18**:68–77.

Bertoni G, Pacchione D, Sassatelli R, Ricci E, Mortilla MG, Gumina C: **A New Protector Device for Safe Endoscopic Removal of Sharp Gastroesophageal Foreign Bodies in Infants.** *J Pediatr Gastroenterol Nutr* 1993, **16**:393–396.

Brown CW, Werlin SL, Geenen JE, Schmalz M: **The Diagnostic and Therapeutic Role of Endoscopic Retrograde Cholangiopancreatography in Children.** *J Pediatr Gastroenterol Nutr* 1993, **17**:19–23.

Chan KL, Saing H: **Balloon Catheter Dilatation of Peptic Pyloric Stenosis in Children.** *J Pediatr Gastroenterol Nutr* 1994, **18**:465–468.

Colombo C, Bertolini E, Assaisso ML, Bettinardi N, Giunta A, Podda M: **Failure of Ursodeoxycholic Acid to Dissolve Radiolucent Gallstones in Patients with Cystic Fibrosis.** *Acta Paediatr* 1993, **82**:562–565.

Crombleholme TM, Jacir NN: **Simplified Push Technique for Percutaneous Endoscopic Gastrostomy in Children.** *J Pediatr Surg* 1993, **28**:1393–1395.

Czinn SJ: **Editorial — Dyspepsia in Children.** *J Pediatr Gastroenterol Nutr* 1993, **17**:237–238.

• De Backer A, Bove T, Vandenplas Y, Peeters S, Deconinck P: **Contribution of Endoscopy to Early Diagnosis of Hypertrophic Pyloric Stenosis.** *J Pediatr Gastroenterol Nutr* 1994, **18**:78–81. **[8].**

• de Boissieu D, Dupont C, Barbet JP, Bargaoui K, Badoual J: **Distinct Features of Upper Gastrointestinal Endoscopy in the Newborn.** *J Pediatr Gastroenterol Nutr* 1994, **18**:334–338. **[3].**

• De Giacomo C, Gianatti A, Negrini R, Perotti P, Bawa P, Maggiore G, *et al.*: **Lymphocytic Gastritis: a positive Relationship with Celiac Disease.** *J Pediatr* 1994, **124**:57–62. **[26].**

Debray D, Pariente D, Urvoas E, Hadchouel M, Bernard O: **Sclerosing Cholangitis in Children.** *J Pediatr* 1994, **124**:49–56.

Dowd MD: **Radiological Cases of the Month — Case 2 — Esophageal Coins.** *Arch Pediatr Adolesc Med* 1994, **148**:423–424.

Ellenhorn JDI, Lambroza A, Lindsley KL, Laquaglia MP: **Treatment-Related Esophageal Stricture in Pediatric Patients with Cancer.** *Cancer* 1993, **71**:4084–4090.

Emblem R, Diseth T, Morkrid L, Stien R, Bjordal R: **Anal Endosonography and Physiology in Adolescents with Corrected Low Anorectal Anomalies.** *J Pediatr Surg* 1994, **29**:447–451.

Faure C, Ategbo S, Ferreira GC, Cargill G, Bellaiche M, Boige N, Viarme F, Aigrain Y, Cezard JP, Navarro J: **Duodenal and Esophageal Manometry in Total Colonic Aganglionosis.** *J Pediatr Gastroenterol Nutr* 1994, **18**:193–199.

Foy TM, Hawkins EP, Peters KR, Shearer WT, Ferry GD: **Colonic Ulcers and Lower GI Bleeding Due to Disseminated Aspergillosis.** *J Pediatr Gastroenterol Nutr* 1994, **18**:399–403.

• Garau P, Orenstein SR, Neigut DA, Putnam PE, Reyes J, Tzakis AG, *et al.*: **Role of Endoscopy Following Small Intestinal Transplantation in Children.** *Transplant Proc* 1994, **26**:136–137. **[27].**

Gilger MA, Jeiven SD, Barrish JO, McCarroll LR: **Oxygen Desaturation and Cardiac Arrhythmias in Children During Esophagogastroduodenoscopy Using Conscious Sedation.** *Gastrointest Endosc* 1993, **39**:392–395.

Grosfeld JL, Rescorla FJ, Skinner MA, West KW, Scherer LR: **The Spectrum of Biliary Tract Disorders in Infants and Children — Experience with 300 Cases.** *Arch Surg* 1994, **129**:513–520.

Guelrud M, Mujica C, Jaen D, Machuca J, Essenfeld H: **Prevalence of Helicobacter-Pylori in Neonates and Young Infants Undergoing ERCP for Diagnosis of Neonatal Cholestasis.** *J Pediatr Gastroenterol Nutr* 1994, **18**:461–464.

•• Guelrud M, Mujica C, Jaen D, Plaz J, Arias J: **The Role of ERCP in the Diagnosis and the Treatment of Idiopathic Recurrent Pancreatitis.** *Gastrointest Endosc* 1994, **40**:428–436. **[38].**

Gunasekaran TS, Hassall EG: **Efficacy and Safety of Omeprazole for Severe Gastroesophageal Reflux in Children.** *J Pediatr* 1993, **123**:148–154.

Hassall E: **Barretts Esophagus — an Unlikely Diagnosis in Infants and Young Children [Letter].** *Am J Gastroenterol* 1994, **89**:287.

Holcomb GW, Naffis D: **Laparoscopic Cholecystectomy in Infants.** *J Pediatr Surg* 1994, **29**:86–87.

Holcomb GW, Sharp KW, Neblett WW, Morgan WM, Pietsch JB: **Laparoscopic Cholecystectomy in Infants and Children: Modifications and Cost Analysis.** *J Pediatr Surg* 1994, **29**:900–904.

•• Israel DM, McLain BI, Hassal E: **Successful Pancolonoscopy and Ileoscopy in Children.** *J Pediatr Gastroenterol Nutr* 1994, **19**:283–289. **[2].**

Kautz G: **Indications, Results and Complications of ERCP in Childhood and Youth.** *Z Gastroenterol* 1993, **31**:742–750.

Kim I-O, Yeon KM, Kim WS, Park KW, Kim JH, Han MC: **Perforation Complicating Balloon Dilation of Esophageal Strictures in Infants and Children.** *Radiology* 1993, **189**:741–744.

Kose G, Ozkan H, Ozdamar F, Kavukcu S, Ozaksoy D: **Cholelithiasis in Cervico-Oculo-Acoustic (Wildervancks) Syndrome.** *Acta Paediatr* 1993, **82**:890–891.

Kozarek RA, Christie D, Barclay G: **Endoscopic Therapy of Pancreatitis in the Pediatric Population.** *Gastrointest Endosc* 1993, **39**:665–669.

Lang T, Berquist W, Rich E, Cox K, Devries P, Cahill J, Baker E, Gish R: **Treatment of Recurrent Pancreatitis by Endoscopic Drainage of a Duodenal Duplication.** *J Pediatr Gastroenterol Nutr* 1994, **18**:494–496.

•• Machida HM, Catto Smith AG, Gall DG, Trevenen C, Scott RB: **Allergic Colitis in Infancy: Clinical and Pathologic Aspects.** *J Pediatr Gastroenterol Nutr* 1994, **19**:22–26. **[32].**

Marin OE, Glassman MS, Schoen BT, Caplan DB: **Safety and Efficacy of Percutaneous Endoscopic Gastrostomy in Children.** *Am J Gastroenterol* 1994, **89**:357–361.

Mohan P, Holcomb GW, Ziegler MM: **Recurrent Jaundice and Pancreatitis in a Child with Pancreatobiliary Duct Anomalies.** *J Pediatr Gastroenterol Nutr* 1994, **18**:386–390.

• Murphy S, Shaw K, Blanchard H: **Report of Three Gastric Tumors in Children.** *J Pediatr Surg* 1994, **29**:1202–1204. **[17].**

Orloff MJ, Orloff MS, Rambotti M: **Treatment of Bleeding Esophagogastric Varices Due to Extrahepatic Portal Hypertension — Results of Portal-Systemic Shunts During 35 Years.** *J Pediatr Surg* 1994, **29**:142–154.

Othersen HB, Ocampo RJ, Parker EF, Smith CD, Tagge EP: **Barrett's Esophagus in Children — Diagnosis and Management.** *Ann Surg* 1993, **217**:676–681.

Pobiel RS, Bissett GS III, Pobiel MS: **Nasojejunal Feeding Tube Placement in Children: Four-Year Cumulative Experience.** *Radiology* 1994, **190**:127–130.

Reyes GA, Fowler CL, Pokorny WJ: **Pancreatic Anatomy in Children — Emphasis on Its Importance to Pancreatectomy.** *J Pediatr Surg* 1993, **28**:712–715.

• Ruuska T, Vaajalahti P, Arajarvi P, Maki M: **Prospective Evaluation of Upper Gastrointestinal Mucosal Lesions in Children with Ulcerative Colitis and Crohn's Disease.** *J Pediatr Gastroenterol Nutr* 1994, **19**:181–186. **[28].**

Sachdeva R, Yapor M, Schwersenz A, Mitty H, Norton K, Rosh J, Borcich A, Benkov K, Leleiko NS: **Massive Variceal Bleeding Caused by a Hepatic-Artery Portal-Vein Fistula — a Manifestation of Hepatocellular Carcinoma in a 12-Year-Old.** *J Pediatr Gastroenterol Nutr* 1993, **16**:468–471.

Stoker J, Lameris JS, Robben SGF, Dees J, Sinaasappel M: **Primary Sclerosing Cholangitis in a Child Treated by Nonsurgical Balloon Dilatation and Stenting.** *J Pediatr Gastroenterol Nutr* 1993, **17**:303–306.

Treem WR, Etienne NL, Hyams JS: **Percutaneous Endoscopic Placement of the Button Gastrostomy Tube as the Initial Procedure in Infants and Children.** *J Pediatr Gastroenterol Nutr* 1993, **17**:382–386.

Tulman S, Holcomb GW, Karamanoukian HL, Reynhout J: **Pediatric Laparoscopic Splenectomy.** *J Pediatr Surg* 1993, **28**:689–692.

Wilson C: **Who Should Perform Pediatric Endoscopic Sedation [Letter].** *J Pediatr Gastroenterol Nutr* 1994, **18**:114.


## Colonoscopy and sigmoidoscopy


Abdulian JD, Santoro MJ, Chen YK, Collen MJ: **Diculafoy-Like Lesion of the Rectum Presenting with Exsanguinating Hemorrhage — Successful Endoscopic Sclerotherapy.** *Am J Gastroenterol* 1993, **88**:1939–1941.

Agre P, Kurtz RC, Krauss BJ: **A Randomized Trial Using Videotape to Present Consent Information for Colonoscopy.** *Gastrointest Endosc* 1994, **40**:271–276.

• Axon ATR: **Cancer Surveillance in Ulcerative Colitis — a Time for Reappraisal.** *Gut* 1994, **35**:587–589. **[31].**

Balthazar EJ, Megibow AJ, Barry M, Opulencia JF: **Histoplasmosis of the Colon in Patients with AIDS — Imaging Findings in 4 Cases.** *AJR Am J Roentgenol* 1993, **161**:585–587.

Barillari P, Calcaterra D, Cesareo S, Cioe I, Bovino A, Cerasi A, Sammartino P: **Colonoscopy in Follow-Up of Patients with Coloredtal Cancer: Results of a Randomised Trial.** *Coloproctology* 1994, **16**:48–55.

•• Bernstein C, Shanahan F, Weinstein WM: **Are we Telling the Truth About Surveillance Colonoscopy in Ulcerative Colitis?** *Lancet* 1994, **343**:71–74. **[29].**

Berry MA, Dipalma JA: **Review Article — Orthograde Gut Lavage for Colonoscopy.** *Aliment Pharmacol Ther* 1994, **8**:391–395.

Botoman VA, Pietro M, Thirlby RC: **Localization of Colonic Lesions with Endoscopic Tattoo.** *Dis Colon Rectum* 1994, **37**:775–776.

Brewster NT, Grieve DC, Saunders JH: **Double-Contrast Barium Enema and Flexible Sigmoidoscopy for Routine Colonic Investigation.** *Br J Surg* 1994, **81**:445–447.

• Cadranel JF, Benhamou Y, Zylberberg P, Novello P, Luciani F, Valla D, *et al.*: **Hypnotic Relaxation: a new Sedative Tool for Colonoscopy.** *J Clin Gastroenterol* 1994, **18**:127–129. **[8].**

Cappell MS: **Safety and Clinical Efficacy of Flexible Sigmoidoscopy and Colonoscopy for Gastrointestinal Bleeding after Myocardial Infarction: a 6-Year Study of 18 Consecutive Lower Endoscopies at 2 University Teaching Hospitals.** *Dig Dis Sci* 1994, **39**:473–480.

• Carbonnel F, Lavergne A, Lemann M, Bitoun A, Valleur P, Hautefeuille P, *et al.*: **Colonoscopy of Acute Colitis.** *Dig Dis Sci* 1994, **39**:1550–1557. **[17].**

Choi PM, Nugent FW, Schoetz DJ, Silverman ML, Haggitt RC: **Colonoscopic Surveillance Reduces Mortality from Colorectal Cancer in Ulcerative Colitis.** *Gastroenterology* 1993, **105**:418–424.

Chun D, Chandrasoma P, Kiyabu M: **Fulminant Amebic Colitis — a Morphologic Study of Four Cases.** *Dis Colon Rectum* 1994, **37**:535–539.

Church JM: **Complete Colonoscopy — How Often — and if Not, Why Not.** *Am J Gastroenterol* 1994, **89**:556–560.

Clarkston WK, Smith OJ: **The use of GoLYTELY and Dulcolax in Combination in Outpatient Colonoscopy.** *J Clin Gastroenterol* 1993, **17**:146–148.

•• Cohen SM, Wexner SD, Binderow SR, Nogueras JJ, Daniel NRN, Ehrenpreis ED, *et al.*: **Prospective, Randomized, Endoscopic-blinded Trial Comparing Precolonoscopy Bowel Cleansing Methods.** *Dis Colon Rectum* 1994, **37**:689–696. **[1].**

Colin R, Hochain P, Czernichow P, Petit A, Manchon N-D, Berkelmans I: **Non-Steroidal Anti-Inflammatory Drugs and Segmental Non-Gangrenous Colitis: a Case-Control Study.** *Eur J Gastroenterol Hepatol* 1993, **5**:715–720.

Corman ML: **Understanding Surveillance Colonoscopy.** *Lancet* 1994, **343**:556.

•• Eckardt VF, Stamm H, Kanzler G, Bernhard G: **Improved Survival after Colorectal Cancer in Patients Complying with a Postoperative Endoscopic Surveillance Program.** *Endoscopy* 1994, **26**:523–527. **[33].**

Eu KW, Teoh TA: **Delayed Perforation of the Colon Following Colonoscopic Biopsy [Letter].** *Br J Surg* 1994, **81**:311.

Ferraro FJ, Livingston DH, Odom J, Swan KG, McCormack M, Rush BF: **The Role of Sigmoidoscopy in the Management of Gunshot Wounds to the Buttocks.** *Am Surg* 1993, **59**:350–352.

Gomezrubio M, Decuenca B, Opio V, Ulloa J, Garcia J: **Colonic Tuberculosis — an Unusual Endoscopic Diagnosis.** *Endoscopy* 1993, **25**:377.

Gostout CJ: **Colonic Findings in Cirrhotics with Portal Hypertension: a Prospective Colonoscopic and Histological Study — Comment.** *J Clin Gastroenterol* 1994, **18**:329.

Harris MT, Laudito A, Waye JD: **Colonoscopic Features of Colonic Anastomoses.** *Gastrointest Endosc* 1994, **40**:554–557.

Heath B, Rogers A, Taylor A, Lavergne J: **Splenic Rupture — an Unusual Complication of Colonoscopy.** *Am J Gastroenterol* 1994, **89**:449–450.

Herman LL, Kurtz RC, McKee KJ, Sun M, Thaler HT, Winawer SJ: **Risk Factors Associated with Vasovagal Reactions During Colonoscopy.** *Gastrointest Endosc* 1993, **39**:388–391.

Itabashi M, Hamano K, Kameoka S, Asahina K: **Self-Expanding Stainless Steel Stent Application in Rectosigmoid Stricture.** *Dis Colon Rectum* 1993, **36**:508–511.

Jayanthi V, Chuah SY, Probert CSJ, Mayberry M, Mayberry JF: **Proctitis and Proctosigmoiditis — a Need to Identify the Extent of Disease in Epidemiological Surveys.** *Digestion* 1993, **54**:61–64.

Jentschura D, Raute M, Winter J, Henkel T, Kraus M, Manegold BC: **Complications in Endoscopy of the Lower Gastrointestinal Tract — Therapy and Prognosis.** *Surg Endosc* 1994, **8**:672–676.

Johnson DL, Lang E: **Technical Aspects of Nonoperative Dilation of a Complex Colon Anastomotic Stricture.** *Dig Dis Sci* 1993, **38**:1929–1932.

Jonsson B, Ahsgren L, Andersson LO, Stenling R, Rutegard J: **Colorectal Cancer Surveillance in Patients with Ulcerative Colitis.** *Br J Surg* 1994, **81**:689–691.

Kasmin FE, Cohen SA, Siegel JH: **Passage of the Colonoscope "over the Forceps" to Achieve Total Colonoscopy in Difficult Cases.** *Endoscopy* 1994, **26**:330–331.

Kim YI, Marcon NE: **Injection Therapy for Colonic Diverticular Bleeding — a Case Study.** *J Clin Gastroenterol* 1993, **17**:46–48.

Kolts BE, Lyles WE, Achem SR, Burton L, Geller AJ, Macmath T: **A Comparison of the Effectiveness and Patient Tolerance of Oral Sodium Phosphate, Castor Oil, and Standard Electrolyte Lavage for Colonoscopy or Sigmoidoscopy Preparation.** *Am J Gastroenterol* 1993, **88**:1218–1223.

Koobatian GJ, Choi PM: **Safety of Surveillance Colonoscopy in Long-standing Ulcerative Colitis.** *Am J Gastroenterol* 1994, **89**:1472–1475.

• Kundrotas LW, Clement DJ, Kubik C, Robinson AB, Phillip AW: **A Prospective Evaluation of Successful Terminal Ileum Intubation During Routine Colonoscopy.** *Gastrointest Endosc* 1994, **40**:544–546. **[13].**

• Lazzoroni M, Petrillo M, Desideri S, Bianchi Porro G: **Efficacy and Tolerability of Polyethylene-glycol-electrolyte Lavage Solution with and Without Simethicone in the Preparation of Patients with Inflammatory Bowel Disease for Colonoscopy.** *Aliment Pharmacol Ther* 1993, **7**:655–659. **[3].**

Lindblom A, Jansson O, Jeppsson B, Tornebrandt K, Benoni C, Hedenbro JL: **Nitrous Oxide for Colonoscopy Discomfort: a Randomized Double-blind Study.** *Endoscopy* 1994, **26**:283–286.

Lo AY, Beaton HL: **Selective Management of Colonoscopic Perforations.** *J Am Coll Surg* 1994, **179**:333–337.

Lycke KG, Gothlin JH, Jensen JK, Philipson BM, Kock NG: **Comparison Between Radiologic and Endoscopic Evaluation of the Continent Ileostomy Reservoir.** *Scand J Gastroenterol* 1993, **28**:1115–1120.

Lynch DAF, Lobo AJ, Sobala GM, Dixon MF, Axon ATR: **Failure of Colonoscopic Surveillance in Ulcerative Colitis.** *Gut* 1993, **34**:1075–1080.

Maciel J, Barbosa J, Junior A: **Endoscopic Nd-YAG Laser Surgery in the Treatment of Villous Adenomas of the Rectum.** *Hepatogastroenterology* 1994, **41**:58–60.

Makela JT, Kiviniemi H, Laitinen S, Kairaluoma MI: **Diagnosis and Treatment of Acute Lower Gastrointestinal Bleeding.** *Scand J Gastroenterol* 1993, **28**:1062–1066.

Markoglou C, Avgerinos A, Mitrakou M, Sava S, Prigouris S, Hatziyoannou J, Raptis S: **Toxic Megacolon Secondary to Acute Ischemic Colitis.** *Hepatogastroenterology* 1993, **40**:188–190.

Marshall JB, Barthel JS: **The Frequency of Total Colonoscopy and Terminal Ileal Intubation in the 1990s.** *Gastrointest Endosc* 1993, **39**:518–520.

Marshall JB, Barthel JS, King PD: **Prospective, Randomized Trial Comparing a Single Dose Sodium Phosphate Regimen with Peg-Electrolyte Lavage for Colonoscopy Preparation.** *Aliment Pharmacol Ther* 1993, **7**:679–682.

Marshall JB, Pineda JJ, Barthel JS, King PD: **Prospective, Randomized Trial Comparing Sodium Phosphate Solution with Polyethylene Glycol Electrolyte Lavage for Colonoscopy Preparation.** *Gastrointest Endosc* 1993, **39**:631–634.

• Matsumoto T, Iida M, Kimura Y, Masatoshi F: **Culture of Colonoscopically Obtained Biopsy Specimens in Acute Infectious Colitis.** *Gastrointest Endosc* 1994, **40**:184–187. **[19].**

McIntyre AS, Long RG: **Prospective Survey of Investigations in Outpatients Referred with Iron Deficiency Anaemia.** *Gut* 1993, **34**:1102–1107.

Mecklin JP, Svendsen LB, Peltomaki P, Vasen HFA: **Hereditary Nonpolyposis Colorectal Cancer.** *Scand J Gastroenterol* 1994, **29**:673–677.

Modigliani R: **Endoscopic Management of Inflammatory Bowel Disease.** *Am J Gastroenterol* 1994, **89** (suppl):S53–S65.

O'Brien TS, Garrido MC, Dorudi S, Collin J: **Delayed Perforation of the Colon Following Colonoscopic Biopsy.** *Br J Surg* 1993, **80**:1204.

Paoluzi OA, Dipaolo MC, Ricci F, Pasquali C, Zarug S, Delibero F, Paoluzi P: **A Randomized Controlled Trial of a New PEG-Electrolyte Solution Compared with a Standard Preparation for Colonoscopy.** *Ital J Gastroenterol* 1993, **25**:174–178.

Park JG, Han HJ, Kang MS, Nakamura Y: **Presymptomatic Diagnosis of Familiar Adenomatous Polyposis Coli.** *Dis Colon Rectum* 1994, **37**:700–707.

Parry BR, Goh HS: **Quality Control in Colonoscopy — a Singapore Perspective.** *Int J Colorectal Dis* 1993, **8**:139–141.

Pitsch RJ, Becker JM, Dayton MT: **The Occurrence of Colon Cancer in Patients with Known Premalignant Colonic Mucosal Diseases.** *J Surg Res* 1994, **57**:293–298.

Rex DK, Lehman GA, Ulbright TM, Smith JJ, Hawes RH: **The Yield of a Second Screening Flexible Sigmoidoscopy in Average-Risk Persons after One Negative Examination.** *Gastroenterology* 1994, **106**:593–595.

• Rolney P: **Anastomotic Strictures in Crohn's Disease: a New Field for Therapeutic Endoscopy.** *Gastrointest Endosc* 1993, **39**:862–864. **[23].**

• Rubio CA, Slezak P, Befrits R: **The Costs of Colonoscopy in Patients with Ulcerative Pancolitis in Sweden.** *Endoscopy* 1994, **26**:228–230. **[27].**

Sachar DB: **Clinical and Colonoscopic Surveillance in Ulcerative Colitis: are we Saving Colons or Saving Lives?** *Gastroenterology* 1993, **105**:587–589.

Salmon P, Shah R, Berg S, Williams C: **Evaluating Customer Satisfaction with Colonoscopy.** *Endoscopy* 1994, **26**:342–346.

• Salomon P, Berner JS, Waye JD: **Endoscopic India Ink Injection: a Method for Preparation, Sterilization and Administration.** *Gastrointest Endosc* 1993, **39**:803–805. **[25].**

•• Saunders BP, Fukumoto M, Halligan S, Masaki T, Love S, Williams CB: **Patient Administered Nitrous Oxide/oxygen Inhalation Provides Effective Sedation and Analgesia for Colonoscopy.** *Gastrointest Endosc* 1994, **40**:418–421. **[7].**

Savides TJ, Jensen DM: **Colonoscopic Hemostasis for Recurrent Diverticular Hemorrhage Associated with a Visible Vessel — a Report of Three Cases.** *Gastrointest Endosc* 1994, **40**:70–73.

Sayer JM, Long RG: **A Perspective on Iron Deficiency Anaemia.** *Gut* 1993, **34**:1297–1299.

Scandalis N, Archimandritis A, Kastanas K, Spiliadis C, Delis B, Manika Z: **Colonic Findings in Cirrhotics with Portal Hypertension — a Prospective Colonoscopic and Histological Study.** *J Clin Gastroenterol* 1994, **18**:325–328.

Schutz SM, Lee JG, Schmitt CM, Almon M, Baillie J: **Clues to Patient Dissatisfaction with Conscious Sedation for Colonoscopy.** *Am J Gastroenterol* 1994, **89**:1476–1479.

Selby JV: **Targeting Colonoscopy.** *Gastroenterology* 1994, **106**:1702–1705.

• Shoenut PJ, Semelka RC, Magro CM, Silverman R, Yafffe CS, Micflikier AB: **Comparison of Magnetic Resonance Imaging and Endoscopy in Distinguishing the Type and Severity of Inflammatory Bowel Disease.** *J Clin Gastroenterol* 1994, **19**:31–35. **[20].**

Smiley DN, Barkin J: **Unusual Endoscopic Appearance of Collagenous Colitis.** *J Clin Gastroenterol* 1993, **17**:84–85.

Steine S: **Which Hurts the Most? A Comparison of Pain Rating During Double-Contrast Barium Enema Examination and Colonoscopy.** *Radiology* 1994, **191**:99–102.

Straub RF, Wilcox CM, Schwartz DA: **Variable Endoscopic Appearance of Colonic Lymphoid Tissue.** *J Clin Gastroenterol* 1994, **19**:158–165.

Surawicz CM, Haggitt RC, Husseman M, McFarland LV: **Mucosal Biopsy Diagnosis of Colitis: Acute Self-limited Colitis and Idiopathic Inflammatory Bowel Disease.** *Gastroenterology* 1994, **107**:755–763.

Thomas AW, Mitre RJ: **Acute Pancreatitis as a Complication of Colonoscopy.** *J Clin Gastroenterol* 1994, **19**:177–178.

• Ueda S, Iishi H, Tatsuta M, Oda K, Osaka S: **Addition of Cisapride Shortens Colonoscopy Preparation with Lavage in Elderly Patients.** *Aliment Pharmacol Ther* 1994, **8**:209–214. **[4].**

Vamosi-Nagy I, Koves I, Szanto I, Banai J: **Intraoperative Colonoscopy.** *Eur J Surg Oncol* 1993, **19**:615–618.

Vemulapalli R, Lance P: **Cancer Surveillance in Ulcerative Colitis: More of the Same or Progress?** *Gastroenterology* 1994, **107**:1196–1199.

Vonherbay A, Herfarth C, Otto HF: **Cancer and Dysplasia in Ulcerative Colitis — a Histologic Study of 301 Surgical Specimen.** *Z Gastroenterol* 1994, **32**:382–388.

• Wallner M, Allinger S, Wiesinger H, Prischl FC, Kramar R, Knoflauch P: **Small Bowel Ileus after Diagnostic Colonoscopy.** *Endoscopy* 1994, **26**:329. **[14].**

Weinstock LB, Shatz BA: **Endoscopic Abnormalities of the Anastomosis Following Resection of Colonic Neoplasm.** *Gastrointest Endosc* 1994, **40**:558–561.

•• Williams CB: **Comfort and Quality in Colonoscopy.** *Gastrointest Endosc* 1994, **40**:769–770. **[9].**


## Colon polyps and cancer


Achord JL: **Polyp Guideline [Editorial].** *Am J Gastroenterol* 1994, **89**:660–661.

• Afridi SA, Jafri SF, Marshall JB: **Do Gastroenterologists Themselves Follow the American Cancer Society Recommendation for Colorectal Cancer Screening?** *Am J Gastroenterol* 1994, **89**:2184–2187. **[74].**

Armbrecht U, Manus B, Bragelmann R, Stockbrugger RW, Stolte M: **Acceptance and Outcome of Endoscopic Screening for Colonic Neoplasia in Patients Undergoing Clinical Rehabilitation for Gastrointestinal and Metabolic Diseases.** *Z Gastroenterol* 1994, **32**:3–7.

• Bapat BV, Parker JA, Berk T, Cohen Z, McLeod RS, Ray PN, *et al.*: **Combined use for Molecular and Biomarkers for Presymptomatic Carrier Risk Assessment in Familial Adenomatous Polyposis: Implications for Screening Guidelines.** *Dis Colon Rectum* 1994, **37**:165–171. **[59].**

Barlow AP, Thompson MH: **Colonoscopic Follow-Up after Resection for Colorectal Cancer — a Selective Policy.** *Br J Surg* 1993, **80**:781–784.

Beck DE, Karulf RE: **Laparoscopic-Assisted Full-Thickness Endoscopic Polypectomy.** *Dis Colon Rectum* 1993, **36**:693–695.

• Bertario L, Presciuttini S, Sala P, Rossetti C, Pietroiusti M: **Causes of Death and Postsurgical Survival in Familial Adenomatous Polyposis: Results from the Italian Registry.** *Semin Surg Oncol* 1994, **10**:225–234. **[57].**

Bond JH: **Polyp Guideline — Diagnosis, Treatment, and Surveillance for Patients with Nonfamilial Colorectal Polyps.** *Ann Intern Med* 1993, **119**:836–843.

Brady PG, Straker RJ, McClave SA, Nord HJ, Pinkas M, Robinson BE: **Are Hyperplastic Rectosigmoid Polyps Associated with an Increased Risk of Proximal Colonic Neoplasms.** *Gastrointest Endosc* 1993, **39**:481–485.

• Brint SL, DiPalma JA, Herrera JL: **Colorectal Cancer Screening: is One-year Surveillance Sigmoidoscopy Necessary?** *Am J Gastroenterol* 1993, **88**:2019–2021. **[33].**

• Bronner CE, Baker SM, Morrison PT, Warren G, Smith LG, Lescoe MK, *et al.*: **Mutation in the DNA Mismatch Repair Gene Homologue HMLH1 is Associated with Hereditary Non-polyposis Colon Cancer.** *Nature* 1994, **368**:258–261. **[61].**

Bulow S, Burn J, Neale K, Northover J, Vasen H: **The Establishment of a Polyposis Register.** *Int J Colorectal Dis* 1993, **8**:34–38.

Burn J, Chapman PD, Eastham EJ: **Familial Adenomatous Polyposis.** *Arch Dis Child* 1994, **71**:103–105.

Carey WD, Achkar E: **Colon Polyps and Cancer in 1994.** *Am J Gastroenterol* 1994, **89**:823–825.

Catnach SM, Rutter KRP, Bown RL: **Colorectal Carcinoma in Patients with Ulcerative Colitis and Recent Colonoscopy.** *Gut* 1993, **34**:1148–1149.

Chapuis PH, Dent OF, Bokey EL, McDonald CA, Newland RC: **Patient Characteristics and Pathology in Colorectal Adenomas Removed by Colonoscopic Polypectomy.** *Aust N Z J Surg* 1993, **63**:100–104.

Chaves DM, Sakai P, Mester M, Spinosa SR, Tomishige T, Ishioka S: **A New Endoscopic Technique for the Resection of Flat Polypoid Lesions.** *Gastrointest Endosc* 1994, **40**:224–226.

• Chen F, Stuart M: **Colonoscopic Follow-up of Colorectal Carcinoma.** *Dis Colon Rectum* 1994, **37**:568–572. **[46].**

Choi PM, Nugent FW, Schoetz DJ, Silverman ML, Haggitt RC: **Colonoscopic Surveillance Reduces Mortality from Colorectal Cancer in Ulcerative Colitis.** *Gastroenterology* 1993, **105**:418–424.

•• Chu KC, Tarone RE, Chow W-H, Hankey BF, Gloeckler Ries LA: **Temporal Patterns in Colorectal Cancer Incidence, Survival, and Mortality from 1950 Through 1990.** *J Natl Cancer Inst* 1994, **86**:997–1006. **[1].**

Cunningham KN, Mills LR, Schuman BM, Mwakyusa DH: **Long-term Prognosis of Well-differentiated Adenocarcinoma in Endoscopically Removed Colorectal Adenomas.** *Dig Dis Sci* 1994, **39**:2034–2037.

Dickinson AJ, Savage AP, Mortensen NJM, Kettlewell MGW: **Long-Term Survival after Endoscopic Transanal Resection of Rectal Tumours.** *Br J Surg* 1993, **80**:1401–1404.

•• Dinning JP, Hixson LJ, Clark LC: **Prevalence of Distal Colonic Neoplasia Associated with Proximal Colon Cancers.** *Arch Intern Med* 1994, **154**:853–856. **[81].**

Driman DK, Riddell RH: **Flat Adenomas and Flat Carcinomas: do You See what I See [Editorial].** *Gastrointest Endosc* 1994, **40**:106–109.

• Eberhart CE, Coffey RJ, Radhika A, Giardiello FM, Ferrenbach S, Dubois RN: **Up-regulation of Cyclooxygenase 2 Gene Expression in Human Colorectal Adenomas and Adenocarcinomas.** *Gastroenterology* 1994, **107**:1183–1188. **[14].**

Eckardt VF, Stamm H, Kanzler G, Bernhard G: **Improved Survival after Colorectal Cancer in Patients Complying with a Postoperative Endoscopic Surveillance Program.** *Endoscopy* 1994, **26**:523–527.

• Eisen GM, Sandler RS: **Are Women with Breast Cancer More Likely to Develop Colorectal Cancer?** *J Clin Gastroenterol* 1994, **19**:57–63. **[6].**

Evans DGR, Guy SP, Thakker N, Armstrong JG, Dodd C, Davies DR, Babbs C, Clancy T, Warnes T, Sloan P, Taylor TV, Harris R: **Non-Penetrance and Late Appearance of Polyps in Families with Familial Adenomatous Polyposis.** *Gut* 1993, **34**:1389–1393.

Forde KA, Treat MR, Tsai JL: **Initial Clinical Experience with a Bipolar Snare for Colon Polypectomy.** *Surg Endosc* 1993, **7**:427–428.

Fruhmorgen P: **Guidelines for Endoscopic Studies on Colorectal Polyps.** *Z Gastroenterol* 1994, **32**:371–374.

• Fuchs CS, Giovannucci EL, Colditz GA, Hunter DJ, Speizer FE, Willett WC: **A Prospective Study of Family History and the Risk of Colorectal Cancer.** *N Engl J Med* 1994, **331**:1669–1674. **[4].**

Fujimura Y, Mizuno M, Takeda M, Sato I, Hoshika K, Uchida J, Kihara T, Mure T, Sano K, Moriya T: **A Carcinoid Tumor of the Rectum Removed by Strip Biopsy.** *Endoscopy* 1993, **25**:428–430.

Geller AJ, Kolts BE, Achem SR, Wears R: **The High Frequency of Upper Gastrointestinal Pathology in Patients with Fecal Occult Blood and Colon Polyps.** *Am J Gastroenterol* 1993, **88**:1184–1187.

• Giardiello FM, Krush AJ, Petersen GM, Booker SV, Kerr M, Tong LL, *et al.*: **Phenotypic Variability of Familial Adenomatous Polyposis in 11 Unrelated Families with Identical APC Gene Mutation.** *Gastroenterology* 1994, **106**:1542–1547. **[52].**

• Giovannucci E, Colditz GA, Stampfer MJ, Hunter D, Rosner BA, Willett WC, *et al.*: **A Prospective Study of Cigarette Smoking and Risk of Colorectal Adenoma and Colorectal Cancer in U.S. Women.** *J Natl Cancer Inst* 1994, **86**:192–199. **[3].**

• Giovannucci E, Rimm EB, Stampfer MJ, Colditz GA, Ascherio A, Kearney J, *et al.*: **A Prospective Study of Cigarette Smoking and Risk of Colorectal Adenoma and Colorectal Cancer in U.S. Men.** *J Natl Cancer Inst* 1994, **86**:183–191. **[2].**

• Giovannucci E, Rimm EB, Stampfer MJ, Colditz GA, Ascherio A, Willett WC: **Aspirin use and the Risk for Colorectal Cancer and Adenoma in Male Health Professionals.** *Ann Intern Med* 1994, **121**:241–246. **[11].**

Green JB, Timmcke AE, Mitchell WT: **Endoscopic Resection of Primary Rectal Teratoma.** *Am Surg* 1993, **59**:270–272.

• Gurbuz AK, Giardiello FM, Petersen GM, Krush AJ, Offerhaus GJ, Booker SV, *et al.*: **Desmoid Tumours in Familiar Adenomatous Polyposis.** *Gut* 1994, **34**:377–381. **[58].**

Hill DH, Mills JOM, Maxwell RJ: **Metachronous Colonic Lymphomas Complicating Chronic Ulcerative Colitis.** *Abdom Imaging* 1993, **18**:369–370.

Hixson LJ, Earnest DL, Fennerty MB, Sampliner RE: **NSAID Effect on Sporadic Colon Polyps [Review].** *Am J Gastroenterol* 1993, **88**:1652–1656.

Hixson LJ, Fennerty MB, Sampliner RE, McGee DL, Garewal H: **Two-Year Incidence of Colon Adenomas Developing after Tandem Colonoscopy.** *Am J Gastroenterol* 1994, **89**:687–691.

•• Hofstad B, Vatn M, Larsen S, Osnes M: **Growth of Colorectal Polyps: Recovery and Evaluation of Unresected Polyps of Less Than 10 Mm, 1 Year after Detection.** *Scand J Gastroenterol* 1994, **29**:640–645. **[40].**

Hough DM, Malone DE, Rawlinson J, Degara CJ, Moote DJ, Irvine EJ, Somers S, Stevenson GW: **Colon Cancer Detection: an Algorithm Using Endoscopy and Barium Enema.** *Clin Radiol* 1994, **49**:170–175.

Iida Y, Miura S, Munemoto Y, Kasahara Y, Asada Y, Toya D, Fujisawa M: **Endoscopic Resection of Large Colorectal Polyps Using a Clipping Method.** *Dis Colon Rectum* 1994, **37**:179–180.

Iishi H, Kitamura S, Nakaizumi A, Tatsuta M, Otani T, Okuda S, Ishiguro S: **Clinicopathological Features and Endoscopic Diagnosis of Superficial Early Adenocarcinomas of the Large Intestine.** *Dig Dis Sci* 1993, **38**:1333–1337.

Isbister WH: **Hyperplastic Polyps.** *Aust N Z J Surg* 1993, **63**:175–180.

• Jacobson JS, Neugut AI, Murray T, Garbowski GC, Forde KA, Treat MR, *et al.*: **Cigarette Smoking and Other Behavioral Risk Factors for Recurrence of Colorectal Adenomatous Polyps (New York City, NY, USA). Cancer Causes.** *Control* 1994, **5**:215–220. **[48].**

Karita M, Cantero D, Okita K: **Endoscopic Diagnosis and Resection Treatment for Flat Adenoma with Severe Dysplasia.** *Am J Gastroenterol* 1993, **88**:1421–1423.

• Kewenter J, Breveinge H, Engares B, Haglind E, Ehrin C: **Results of Screening, Rescreening, and Follow-up in a Prospective Randomized Study for Detection of Colorectal Cancer by Fecal Occult Blood Testing.** *Scand J Gastroenterol* 1994, **29**:468–473. **[73].**

Khanduja KS, Pons R: **Efficient Technique for Retrieving Small Polyps from the Colon and Rectum Following Snare Polypectomy.** *Dis Colon Rectum* 1994, **37**:190.

Krevsky B, Fisher RS: **Yield of Rescreening for Colonic Polyps Using Flexible Sigmoidoscopy.** *Am J Gastroenterol* 1994, **89**:1165–1168.

Krukemeyer MG: **Colorectal Carcinoma — Epidemiology, Diagnosis and Treatment.** *Coloproctology* 1993, **15**:176–179.

• Lang CA, Ransohoff DF: **Fecal Occult Blood Screening for Colorectal Cancer.** *JAMA* 1994, **271**:1011–1013. **[72].**

• Lanspa SJ, Jenkins JX, Cavalieri RJ, Smyrk TC, Watson P, Lynch J, *et al.*: **Surveillance in Lynch Syndrome: How Aggressive?** *Am J Gastroenterol* 1994, **89**:1978–1980. **[36].**

Latt TT, Nicholl R, Domizio P, Walkersmith JA, Williams CB: **Rectal Bleeding and Polyps.** *Arch Dis Child* 1993, **69**:144–147.

Lautenbach E, Forde KA, Neugut AI: **Benefits of Colonoscopic Surveillance after Curative Resection of Colorectal Cancer.** *Ann Surg* 1994, **220**:206–211.

• Liu B, Parsons RE, Hamilton SR, Petersen GM, Lynch HT, Watson P, *et al.*: **hMSH2 Mutations in Hereditary Nonpolyposis Colorectal Cancer Kindreds.** *Cancer Res* 1994, **54**:4590–4594. **[64].**

Lynch HT, Smyrk TC, Cavalieri J, Lynch JF: **Identification of an HNPCC Family.** *Am J Gastroenterol* 1994, **89**:605–609.

Marshall JB, Diazarias AA, Barthel JS, King PD, Butt JH: **Prospective Evaluation of Optimal Number of Biopsy Specimens and Brush Cytology in the Diagnosis of Cancer of the Colorectum.** *Am J Gastroenterol* 1993, **88**:1352–1354.

Matsui K, Iwase T, Kitagawa M: **Small, Polypoid-Appearing Carcinoid Tumors of the Rectum — Clinicopathologic Study of 16 Cases and Effectiveness of Endoscopic Treatment.** *Am J Gastroenterol* 1993, **88**:1949–1953.

Maule WF: **Screening for Colorectal Cancer by Nurse Endoscopists.** *N Engl J Med* 1994, **330**:183–187.

• McAfee JH, Katon RM: **Tiny Snares Prove Safe and Effective for Removal of Diminutive Colorectal Polyps.** *Gastrointest Endosc* 1994, **40**:301–303. **[23].**

• McFarlane MJ, Welch KE: **Gallstones, Cholecystectomy, and Colorectal Cancer.** *Am J Gastroenterol* 1994, **88**:1994–1999. **[8].**

McGahan RP, Gilinsky NH: **Colonic Tumors.** *Endoscopy* 1994, **26**:70–87. **[85].**

• Meagher AP, Stuart M: **Does Colonoscopic Polypectomy Reduce the Incidence of Colorectal Carcinoma?** *Aust N Z J Surg* 1994, **64**:400–404. **[47].**

• Minamoto T, Sawaguchi K, Ohta T, Itoh T, Mai M: **Superficial-type Adenomas and Adenocarcinomas of the Colon and Rectum: a Comparative Morphological Study.** *Gastroenterology* 1994, **106**:1436–1443. **[37].**

• Moore JW, Hoffmann DC, Rowland R: **Management of the Malignant Colorectal Polyp: the Importance of Clinicopathological Correlation.** *Aust N Z J Surg* 1994, **64**:242–246. **[42].**

Mulloy JP, Scott RL: **Technical Note. Differentiating Colonic Polyps from Air Bubbles on Barium Enema: The "Arpenter's Level Sign".** *Am J Roentgenol* 1994, **163**:84–86.

Neugut AI, Garbowski GC, Waye JD, Forde KA, Treat MR, Tsai JL, Lee WC: **Diagnostic Yield of Colorectal Neoplasia with Colonoscopy for Abdominal Pain, Change in Bowel Habits, and Rectal Bleeding.** *Am J Gastroenterol* 1993, **88**:1179–1183.

•• Nicolaides NC, Papadopoulos N, Liu B, Wei YF, Carter FC, Ruben SM, *et al.*: **Mutations of Two PMS Homologues in Hereditary Nonpolyposis Colon Cancer.** *Nature* 1994, **371**:75–80. **[63].**

• Nystrom-Lahti M, Sistonen P, Mecklin JP, Pylkkdnen L, Aaltonen LA, Jdrvinen H, *et al.*: **Close Linkage to Chromosome 3p and Conservation of Ancestral Founding Haplotype in Hereditary Nonpolyposis Colorectal Cancer Families.** *Proc Natl Acad Sci U S A* 1994, **91**:6054–6058. **[60].**

Ottenjann R: **Endoscopic Polypectomy — Sense and Nonsense.** *Z Gastroenterol* 1994, **32**:412–415.

• Paganini-Hill A: **Aspirin and the Prevention of Colorectal Cancer: a Review of the Evidence.** *Semin Surg Oncol* 1994, **10**:158–164. **[12].**

• Papadopoulos N, Nicolades NC, Wei YF, Ruben SM, Carter KC, Rosen CA, *et al.*: **Mutation of MutL Homolog in Hereditary Colon Cancer.** *Science* 1994, **263**:1625–1629. **[62].**

Patchett SE, Mulcahy HE, Odonoghue DP: **Colonoscopic Surveillance after Curative Resection for Colorectal Cancer.** *Br J Surg* 1993, **80**:1330–1332.

• Penman ID, El-Omar E, Ardill JES, McGregor JR, Galloway DJ, O'Wyer PJ, *et al.*: **Plasma Gastrin Concentrations are Normal in Patients with Colorectal Neoplasia and Unaltered Following Tumor Resection.** *Gastroenterology* 1994, **106**:1263–1270. **[83].**

Pennazio M, Arrigoni A, Risio M, Spandre M, Rossini FP: **Small Rectosigmoid Polyps as Markers of Proximal Neoplasms.** *Dis Colon Rectum* 1993, **36**:1121–1125.

• Petersen GM: **Knowledge of the Adenomatous Polyposis Coli Gene and Its Clinical Application.** *Ann Med* 1994, **26**:205–208. **[54].**

Pidala MJ, Slezak FA, Hlivko TJ: **Delayed Presentation of an Inflammatory Polyp Following Colonic-Ischemia.** *Am Surg* 1993, **59**:315–318.

Porschen R: **Endoscopic Diagnosis in the Prevention and Early Diagnosis of Colorectal Cancer.** *Dtsch Med Wochenschr* 1994, **119**:1001–1003.

Post AB, Achkar E, Carey WD: **Prevalence of Colonic Neoplasia in Patients with Barrett's Esophagus.** *Am J Gastroenterol* 1993, **88**:877–880.

• Potter JD, Slattery ML, Bostick RM, Gapstur SM: **Colon Cancer: a Review of the Epidemiology.** *Colon Cancer* 1993, **15**:499–545. **[84].**

•• Powell SM, Petersen GM, Krush AJ, Booker S, Jen J, Giardiello FM, *et al.*: **Molecular Diagnosis of Familial Adenomatous Polyposis.** *N Engl J Med* 1993, **329**:1982–1987. **[53].**

Radin DR: **Hereditary Generalized Juvenile Polyposis — Association with Arteriovenous Malformations and Risk of Malignancy.** *Abdom Imaging* 1994, **19**:140–142.

Reiser JR, Waye JD, Janowitz HD, Harpaz N: **Adenocarcinoma in Strictures of Ulcerative Colitis Without Antecedent Dysplasia by Colonoscopy.** *Am J Gastroenterol* 1994, **89**:119–122.

Rex DK: **Determining Indications for Primary Colonoscopy — How can we Predict the Need for Polypectomy [Editorial].** *Am J Gastroenterol* 1993, **88**:1154–1156.

• Rex DK, Lehman GA, Ulbright TM, Smith JJ, Hawes RH: **The Yield of a Second Screening Flexible Sigmoidoscopy in Average-risk Persons after One Negative Examination.** *Gastroenterology* 1994, **106**:593–595. **[32].**

Rex DK, Lehman GA, Ulbright TM, Smith JJ, Pound DC, Hawes RH, Helper DJ, Wiersema MJ, Langefeld CD, Li W: **Colonic Neoplasia in Asymptomatic Persons with Negative Fecal Occult Blood Tests — Influence of Age, Gender, and Family History.** *Am J Gastroenterol* 1993, **88**:825–831.

• Rex DK, Sledge GW, Harper PA, Ulbright TM, Loehrer PJ, Helper DJ, *et al.*: **Colonic Adenomas in Asymptomatic Women with a History of Breast Cancer.** *Am J Gastroenterol* 1993, **88**:2009–2014. **[7].**

• Rodriguez-Bigas MA, Mahoney MC, Karakousis CP, Petrelli NJ: **Desmoid Tumors in Patients with Familial Adenomatous Polyposis.** *Cancer* 1994, **74**:1270–1274. **[56].**

• Rogge JD, Elmore MF, Mahoney SJ, Brown ED, Troiano FP, Wagner DR, *et al.*: **Low-cost, Office-based, Screening Colonoscopy.** *Am J Gastroenterol* 1994, **89**:1775–1780. **[76].**

Rokkas T, Karameris A, Mikou G: **Small Polyps Found at Sigmoidoscopy — are they Significant.** *Hepatogastroenterology* 1993, **40**:475–477.

Rosen L, Bub DS, Reed JF, Nastasee SA: **Hemorrhage Following Colonoscopic Polypectomy.** *Dis Colon Rectum* 1993, **36**:1126–1131.

• Rustgi AK: **Hereditary Gastrointestinal Polyposis and Nonpolyposis Syndromes.** *N Engl J Med* 1994, **331**:1694–1701. **[86].**

Safi F, Link KH, Beger HG: **Is Follow-Up of Colorectal Cancer Patients Worthwhile.** *Dis Colon Rectum* 1993, **36**:636–642.

Salomon P, Berner JS, Waye JD: **Endoscopic India Ink Injection — a Method for Preparation, Sterilization, and Administration.** *Gastrointest Endosc* 1993, **39**:803–805.

• Schoen RE, Weissfeld JL, Kuller LH: **Are Women with Breast, Endometrial, or Ovarian Cancer at Increased Risk for Colorectal Cancer?** *Am J Gastroenterol* 1994, **89**:835–842. **[5].**

Schrock TR: **Colonoscopy for Colorectal Cancer — Too Much, Too Little, Just Right [Editorial].** *Gastrointest Endosc* 1993, **39**:848–851.

Schusdziarra V: **Prevention of Colorectal Carcinoma: Sigmoidoscopy or Colonoscopy.** *Z Gastroenterol* 1993, **31**:758–759.

Shirai M, Nakamura T, Matsuura A, Ito Y, Kobayashi S: **Safer Colonoscopic Polypectomy with Local Submucosal Injection of Hypertonic Saline-Epinephrine Solution.** *Am J Gastroenterol* 1994, **89**:334–338.

Siegers CP, Vonhertzberglottin E, Otte M, Schneider B: **Anthranoid Laxative Abuse — a Risk for Colorectal Cancer.** *Gut* 1993, **34**:1099–1101.

Slivka A, Parsons WG, Carrlocke DL: **Endoscopic Band Ligation for Treatment of Post-polypectomy Hemorrhage.** *Gastrointest Endosc* 1994, **40**:230–232.

• Spagnesi MT, Tonelli F, Dolara P, Caderni G, Valanzano R, Anastasi A, *et al.*: **Rectal Proliferation and Polyp Occurrence in Patients with Familial Adenomatous Polyposis after Sulindac Treatment.** *Gastroenterology* 1994, **106**:362–366. **[17].**

Squillace S, Berggreen P, Jaffe P, Fennerty MB, Hixson L, Garewal H, Sampliner RE: **A Normal Initial Colonoscopy after Age 50 Does not Predict a Polyp-free Status for Life.** *Am J Gastroenterol* 1994, **89**:1156–1159.

Stevenson GW: **Radiology and Endoscopy in the Pretreatment Diagnostic Management of Colorectal Cancer.** *Cancer* 1993, **71** (suppl):4198–4206.

Sturniolo GC, Montino MC, Dalligna F, Dinca R, Messineo A, Cecchetto A, Previtera C, Riddell RH: **Familial Juvenile Polyposis-Coli — Results of Endoscopic Treatment and Surveillance in Two Sisters.** *Gastrointest Endosc* 1993, **39**:561–565.

Swaroop VS, Desai D, Mohandas KM, Dhir V, Dave UR, Gulla RI, Dinshaw KA, Deshpande RK, Desai PB: **Dilation of Esophageal Strictures Induced by Radiation Therapy for Cancer of the Esophagus.** *Gastrointest Endosc* 1994, **40**:311–315.

Tsang TK, Buto SK, Sadowitz RH: **Colonoscopic Relief of Small Bowel Obstruction.** *Gastrointest Endosc* 1993, **39**:426–429.

• Uno Y, Munakata A, Tanaka M: **The Discrepancy of Histologic Diagnosis Between Flat Early Colon Cancers and Flat Adenomas.** *Gastrointest Endosc* 1994, **40**:1–5. **[39].**

• Vernava III AM, Longo WE, Virgo KS, Coplin MA, Wade TP, Johnson FE: **Current Follow-up Strategies after Resection of Colon Cancer.** *Dis Colon Rectum* 1994, **37**:573–583. **[45].**

Watanabe T, Sawada T, Kubota Y, Adachi M, Saito Y, Masaki T, Muto T: **Malignant Potential in Flat Elevations.** *Dis Colon Rectum* 1993, **36**:548–553.

Waye JD: **Saline Injection Colonoscopic Polypectomy.** *Am J Gastroenterol* 1994, **89**:305–306.

Wetherall AP, Williams NMA, Kelly MJ: **Endoscopic Transanal Resection in the Management of Patients with Sessile Rectal Adenomas, Anastomotic Stricture and Rectal Cancer.** *Br J Surg* 1993, **80**:788–793.

Wherry DC, Thomas WM: **The Yield of Flexible Fiberoptic Sigmoidoscopy in the Detection of Asymptomatic Colorectal Neoplasia.** *Surg Endosc* 1994, **8**:393–395.

Williams B, Saunders BP: **The Rationale for Current Practice in the Management of Malignant Colonic Polyps.** *Endoscopy* 1993, **25**:469–474.

Winawer SJ, Et Al: **Prevention of Colorectal Cancer by Colonoscopic Polypectomy.** *N Engl J Med* 1993, **329**:1977–1981.

Yamaguchi A, Nakagawara G, Kurosaka Y, Nishimura G, Yonemura Y, Miyazaki I: **p53 Immunoreaction in Endoscopic Biopsy Specimens of Colorectal Cancer, and Its Prognostic Significance.** *Br J Cancer* 1993, **68**:399–402.

•• Zarchy TM, Ershoff D: **Do Characteristics of Adenomas on Flexible Sigmoidoscopy Predict Advanced Lesions on Baseline Colonoscopy?** *Gastroenterology* 1994, **106**:1501–1504. **[41].**


## General topics


Anon: **Nurse Practitioners as Endoscopists [Letter].** *N Engl J Med* 1994, **330**:1534–1535.

Classen M, Maratka Z: **Report on the Symposium on Endoscopic Terminology and Computerisation Held in Athens in September 1992.** *Endoscopy* 1993, **25**:258.

•• Cotton PB: **Interventional Gastroenterology (endoscopy) at the Crossroads: a Plea for Restructuring in Digestive Diseases.** *Gastroenterology* 1994, **107**:294–299. **[1].**

Keeffe EB: **Determinants of Safe Endoscopy.** *Gastrointest Endosc* 1994, **40**:379–382.

• Lazzaroni M, Bianchi Porro G: **Preparation, Premedication and Surveillance in Gastrointestinal Endoscopy.** *Endoscopy* 1994, **26**:3–8. **[6].**

Lynch DAF, Parnell P, Porter C, Axon ATR: **Patient and Staff Exposure to Glutaraldehyde from Keymed Auto-Disinfector Endoscope Washing Machine.** *Endoscopy* 1994, **26**:359–361.

Mallinson CN: **Special Training in Gastroenterology in the European Community: the Case for European Boards.** *Gut* 1994, **35**:135–138.

McGill DB, Moody FG: **Invasive Endoscopy and the Medical/surgical Divide.** *Gastroenterology* 1994, **107**:306–308.

Nagengast FM: **Sedation and Monitoring in Gastrointestinal Endoscopy.** *Scand J Gastroenterol* 1993, **28** (suppl 200):28–32.

Rosch T, Allescher HD: **Update in Gastroenterologic Endoscopy — a Review of Endoscopy Abstracts Presented at the 1993 DDW in Boston.** *Endoscopy* 1993, **25**:401–422.

•• Schembre D, Bjorkman DJ: **Review Article: Endoscopy-related Infections.** *Aliment Pharmacol Ther* 1993, **7**:347–355. **[8].**

# List of journals scanned

The *Index Medicus* abbreviation is given in parentheses

Abdominal Imaging (Abdom Imaging)
Acta Paediatrica (Acta Paediatr)
AIDS (AIDS)
Alimentary Pharmacology and Therapeutics (Aliment Pharmacol Ther)
American Journal of Clinical Nutrition (Am J Clin Nutr)
American Journal of Clinical Pathology (Am J Clin Pathol)
American Journal of Epidemiology (Am J Epidemiol)
American Journal of Gastroenterology (Am J Gastroenterol)
American Journal of Medicine (Am J Med)
American Journal of Pathology (Am J Pathol)
American Journal of Physiology - Cell Physiology (Am J Physiol - Cell Physiol)
American Journal of Physiology - Gastrointestinal and Liver Physiology (Am J Physiol - Gastrointest Liver Physiol)
American Journal of Physiology - Regulatory Integrative and Comparative Physiology (Am J Physiol - Regul Intergr Comp Physiol)
American Journal of Roentgenology (AJR Am J Roentgenol)
American Journal of Surgery (Am J Surg)
American Journal of Surgical Pathology (Am J Surg Pathol)
American Journal of Tropical Medicine and Hygiene (Am J Trop Med Hyg)
American Surgeon (Am Surg)
Annals of Internal Medicine (Ann Intern Med)
Annals of Surgery (Ann Surg)
Annals of the Royal College of Surgeons of England (Ann R Coll Surg Engl)
Annals of Thoracic Surgery (Ann Thorac Surg)
Archives of Disease in Childhood (Arch Dis Child)
Archives of Internal Medicine (Arch Intern Med)
Archives of Pediatrics & Adolescent Medicine (Arch Pediatr Adolesc Med)
Archives of Surgery (Arch Surg)
Australian and New Zealand Journal of Surgery (Aust N Z J Surg)
Biochemical Journal (Biochem J)
Biochimica et Biophysica Acta — Bioenergetics (Biochim Biophys Acta)
Biochimica et Biophysica Acta — Biomembranes (Biochim Biophys Acta)
Biochimica et Biophysica Acta — Gene Structure and Expression (Biochim Biophys Acta)
Biochimica et Biophysica Acta — General Subjects (Biochim Biophys Acta)
Biochimica et Biophysica Acta — Lipids and Lipid Metabolism (Biochim Biophys Acta)
Biochimica et Biophysica Acta — Molecular Basis of Disease (Biochim Biophys Acta)
Biochimica et Biophysica Acta — Molecular Cell Research (Biochim Biophys Acta)
Biochimica et Biophysica Acta — Protein Structure and Molecular Enzymology (Biochim Biophys Acta)
Biochimica et Biophysica Acta — Reviews on Biomembranes (Biochim Biophys Acta)
Biochimica et Biophysica Acta — Reviews on Cancer (Biochim Biophys Acta)
British Journal of Cancer (Br J Cancer)
British Journal of Radiology (Br J Radiol)
British Journal of Surgery (Br J Surg)

British Medical Journal (BMJ)
Cancer (Cancer)
Cancer Research (Cancer Res)
Carcinogenesis (Carcinogenesis)
Cell (Cell)
Clinica Chimica Acta (Clin Chim Acta)
Clinical and Experimental Immunology (Clin Exp Immunol)
Clinical Chemistry (Clin Chem)
Clinical Nutrition (Clin Nutr)
Clinical Radiology (Clin Radiol)
Clinical Science (Clin Sci (Colch))
Colo-Proctology (Coloproctology)
Deutsche Medizinische Wochenschrift (Dtsch Med Wochenschr)
Digestion (Digestion)
Digestive Diseases and Sciences (Dig Dis Sci)
Diseases of the Colon and Rectum (Dis Colon Rectum)
Endoscopy (Endoscopy)
Epidemiology and Infection (Epidemiol Infect)
European Journal of Clinical Investigation (Eur J Clin Invest)
European Journal of Clinical Microbiology and Infectious Diseases (Eur J Clin Microbiol Infect Dis)
European Journal of Gastroenterology and Hepatology (Eur J Gastroenterol Hepatol)
European Journal of Surgery (Eur J Surg)
European Journal of Surgical Oncology (Eur J Surg Oncol)
FASEB Journal (FASEB J)
Gastroenterologie Clinique et Biologique (Gastroenterol Clin Biol)
Gastroenterology (Gastroenterology)
Gastroenterology Clinics of North America (Gastroenterol Clin North Am)
Gastrointestinal Endoscopy (Gastrointest Endosc)
Gut (Gut)
Hepato-Gastroenterology (Hepatogastroenterology)
Hepatology (Hepatology)
Histopathology (Histopathology)
Human Pathology (Hum Pathol)
Immunology (Immunology)
Infection and Immunity (Infect Immun)
International Journal of Colorectal Disease (Int J Colorectal Dis)
International Journal of Pancreatology (Int J Pancreatol)
Italian Journal of Gastroenterology (Ital J Gastroenterol)
JAMA — Journal of the American Medical Association (JAMA)
Journal of Biological Chemistry (J Biol Chem)
Journal of Clinical Gastroenterology (J Clin Gastroenterol)
Journal of Clinical Investigation (J Clin Invest)
Journal of Clinical Microbiology (J Clin Microbiol)
Journal of Clinical Oncology (J Clin Oncol)
Journal of Clinical Pathology (J Clin Pathol)
Journal of Computer Assisted Tomography (J Comput Assist Tomogr)
Journal of Experimental Medicine (J Exp Med)
Journal of Gastroenterology and Hepatology (J Gastroenterol Hepatol)
Journal of Hepatology (J Hepatol)
Journal of Immunology (J Immunol)
Journal of Infectious Diseases (J Infect Dis)

Journal of Laboratory and Clinical Medicine (J Lab Clin Med)
Journal of Lipid Research (J Lipid Res)
Journal of Medical Virology (J Med Virol)
Journal of Membrane Biology (J Membr Biol)
Journal of Nuclear Medicine (J Nucl Med)
Journal of Parenteral and Enteral Nutrition (JPEN J Parenter Enteral Nutr)
Journal of Pathology (J Pathol)
Journal of Pediatric Gastroenterology and Nutrition (J Pediatr Gastroenterol Nutr)
Journal of Pediatric Surgery (J Pediatr Surg)
Journal of Pediatrics (J Pediatr)
Journal of Pharmacology and Experimental Therapeutics (J Pharmacol Exp Ther)
Journal of Surgical Oncology (J Surg Oncol)
Journal of Surgical Research (J Surg Res)
Journal of the American College of Surgeons (J Am Coll Surg)
Journal of the Royal College of Surgeons of Edinburgh (J R Coll Surg Edinb)
Journal of the Royal Society of Medicine (J R Soc Med)
Lancet (Lancet)
Liver (Liver)
Mayo Clinic Proceedings (Mayo Clin Proc)
Medical Science Research (Med Sci Res)

Medicinal Research Reviews (Med Res Rev)
Metabolism: Clinical and Experimental (Metabolism)
Nature (Nature)
New England Journal of Medicine (N Engl J Med)
Pancreas (Pancreas)
Pediatric Research (Pediatr Res)
Pediatrics (Pediatrics)
Peptides (Peptides)
Postgraduate Medical Journal (Postgrad Med J)
Proceedings of the National Academy of Sciences of the United States of America (Proc Natl Acad Sci U S A)
Quarterly Journal of Medicine (Q J Med)
Radiology (Radiology)
Regulatory Peptides (Regul Pept)
Scandinavian Journal of Gastroenterology (Scand J Gastroenterol)
Scandinavian Journal of Infectious Diseases (Scand J Infect Dis)
Science (Science)
Surgery (Surgery)
Transactions of the Royal Society of Tropical Medicine and Hygiene (Trans R Soc Trop Med Hyg)
Transplantation (Transplantation)
World Journal of Surgery (World J Surg)
Zeitschrift fur Gastroenterologie (Z Gastroenterol)

# Index to subjects

# SLIDE ATLAS OF
# Gastrointestinal Endoscopy 1995

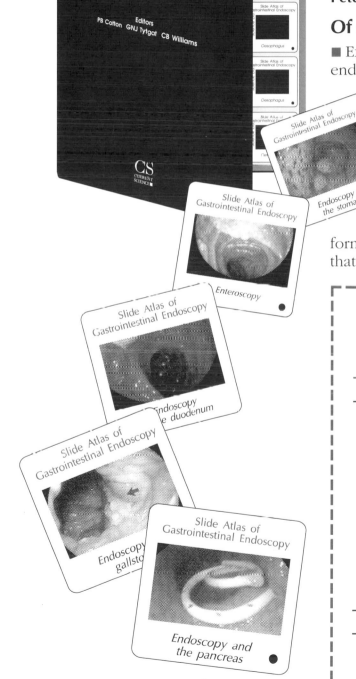

## THE ULTIMATE SLIDE COLLECTION

## Approximately 85 full-color slides

## Edited by
Peter B Cotton, Guido NJ Tytgat, and Christopher B Williams

## Of special interest to Lecturers & Teachers

■ Expert reviewers from all areas of gastrointestinal endoscopy evaluate the latest literature and select the most relevant new images to be included in this slide atlas.

■ Top quality color and b&w slides — consisting of original photographs and specially designed diagrams and tables — are presented in durable plastic mounts, clearly marked and displayed in a special ring binder.

■ Each year, you will receive 85 slides accompanied by detailed descriptions. The slides form a growing collection of up-to-date visual material that will significantly enhance your existing collection.

**Slide Atlas of Gastrointestinal Endoscopy 1995**
Price: £135.00 / $195.00

ISBN: 1-85922-238-2

*Also available:*

**Slide Atlas of Gastrointestinal Endoscopy 1994**
ISBN: 1-85722-166-1

**Slide Atlas of Gastrointestinal Endoscopy 1993**
ISBN: 1-85922-163-7

**Slide Atlas of Gastrointestinal Endoscopy 1992**
ISBN: 1-85922-252-8

All previous slide atlases were produced under the expert guidance of PB Cotton, GNJ Tytgat, & CB Williams.

*Available through your local bookshop.*

For further information contact:
**Current Science Ltd, Middlesex House, 34-42 Cleveland Street, London W1P 6LB**.

Freephone: **0800 212530 (UK only)**
Tel: **+44 (0) 171 323 0323**
Fax: **+44 (0) 171 636 6911**

The **Slide Atlas of GASTROINTESTINAL ENDOSCOPY** is prepared in conjunction with the leading international review publication, **Annual of GASTROINTESTINAL ENDOSCOPY**.

CS
CURRENT SCIENCE ■

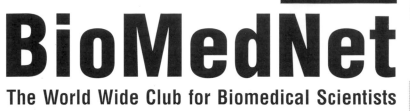
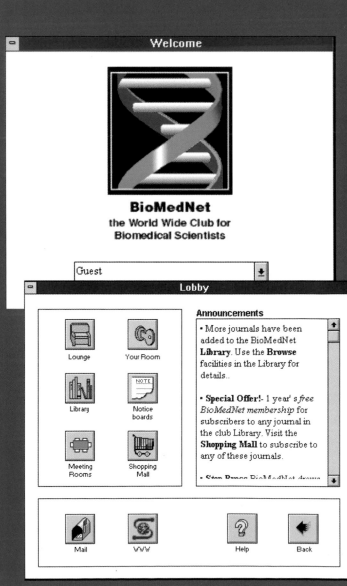